D1290119

Fertility, Cycles & Nutrition

Self-care for improved cycles and fertility
...naturally!

Fertility, Cycles & Nutrition

Self-care for improved cycles and fertility
...naturally!

By Marilyn M. Shannon

COUPLE TO
COUPLE LEAGUE

The Couple to Couple League International, Inc.
5440 Moeller Ave., Suite 149 • Norwood, OH 45212-1211

Published by:

The Couple to Couple League International, Inc.
5440 Moeller Ave., Suite 149
Norwood, Ohio 45212-1211
U.S.A.
800-745-8252
www.ccli.org
info@ccli.org

Cataloging data:

      L.C.: 2019909090
      ISBN: 978-0-926412-05-7

Shannon, Marilyn M.
Fertility, Cycles & Nutrition: Self-care for improved cycles and fertility...naturally!, 5th ed.

Nutrition
Health, reproductive
Menstrual cycles
Natural family planning
Infertility
Pregnancy

Printed in the United States
10 9 8 7 6 5 4 3 2

ACKNOWLEDGEMENTS

As with the original edition of this book, thanks go first to John F. Kippley, a founder of The Couple to Couple League for natural family planning. Having the privilege of teaching natural family planning through this organization since 1982 originally sparked my interest in the relationship between nutrition and reproductive health, and it was he who suggested that I undertake the original edition.

Special thanks go to my husband and best friend, Ron, who not only suggested the very popular "80-20" rule for better nutrition (Rule 12, Chapter 1), but who has also been involved with this project from every angle. He has buoyed me up with the inherent moral support that comes from an equal interest in nutrition, as well as with the practical support with our family activities during this busy time.

Our daughter, Rosemary Shannon Imrick, has again assisted me in the daunting task of identifying and selecting relevant new research articles. Her fast and efficient response to my many requests was essential to this completely updated book. She is also responsible for the recipe for extra-thick yogurt, made at home in a crock pot (see Chapter 2).

I gratefully acknowledge the assistance and dedication of our Couple to Couple League editor, Ann Gundlach, who has patiently, professionally and cheerfully worked with me, beginning with the first edition in 1990, and continuing with this updated fifth edition. This time, I tried to accept her advice, "Marilyn, you can't edit 'til the cows come home!" with fewer writes and rewrites. Likewise, I thank Rachel Schenck of RS Creative&Design, for giving this book a fresh new layout and design, including the attractive new cover.

Thank you to the Couple to Couple League teachers and members who have offered so many encouraging words about the previous editions. I am truly humbled by your passion for "fertility, cycles and nutrition," your interest in learning more about these relationships, and in sharing what you have learned. I also wish to express my gratitude to those men and women who permitted me to relate their experiences with nutrition and reproductive health. Their anecdotes are contained within these pages, though their names have been changed.

Many thanks also go to Indiana University Purdue University Fort Wayne (now Purdue University Fort Wayne) for granting me a sabbatical in order to update *Fertility, Cycles & Nutrition* to this fifth edition. I have just retired after thirty-five years as a part-time, tenured instructor of human anatomy and physiology, and have been grateful for Indiana U. Purdue U.'s support of the update of the previous editions as well.

Grateful acknowledgment is also given for the quoted materials on pages 92 and 93, which are excerpts from *Vitamin B6: The Doctor's Report*, © 1973 by John M. Ellis and James Presley. Reprinted by permission of Harper and Row, Publishers, Inc.

All Bible verses at the start of each chapter are from The New American Bible, 1972-1973 edition, except where noted.

TABLE OF CONTENTS

FOREWORD

I firmly believe that a patient is her own best health care advocate. As such, I look at myself not only as a doctor, but also as an educator. One of my favorite resources is Marilyn Shannon's *Fertility, Cycles & Nutrition* because it is so pertinent to women's health from a medical perspective. I particularly like the fact that Marilyn first emphasizes good nutrition, before she targets particular problems such as painful cycles, PMS, polycystic ovary syndrome, infertility, thyroid or any of a number of other issues. It is amazing for me to see the number of problems that simply resolve with good nutrition and a healthy lifestyle. What a blessing it is for my patients to learn that they do not have to rely on powerful drugs or hormones to effectively manage their health.

I work with many couples who use Natural Family Planning (NFP). The quality of a woman's cycle is foundational. Clear and consistent fertility observations provide the basis for achieving pregnancy if that is desired, or a reasonable amount of abstinence if it is not. For women with healthy fertility and menstrual cycles, the practice of NFP is relatively easy. However, among young women today it is common to see less than ideal cycles due to a combination of poor diet and lifestyle factors, the effects of contraceptive hormone use, and even environmental influences. I see charts that indicate various problems which can make NFP more difficult for a couple, as well as interfere with the conception of a much-desired child. As a couple begins to chart, NFP observations frequently raise suspicions for underlying illness which may have been longstanding. I find this information essential to my medical practice.

For these reasons, Marilyn Shannon's *Fertility, Cycles & Nutrition* is now a valued "partner" in my OB/GYN practice. The book covers such a wide range of issues related to female and male fertility that I find myself recommending it often. Marilyn has thoroughly examined the research and cites reliable, up-to-date references which demonstrate the positive impact of improved nutrition and lifestyle on health, both reproductive and general. I heartily recommend it to my patients for advice targeted to the issues they experience, or for anyone who simply wants to live more healthfully.

Marie A. Anderson, M.D. FACOG
Tepeyac OB/GYN
Fairfax, Virginia

INTRODUCTION

UPDATE FOR THE 5TH EDITION

It has been nearly 30 years since the very first edition of *Fertility, Cycles & Nutrition* was published by the Couple to Couple League. Yet the original intent of the first edition holds true with this latest edition: To enable women to have more regular cycles, to enable couples to improve their fertility through natural means, and ultimately to have the children their hearts desire. The fifth edition that you are now reading reflects the amazing changes which are occurring in the field of human nutrition over that time span. Daily we learn about new links between nutrition and health, whether it is the role of vitamin D in reducing the risk of endometriosis, the effect of the omega-3 fatty acids on male fertility, or the antioxidant properties of the hundreds of newly-discovered nutrients in brightly-colored plant foods. For sure, when it comes to "fertility, cycles, and nutrition," there has been an explosion of interest and new research. Because of the exponential increase in relevant information, the fifth edition of this book has been rewritten from beginning to end. While many of the chapter subjects are the same, virtually every topic has been expanded as well as updated, and some new topics have been added.

A sampling of some updates to the fifth edition:

Chapter 1, "Twelves Rules for Better Nutrition": The role of food sensitivities has been addressed, and strategies for improving digestion have been added.

Chapter 2, "Obtaining and Preparing Nutritious Food": A sidebar has been added encouraging readers to consider homesteading; that is, raising their own chickens and perhaps other small livestock. This perspective comes right from the Shannon family's long-time experience with poultry, dairy goats, and sheep.

Chapter 4, "Increasing Your Energy and Decreasing Your Stress," has been moved from Part 2 to Part 1. Why? This topic is more vital than ever to women's health. It features an expanded discussion of sleep, how it rests the brain, and how to improve the quality and quantity of sleep. A full-page sidebar offers tips to improve sleep.

Chapter 5, "Questions and Answers, Part 1": A comprehensive question and answer deals with the role of body weight—really body fat—on the female fertility cycle and female fertility. A second new Q & A reviews many possible strategies to lose weight if that's necessary.

Chapter 7, "Shorter, Lighter, and Pain-free Periods": A new discussion on possibly *preventing* endometriosis completes this chapter.

Chapter 8, "Four Common Causes of Cycle Irregularity and Infertility": The possibility of excess iodine on thyroid function is addressed, and frequent eating out at fast-food and sit-down restaurants is suggested as a common source of *excess* iodine in iodized salt.

Chapter 10, "Other Factors That May Affect Cycle Regularity or Fertility": Periodontal disease has been added as a topic, as it may be related to cycle irregularity, infertility, and pregnancy problems. Under the topic "Age-Related Infertility/Fertility of Unknown Cause" CoEnzyme Q10, in the form ubiquinol, has been added to the list of supplements recommended for this topic.

Chapter 12, "Repeated Miscarriage and Birth Defects": Though a large number of major research studies have conclusively shown that the supplement, folic acid, reduces the incidence of miscarriage, birth defects including spina bifida, anencephaly, heart defects, abdominal defects and others, folic acid is synthetic. New research shows that many people have a genetic variation that causes their metabolism of folate, the natural vitamin, to be suboptimal. Though research studies on the value of methyl folate, the natural B vitamin, in preventing miscarriage and birth defects, is not yet available, Chapter 12 recommends the natural methyl folate instead of folic acid. In addition, ovum quality, that is, the ability of the unfertilized ovum to complete its cell division (meiosis) shortly before ovulation, is explained in this chapter, and the nutrients needed for optimal ovum quality are recommended.

Chapter 13, "Perimenopause, Menopause, and Beyond": A new discussion of two types of bladder problems that can occur in women as they age in included. The problem of sleep quality is also addressed.

Chapter 14, "Miscellaneous Problems That Affect Women": The section on low sexual desire in women has been expanded along many fronts, with more suggestions offered compared to the previous editions.

Chapter 15, "Men's Fertility and Reproductive Health": A discussion of the amazing process of sperm development has been added. New studies adding evidence that daily diet makes a difference to male sperm quality and quantity are reviewed. The omega-3 oils have been studied, using daily intake of raw walnuts, to improve male fertility. New research is also uncovering what should be avoided, including regular intake of ibuprofen and perhaps other over-the-counter anti-inflammatory medications.

It has been most heartening to see that without exception, the new research confirms, extends, and strengthens older studies that formed the basis of the first four editions of *Fertility, Cycles & Nutrition*. This means that the new is consistent with the old, but now there are many more options as you attempt to overcome specific reproductive problems. The newest *Fertility, Cycles & Nutrition*, like the old one, has an inherently Catholic outlook, since the publisher, Couple to Couple League, is a Catholic organization that teaches natural family planning. But whether or not you are Catholic or Christian, you will still find it a gentle, encouraging, and practical book, whether you are using it to overcome irregular cycles or to increase your chances of having a baby.

Among the nicest and most common compliments I receive about *Fertility, Cycles & Nutrition* are comments like these: "I loaned it to my friend. She never gave it back!" Or, "I've had to buy three or four copies because I keep giving it to my sisters and my friends!" When women lend their books to their sisters and friends, it is because they believe that the book will make a positive difference in their lives. With all my heart, I hope that this edition of *Fertility, Cycles & Nutrition* will make an even bigger difference in your life and health, and in that of your friends and family. I am excited and optimistic that it will do so.

PART 1
GOOD NUTRITION FOR GOOD HEALTH

Most likely you have picked up this book to help solve a problem involving your cycles or your fertility. Perhaps you would like to overcome PMS, or have lighter periods or more regular cycles. Perhaps you are having difficulty achieving a pregnancy. In any case, it is tempting to go right to the specifics of Part 2 to do so, but first, please take some time to review the basics of good nutrition and to consider the benefits of vitamin and mineral supplements. You will gain much more from the recommendations of Part 2 if you are well on your way to a more natural, holistic diet and balanced supplementation.

Part 1 of this book encourages you to improve your overall nutrition on a day-to-day basis. You will see that drastic alterations in the foods you eat are not necessary, and that the much-maligned American diet can be used as the foundation for excellent nutrition. Good nutrition is far more a matter of careful selection and emphasis than wholesale change from, say, meat and potatoes to chick peas on rye! Part 1 also emphasizes that good food does not require hours of time to find or to prepare. Once you know where to shop and what to shop for, it doesn't take any more time than you are now accustomed to. Once you have the food, there are some wonderful appliances that can even reduce your food preparation in some cases to one-tenth the effort it would take otherwise.

The first chapter consists of some practical guidelines that will help you to substantially increase the value of your family's meals while continuing to "cook American." The rationale behind each guideline is briefly explained, because I believe that you will be more motivated to make improvements when you understand the value of doing so. Chapter 2 focuses on ways to source and prepare great-tasting food conveniently and quickly. Chapter 3 looks at vitamin and mineral supplements and their value to overall health. Chapter 4 tackles a preliminary problem that is all too common: low energy and high stress. Strategies to improve your sleep and increase your energy are presented there. Chapter 5 answers common questions about practical matters involving nutrition.

My sincere hope is that you will implement the general health improvements of Part 1 before you attempt to apply the more specific recommendations of Part 2. Best wishes on your journey toward a healthier you, a healthier family, and a healthier future!

TWELVE RULES FOR BETTER NUTRITION

1

Those who are cheerful and merry at table benefit from their food.

— Sirach 30:25

What kinds of food choices contribute to regular cycles, better fertility, as well as postmenopausal health and even men's health? The answer is very positive: The same choices that support high energy, a feeling of well-being, mental sharpness, and long-term good health. Such a "diet" should be tasty and rich in nutrients, but also highly flexible and absolutely practical for today's busy families. In a nutshell (to make a pun!), the keys are whole, natural foods and related lifestyle choices that maintain steady blood sugar levels. When all nutrients are abundantly available and when blood sugar levels are stable, you feel energetic, your moods are positive, and your hormonal balance is more likely to approach the ideal for healthy cycles and fertility. As a welcome side effect, when you eat with a focus on nutritious foods and steady blood sugar levels, weight control is easier. And a healthy weight contributes importantly to better cycles and better fertility in women. Below are some practical guidelines to increase the value of your food choices and to maintain that all-important blood sugar level.

1: MAKE PROTEIN THE FOUNDATION OF YOUR MEALS

Protein that you eat enables you to make protein that you need. Muscle tissue contains protein, of course. Connective tissue is formed from thread-like proteins called collagen. Skin cells are waterproofed by a special protein. Even your bones are one-third protein. Cells make a huge variety of different proteins for use as enzymes, hormones, antibodies, clotting elements, and many other functions.

The body's proteins are long but intricately folded chains whose links are hundreds of amino acids. Human proteins are made of specific combinations of about twenty different amino acids. Nine of the amino acids are **essential**, which means they must be available in the diet. The other **nonessential** amino acids can be made by the body from the essential ones.[1]

All the essential amino acids must be present in your food in order for your body first to produce the nonessential amino acids, and then to make the various proteins that it needs. **Complete proteins** are foods that contain all of the essential amino acids.

 Animal products—milk, cheese, yogurt, eggs, fish, poultry, and red meat—are all high-quality, complete protein foods.

PLANT-BASED PROTEIN

Those who practice a strict vegetarian diet know that beans and grains together provide all the essential amino acids. While it is not necessary to eat grains and beans at the same meal, there are many traditional dishes that do combine them, perhaps because they taste so good together! For example, beans on a cornmeal taco provide complete protein. A side of rice and beans forms complete protein, as in Mexican cuisine. So does succotash, which is a Native American dish of corn and lima beans. Even the humble peanut butter sandwich is a complete protein food, since the peanut is actually a bean and wheat is a grain.

A small amount of animal protein eaten with a grain food or beans also provides high quality protein dishes. Pasta dishes made with cheese, chili beans with meat sauce, beef and noodles, chicken chop suey over rice, pork and beans, and cereal with milk are all examples of the practical application of this principle, which has been used around the world since antiquity.

Protein is fairly hard to digest, but that's a plus. Why? Eaten with whole carbohydrate foods, protein greatly slows down the release of glucose into the blood, contributing to steady blood sugar levels over several hours. That's why, if your blood glucose tends to be low (hypoglycemia), you may find that extra protein, especially for breakfast, helps to stabilize your blood sugar levels. That's also why more protein and fewer starchy carbohydrates is a helpful approach if you are attempting to lose weight. For the same reason, more protein may help you out if you are trying to overcome a craving for s ugary or starchy junk foods. The slow digestion of protein makes you feel satisfied longer. In addition, protein foods—whether from plant or animal foods—are rich sources of vitamins and minerals.

HOW MUCH PROTEIN DO YOU NEED? There is a wide range of protein intake that is healthy. Many Americans eat more than is necessary for good health, but as the examples above suggest, extra protein is beneficial to some people. If you are pregnant, you need to be careful to get enough protein in the earlier months to combat morning sickness, and during the later months to support your own increasing needs as well as your baby's brain development. You need more protein when you are breastfeeding than when you are not. Growing children need proportionally more protein compared to adults.

Table 1, "Suggested Daily Food Goals" (pages 6-7), provides a means of checking up on your daily servings of all major food groups, including the proteins. If you are pregnant or breastfeeding, Table 13, "Suggested Daily Food Goals for Pregnant and Nursing Women" (pages 204-205 in Chapter 11), provides a checklist to make sure you are getting enough servings of protein each day.

2: EAT PLENTY OF WHOLE PLANT FOODS: GRAINS, BEANS, NUTS, VEGETABLES, SEEDS, AND FRUITS

Whole plant foods provide so much good nutrition and such good taste that they're a great place to focus as you improve your nutrition. Of the three major food classes— proteins, carbohydrates, and natural fats—plant foods are best known as members of the carbohydrate class. However, grains, beans, nuts, and seeds are also good sources of protein, and the nuts and seeds especially contribute healthy natural fats to the diet. All whole plant foods provide an abundance of vitamins, minerals, and other healthful nutrients. When the carbohydrate content is considered, plant foods can be informally subdivided into three groups: starchy carbohydrates, non-starchy garden vegetables, and fruits.

STARCHY CARBOHYDRATES. Whole grains, beans, and a few vegetables are t raditionally called "starchy" foods. Some examples of these basic foods are wholegrain bread, whole-wheat pasta, oatmeal, brown rice, granola, peas, navy beans, kidney beans, sweet potatoes, and white potatoes. During digestion, they gradually release the sugar glucose, providing a major source of energy for the body. Gradual release of glucose is the key, though. When these foods are refined, many of their vitamins and minerals are removed, as well as their valuable fiber. Refined carbohydrates are digested too rapidly, disrupting the blood glucose levels without even furnishing the vitamins and minerals that nature intended. That's why your emphasis should be on whole, unrefined starchy foods, rather than on white bread, white pasta, or white rice.

NON-STARCHY GARDEN VEGETABLES. Most of the plant foods that we call garden vegetables are non-starchy, and are not high energy-producing foods. Instead, they contain a tremendous wealth of vitamins, minerals, fiber, and other nutrients. Spinach, lettuce, green beans, cucumbers, zucchini, Brussels sprouts, asparagus, peppers, cabbage, celery, tomatoes, and onions are common examples of the garden vegetables. It's hard to find an unhealthy example!

FRUITS. Delicious, nutritious fruits, such as apples, oranges, grapefruits, grapes, cherries, peaches, kiwis, pomegranates, and cantaloupes are sweet because they contain natural sugars. Fresh, ripe, and raw, they contain an abundance of fiber, vitamins, minerals, and other nutrients. But sweet fruits eaten on an empty stomach may release their sugars too rapidly, causing blood sugar swings, just like refined starchy foods.

TABLE 1
SUGGESTED DAILY FOOD GOALS

WHOLE GRAINS

3 servings daily

(1 serving = 1 slice bread or ½ cup cooked cereal)

Whole grain bread	Whole grain breakfast cereal	Whole grain pancakes	Tortillas
Oatmeal	Quinoa	Whole grain pasta	Bagels
Brown rice			

DAIRY/EGGS

3 servings daily

(1 serving = 6 oz. milk, 2 oz. cheese, 1 egg)

Whole milk	Cheese	Kefir
Yogurt	Ice cream	Eggs

COMPLETE PROTEIN

1 serving daily

(1 serving = 3-4 oz. meat)

Poultry	Pork	Dairy + Grain
Fish (preferably twice weekly)	Lamb	Dairy + Legume
Beef, including liver and heart	Grain + Legume (Peas, beans, peanut butter, nuts, lentils)	

YELLOW FRUITS AND VEGETABLES

1 serving daily

(1 serving = ½ cup cooked or 1 cup raw)

Carrots	Sweet potatoes	Mangos	Peaches
Squash	Pumpkin	Apricots	Cantaloupe

TABLE 1 (CONT.)
SUGGESTED DAILY FOOD GOALS

LEAFY GREEN VEGETABLES

3 servings daily

(1 serving = ½ cup cooked or 1 cup raw)

Lettuce (leaf, Romaine, Bibb, iceberg)	Endive	Cole crops (cabbage, broccoli, Brussels sprouts, cauliflower, kohlrabi)
Spinach	Beet greens	
	Alfalfa sprouts	
Escarole	Asparagus	Kale
	Chard	

VITAMIN C SOURCE

1 serving daily

(1 serving = 1 medium fruit or ½ cup berries)

Citrus fruits (oranges, grapefruits, tangerines)	Tomatoes	Peppers
	Melons	Potatoes
	Berries	

UNSATURATED OILS

1 serving daily

(1 serving = 1–2 tablespoons)

Monounsaturated	**Polyunsaturated**	**Both**
Olive oil	Soy oil *	Canola oil *
		Sesame oil
Peanut oil	Walnut oil *	
Unprocessed peanut butter	Safflower oil	
	Sunflower oil	* Source of the essential
Avocado oil	Corn oil	omega-3 alpha-linolenic acid.

This table may be photocopied, covered with adhesive backed clear plastic and taped to your refrigerator. Check off the boxes daily with a dry erase marker.

PHYTONUTRIENTS. Plant foods, especially the brightly-colored fruits and garden vegetables such as tomatoes, carrots, pineapple, broccoli, blueberries, beets, and grapes, are full of hundreds of wonderful natural chemicals called **phytonutrients**. Some phytonutrients act as powerful antioxidants, preventing the kind of damage to cells that ultimately results in degenerative diseases, including cardiovascular disease and cancer. Others provide materials for the body's cells that improve the immune system, the eyes' delicate structures, brain function, and even reproductive function.

> **Antioxidants are currently under intense study for their beneficial effect on both male and female fertility.**

FIBER. The presence of fiber is another huge benefit of eating whole plant foods. Fiber is the indigestible material that makes foods such as almonds, celery, carrots, and granola so delightfully crunchy. Fiber takes some chewing, and it makes you feel full, both of which are helpful to appetite control. It slows down the release of glucose from the intestines into the blood, contributing importantly to steady blood sugar levels. It stimulates the contractions of the large intestine, so that waste products and toxins are moved out of the body quickly. **Soluble fiber**, such as the sticky stuff that makes oatmeal pans so hard to clean, is especially healthful. Some fiber-rich foods contain **prebiotics**, soluble fiber components which feed the healthy bacteria that inhabit the intestines.

WHAT ARE PREBIOTICS?

You have no doubt heard of *pro*biotics, which are the friendly bacteria found in fermented foods such as yogurt and sauerkraut. *Pre*biotics are specific molecules found in soluble fiber. They are indigestible to us, but serve as ideal food for the friendly bacteria in the intestines. Sources of prebiotics include onions, whole grains, asparagus, Jerusalem artichoke, garlic, bananas, flax seed, and sweet potatoes.

HOW MUCH OF THE WHOLE PLANT FOODS SHOULD YOU EAT? There is no single answer that suits every individual. But most everyone can—and should—eat the non-starchy garden vegetables plentifully. Because they are so low in calories and so high in fiber, vitamins, minerals, and phytonutrients, aiming to add them to every meal and snack is a good goal. Eaten raw, their crispness gives you something enjoyable to munch on instead of packaged chips or pretzels. Nuts and seeds, with their proteins and natural fats, are a satisfying substitute for chips and dips as well.

Most people can eat whole, raw fresh fruits daily. In moderation, their tangy sweetness and fiber will really help you if you are trying to overcome a craving for sugary junk foods and drinks. Sweet fruits are best eaten with proteins and fats, though, because on an empty stomach many of them release their sugars too fast for the stable blood glucose levels that you are aiming for.

Try having fruit for dessert following a meal. That's a satisfying way to enjoy the benefits of fruits without the blood sugar swings. As an added bonus, you won't miss the typical desserts that provide mostly empty calories.

When it comes to the grains, beans, and starchy vegetables such as potatoes, many people can enjoy these foods as long as they are truly whole and natural, and are eaten with other protein and fatty foods. However, if you are fighting weight gain, polycystic ovary syndrome symptoms (discussed in Chapter 9), water retention, or blood sugar swings caused by a diet of refined sugary and starchy foods, you may need to limit the starchy plant foods such as potatoes, bread, corn, and pasta. If that's the case, don't forget about the seeds, nuts, and the many delicious non-starchy garden vegetables!

3: CHOOSE HEALTHFUL FATS AND OILS

In the not-too-distant past, fats and oils were singled out as foods to avoid. Yes, they are definitely the food group highest in calories. But natural fats provide a large number of nutrients that promote every aspect of health. They are needed in the diet for the fat-soluble vitamins A, D, E, and K to be absorbed. Fats and oils powerfully slow down stomach emptying, providing a feeling of fullness that helps with appetite control.

Sufficient body fat in women is absolutely essential for healthy fertility cycles.

You are probably already well aware that the artificially produced *trans* fats are harmful to your health. Many people, though, are unaware that human beings require specific fats which the human body must have.

ESSENTIAL FATTY ACIDS. The **essential fatty acids** are only two in number: linoleic acid and alpha-linolenic acid. Linoleic acid, called the "omega-6" essential fatty acid because of its biochemistry, is needed in the greater amount. It is abundant in most vegetable oils, especially sunflower oil, corn oil, soy oil, and sesame oil. The omega-6 essential fatty acid is found in excess in the typical American diet, and so restricting these vegetable oils is a healthy strategy.

The wonderfully health-promoting alpha-linolenic acid, often termed the "omega-3" essenttial fatty acid, is needed in lesser amounts, but is considerably harder to get. Small but significant amounts are present in canola oil. Commonly used food oils such as olive oil, corn oil, and peanut oil contain virtually none. Flax oil (also called flaxseed oil) is by far the richest source, since it is more than 50 percent alpha-linolenic acid. However, flax oil is too fragile to be heated, and is better used as a supplement in capsule or liquid form. It has several benefits to reproductive health, and its role as a supplement is explained in Chapter 3.

Because light, oxygen, and heat progressively damage both of the essential fatty acids, it's a good practice to purchase only **expeller-pressed** oils, which are processed at low temperatures and which are available at natural groceries and health food shops. These oils should be bought in small containers, capped tightly and stored in the refrigerator, as much for the darkness as for the cold.

MONOUNSATURATED OILS. Monounsaturated fats are not essential because the body can manufacture them, but they are healthful in the diet. In fact, you may have seen them promoted as the "omega-9" fatty acids. They help to normalize both the blood fats and the blood sugar. Olive oil and canola oil are rich sources of the major monounsaturated fatty acid, oleic acid. Extra-virgin olive oil, valued for its monounsaturated fatty acids, has a zippy taste and many phytonutrients, though it lacks the hard-to-get alpha-linolenic acid. It's a tasty choice for your own homemade vinegar-and-oil salad dressings. For cooking or frying at moderate temperatures, mild-tasting "pure" or "virgin" olive oil can be used.

TRANS FATS

When the unsaturated vegetable oils are converted to margarine or shortening to make them solid at room temperature, the essential fatty acids are destroyed. What's worse, they are converted to unhealthy *trans* fats which interfere with the function of the essential fatty acids. The same occurs when natural peanut butter is partially hydrogenated. As much as possible, avoid these major sources of *trans* fats: margarine, shortening, peanut butter not labeled "natural," prepackaged pastries, and deep-fried fast foods such as french fries and breaded chicken or fish. Examine labels and avoid packaged foods containing any of the following: "*trans* fats" or "hydrogenated" or "partially hydrogenated" oils. Be aware that some foods labeled "0 *trans* fats" actually do contain *trans* fats.[2] Avoiding *trans* fats may improve your cycles or fertility, as research has shown that intake of *trans* fats contributes to endometriosis[3] and infertility.[4]

SATURATED FATS AND CHOLESTEROL. Saturated fats and cholesterol are found together in animal products such as poultry, red meat, whole milk, butter, cheese, and eggs. Because they are used to form part of all cell membranes, these natural fats have important health benefits. They are involved in the maintenance of the fatty coverings that insulate neurons. They strengthen the hard-working gastrointestinal lining, through which digested food molecules must travel. Animal fats are stable when heated, so that lard or bacon grease can be used for frying.

Butter and coconut oil contain saturated fats which offer special benefits. They contain **medium chain fatty acids**, which are absorbed more easily than the ordinary **long chain fatty acids** found in most fats and oils. These medium chain fatty acids are used for energy rather than stored, and unlike carbohydrates, they do not raise insulin. Similar to animal fat, coconut oil is stable when used for frying. It has a distinctive flavor that works with many foods.

Cholesterol is found in animal fats, and is also made by the body's cells. It is the precursor of the sex hormones estrogen, progesterone, and testosterone, as well as the other steroid hormones. It is the precursor of vitamin D, which the body can make if the skin is exposed to sufficient sunshine. It stabilizes all cell membranes.

Both fats and oils powerfully affect the digestive hormones, slowing down the emptying of the stomach and the absorption of glucose into the blood, and therefore stabilizing blood sugar levels.

> When digestive processes occur gradually, the meal "sticks to your ribs,"
> an old expression that means it digests slowly, releasing nutrients
> and satisfying hunger over a long period of time.

If you have a hard time believing that saturated fats or cholesterol can be healthy, here is an important finding: In the very large Nurses' Health Study, having one or two servings of whole milk products daily correlated with significantly higher fertility in women compared to using skim (low fat) milk products.[5] While most likely there are several different explanations for this finding, it should at least reassure those who are nervous about consuming naturally saturated fats and cholesterol, even in moderation.

BUTTER IS BETTER

Butter contains both medium chain and short chain fatty acids which are able to be used as fuel rather than stored in the fat cells. Butter is a rich source of the fat-soluble vitamins A, D, and K, so essential to many bodily functions, including reproductive function in men and women. Butter is easily substituted in most recipes that call for cooking oil or shortening. It is just the right topping for steamed vegetables. It can also be used for sautéing at low temperatures. Best of all, butter tastes delicious!

FISH OIL AND KRILL OIL

What about the healthy fatty acids abundant in fish oil or krill oil, abbreviated DHA and EPA? Your body can actually make DHA (docosahexaenoic acid) and EPA (eicosapentaenoic acid) if you have the hard-to-get omega-3 alpha-linolenic acid discussed above, along with several vitamins and minerals. EPA and DHA are best known for their heart-healthy effects, but they also stimulate the immune system, promote proper brain function, decrease inflammation, and perform other vital functions in virtually every cell. Eating fatty fish regularly is one way to obtain these wonderful nutrients, but now that contaminant-free fish oil and krill oil are available as a fruit-flavored liquid or in capsules, they are recommended as supplements in Chapter 3.

HOW MUCH OF THE FATS AND OILS SHOULD YOU EAT? As with proteins and carbohydrates, the amount of fat in the diet is individual. That said, if you have been avoiding fats and oils, perhaps as part of a vegan diet, consider the many benefits of this food group to your overall health. Your cycles, fertility, and sense of well-being will be helped by adding in small amounts of the healthy salad oils, whole milk, eggs, butter, and/or the natural fat that comes with meat and fish. Oppositely, even if you are fighting a weight problem, please remember that the natural fats and oils really put the brakes on appetite and stomach emptying. Despite higher calories, in moderation they will help with weight control.

4: SUBSTITUTE MORE NUTRITIOUS INGREDIENTS FOR LESS NUTRITIOUS INGREDIENTS IN YOUR FAVORITE RECIPES AND DISHES

More nutritious foods are simply fresher and closer to their natural state than are other less healthful foods. Whole, unprocessed foods, whether from animal or plant sources, are rich in vitamins and minerals. Since they do not contain additives, they minimize the problem of harmful chemicals. Their natural fats satisfy the appetite and supply the body with fuel and essential fatty acids as well. Their starches and sugars, snugly wrapped in the natural packaging called fiber, are slowly digested and released to the blood. Table 2, "Foods to Emphasize" (page 14), lists such foods, and Table 3, "Food Substitutions" (pages 14-15), gives examples of many nutritious foods that can easily be used in place of nutritionally inferior foods in your familiar recipes, salads, and other dishes.

Nutritionally inferior ingredients are those that contain *trans* fats, added sugar, white flour, excess salt, or artificial colors, sweeteners, flavorings, and preservatives. These ingredients are all too common in prepackaged or processed foods. Vitamins, minerals, essential fatty acids, and fiber have been lost from such foods during processing. Food additives may disrupt blood sugar levels, essential fatty acid metabolism, or vitamin and mineral balance. Table 4, "Foods to Limit" (page 15), lists such foods.

WHAT'S COOKING?

Cooking has a value beyond making food taste good. Heating food kills bacteria and parasites, makes the food easier to digest, and makes certain nutrients more available. Unfortunately, it also destroys some vitamins. For example, several B vitamins, vitamins C and E, and the essential fatty acids are all harmed by cooking.

Vegetables that do need cooking can be steamed or heated in a little boiling water. Leave vegetables such as green beans, cauliflower, and asparagus a little crisp when you cook them. You will add a gourmet touch as well as better nutrition by doing so.

When it comes to fish, poultry, and red meat, thorough cooking is necessary for tenderness, good taste, and safety. When meats are cooked, it's healthier to use longer cooking times with lower temperatures rather than higher temperatures. Longer, slower cooking is also the secret to juicy, tender roasts.

5: EAT A GREATER VARIETY OF FOODS (BUT AVOID FOODS YOU ARE SENSITIVE TO)

The best, freshest, most toxin-free natural food cannot build health alone. Other than mother's milk for a young baby, no complete food exists. The dozen or so basic foods that Americans eat—beef, chicken, milk, potatoes, bread, pasta, and so forth—simply don't supply all the dietary factors that produce optimal health. Ongoing research identifying hundreds of beneficial molecules in whole plant and animal foods indicates that there are many more nutrients which have not yet been discovered. The greater the variety of nutritious foods you eat, the greater the chance you have of acquiring such beneficial dietary factors, even those yet undiscovered. Use Tables 2 and 3 (pages 14-15) as well as the information on shopping for food in Chapter 2 for ideas for new foods that you may wish to try.

While you're at it, don't forget to expand the number of raw fruits and vegetables foods that you eat. Fruits, vegetables, seeds, and nuts are foods that can be eaten raw, and they are ideal to satisfy your sweet tooth or your need to munch on something satisfyingly crunchy. In general, eat your fruits raw, not cooked or bottled as a juice. This is one of the simplest and tastiest pieces of nutritional advice around! For example, a raw apple is a delicious food which provides fiber that slows down the release of its natural sugars. Prefer that juicy, crispy apple instead of apple sauce or bottled apple juice, both of which are likely to contain added sugar. Similarly, a real orange contains many more nutrients than pasteurized orange juice. A number of vegetables are good eaten raw, either alone or in big salads. Table 5, "Foods to Eat Raw" (page 15), lists foods that are delicious as

TABLE 2
Foods to Emphasize

Whole grain cereals, breads and pasta	Butter
Brown rice	Expeller pressed oils
Kidney beans, navy beans, pinto beans, lima beans, peas, and lentils	Herbal teas
Nuts and edible seeds	Poultry
Natural peanut butter	Ocean fish
Quinoa	Eggs
Fresh vegetables	Milk
Fresh fruits	Yogurt
Red meats	Natural cheese

TABLE 3
Foods Substitutions

PREFER	INSTEAD OF
100% whole grain bread, sour dough bread, or bread made with rye, oats, barley, or small amounts of other flours	White bread or "wheat" bread
Brown rice or quinoa	White rice or instant rice
"Old-fashioned" rolled oats	Quick-cooking or instant oatmeal
Granola	Boxed breakfast cereals
Bran muffins	Sweet rolls
Whole grain pasta (wheat, rice, or vegetable)	White pasta
Sweet potatoes, acorn squash, butternut squash, turnips	White potatoes
White potatoes	Frozen or boxed potato foods
Dark green leafy vegetables	Light green vegetables
Romaine lettuce, leaf lettuce, Bibb lettuce, endive, spinach, or escarole	Iceberg lettuce
Fresh vegetables	Frozen vegetables
Frozen vegetables	Canned vegetables
Deep yellow, orange, red, or purple vegetables	Pale-colored vegetables
Freshly made salads	Packaged salads
Homemade coleslaw	Packaged coleslaw
Whole, ripe, raw fruits	Canned fruits, fruit juices
Natural cheese	Processed "cheese food"

TABLE 3 (CONT.)
Foods Substitutions

PREFER	INSTEAD OF
Brussels sprouts, broccoli, lima beans, beets, or peas	Green beans
Poultry, beef, lamb, ocean fish, organic liver or heart	Processed meats
Natural peanut butter	Processed peanut butter
Olive oil, canola oil	Shortening
Butter	Margarine
Fruits	Sugary desserts
Air-popped popcorn, trail mix	Packaged chips
Herbs and spices	Salt or monosodium glutamate (MSG)

TABLE 4
Foods To Limit

Sugar	Shortening
Artificial sweeteners	Processed peanut butter
Soft drinks	Processed cheese
Fruit juices	Bacon, wieners, ham, lunch meat, sausage
White flour	Soy foods and soy milk
Refined vegetable oils	Prepackaged foods
Margarine	Aluminum-containing baking powder

TABLE 5
Foods To Eat Raw

VEGETABLES	Leaf lettuce	Tangerines	Watermelon
Carrots	Endive	Nectarines	Honeydew melon
Celery	Mung bean sprouts	Blueberries	Cantaloupe
Cucumbers	Broccoli	Blackberries	**SEEDS & NUTS**
Green peppers	Cauliflower	Raspberries	Pumpkin seeds
Tomatoes	Green or red cabbage	Pears	Sunflower seeds
Snap peas	Mushrooms	Plums	Almonds
Green onions	**FRUITS**	Grapes	Walnuts
Radishes	Apples	Cherries	Brazil nuts
Spinach	Oranges	Peaches	Hazelnuts
Romaine lettuce	Grapefruits	Apricots	Pecans

well as healthy when eaten raw. Notice also how many raw foods are brightly colored. Naturally colorful fruits and vegetables contain a wealth of wonderful phytonutrients.

WHAT IF YOU HAVE FOOD SENSITIVITIES?

Eating a greater variety of foods is an especially good idea if you are sensitive to dairy foods, gluten-containing foods, the tomato family, peanuts, eggs, or seafood. Expanding your grocery list to include new types of basic foods can compensate for those you must avoid.

6: SHARPLY LIMIT YOUR SUGAR INTAKE

Table sugar and brown sugar are calorie-rich, vitamin-poor, and rapidly absorbed. When you snack on a candy bar or soft drink, especially on an empty stomach, your blood sugar is suddenly jolted upward. Your pancreas reacts immediately to this stress by secreting the hormone *insulin*. Insulin quickly lowers blood sugar levels by allowing glucose entry into the body cells (especially the fat cells, where any excess is stored as saturated fat). When this blood sugar jolt is repeated again and again, the pancreas overreacts. It becomes overly efficient, and the stress of high blood glucose brought on by the rapid absorption of sugar results in insulin overproduction and low blood glucose in a short time. This is **reactive hypoglycemia**. Its symptoms include fatigue, irritability, depression, migraine headaches, and the inevitable craving for more sugar.

> As you will see in Part 2, hypoglycemia contributes to PMS (Chapter 6), and high insulin levels adversely affect the ovaries, interfering with cycle regularity and promoting polycystic ovary syndrome (Chapter 9). Sugar craving may also be a sign of low thyroid function (Chapter 8), and adrenal hormone imbalances (Chapter 4).

Sugar depletes the body of hard-to-get B vitamins as well as the minerals chromium, zinc, manganese, and magnesium, all of which are necessary to metabolize it. It lacks the soluble and insoluble fiber found in whole, unrefined carbohydrate foods. It feeds yeast organisms, promoting vaginal yeast infections and **gut dysbiosis** problems, which means the wrong kind of microorganisms in the intestines (discussed in Chapter 10).

Even though fruits do provide vitamins, minerals, fiber, and phytonutrients, very sweet fruits such as ripe bananas, ripe peaches, or grapes may trigger reactive hypoglycemia, especially if you eat them on an empty stomach. Sweet fruit juices and canned fruits are even more likely to do so. Honey is sweeter than table sugar and contains some vitamins and minerals, but it also can interfere with blood sugar levels.

Used in small amounts, however, sugar, honey, and molasses do serve a useful role, because they encourage you to eat healthy foods that you otherwise might not enjoy. For example, health-building foods such as yogurt or cooked oatmeal are rather grim without a little sweetener. The goal should be to link sugar to nutritious foods—to bran in bran muffins, to beans in baked beans, to fresh greens in salad dressings, to cranberries in cranberry relish, and so forth.

JUST A LITTLE SUGAR

Sugar is less harmful on a full stomach since other foods, especially protein and fats, slow down its absorption out of the intestines and into the blood. Because of this, a useful guideline that allows you to "cheat" a bit is to serve your treats and sweet fruits as desserts after a meal, not as snacks by themselves. You can also choose small servings of desserts that have plenty of protein and natural fat in them, such as ice cream, custard pudding, pumpkin pie, or dark chocolate-covered almonds, cashews, or Macadamia nuts.

It's better to prepare your meals starting with whole basic foods such as vegetables, pasta, meat, fish, grains, or dairy products, but when you do buy packaged items be careful to read the labels. Processed and prepackaged foods contain more sugar than you would ever pour into your home-cooked dishes! The amount of sugar in prepared foods is often disguised by adding several different types of sugar; for example, high fructose corn syrup, corn syrup, and fructose.

Watch out also for artificial sweeteners, which may be added to otherwise healthy foods such as yogurt. Artificial sweeteners may actually increase your craving for sugar, and can cause weight gain, elevated blood glucose levels, elevated insulin levels, and related problems knows as **metabolic syndrome**.[6] Amazing new research explains this seeming paradox: artificial sweeteners can cause gut dysbiosis; that is, they favor the growth of unfriendly bacteria that contribute to metabolic syndrome.[7]

If you feel like your sugar craving is a real issue that you are having trouble controlling, please read *Beat Sugar Addiction Now!* by Jacob Teitelbaum, M.D. In the most compassionate yet practical way, Dr. Teitelbaum helps you identify the root cause of your sugar craving, and he offers targeted nutritional and sometimes medical suggestions to overcome your root cause. Better yet, he suggests numerous tips to satisfy that craving with less sugar. For example, he thinks that small amounts of dark chocolate are not just permissible, but helpful to overcoming sugar craving. (See "Further Reading.")

7. DRINK PLENTY OF PURE WATER INSTEAD OF SOFT DRINKS AND CAFFEINATED BEVERAGES

Water can be correctly called the number one nutrient. Water is the solvent of life and is needed more frequently and in far higher amounts than any class of food. Drinking enough water energizes you, since it helps maintain normal blood pressure. Yet it doesn't contribute to elevated blood pressure, because water is a natural diuretic. It affects certain hormones, which in turn signal the kidneys to excrete water as urine. Drinking enough water to ensure that you empty your bladder regularly is one of the most effective ways to prevent bladder infections.

 Drinking extra water around the time of your menstrual period can reduce menstrual pain.

The mucus produced in the respiratory passages, as well as in the reproductive tract, is water based. Being well hydrated, therefore, helps prevent respiratory infections—you've probably learned to drink plenty of water if you are catching a cold. Finally, water can curb your appetite; often what you may think is hunger is really thirst.

How much water should you drink, and when should you drink it? The answer is individual, because people vary in size, activity level, and the amount of water they lose as sweat. But just about no one needs more water than a breastfeeding mother! Those eight glasses of water you often hear about can serve as a guideline; that's about a half-gallon a day. Even a little less (six glasses) is fine for many adults. Enough water input to have plenty of water output is a good guideline. Water is wonderful first thing in the morning, and is a great "snack" between meals. Drinking your water with meals is certainly fine, but drinking large amounts as you eat dilutes your digestive enzymes. For many people, limiting water before bed can help ensure a restful night's sleep.

Given the role of water as the number one nutrient, it's necessary to ask yourself, what's in your water? Or in the water where you work? It's hard to generalize, but depending on where your water comes from, agricultural runoffs, industrial wastes, or bacterial contamination could affect your drinking water. Despite these problems, it's become much easier to acquire purified drinking water conveniently and economically. The popular habit of carrying drinking water is an excellent and encouraging trend. Carrying ice-cold water is also the best way to overcome the bad habit of relying on soft drinks to quench your thirst. But what about the quality of that water?

One possibility to improve the water you drink is to purchase it in three or five-gallon containers from a water dealer or from the grocery store. Just be sure you know exactly what process has been used to purify the water.

There are also a number of options for filtering your own home water. All have some advantages and disadvantages, so it's wise to have your water tested to see exactly what the contaminants are. Depending on your needs and your budget, you may choose a reverse osmosis unit, which can be installed under the kitchen sink, or an activated particulate carbon filter under the faucet or on a carafe. Solid carbon block filters for home drinking water may be the best option of all. Such units filter a great variety of impurities and are modest in cost. They do take up space on the countertop, probably their biggest drawback.

Before you dismiss the idea of paying for healthful drinking water, consider the price of soft drinks: $3.00 to $11.00 per gallon! But you pay much more for soft drinks with your health. Sugar dissolved in water is absorbed extremely rapidly, especially on an empty stomach. That triggers a rapid insulin spike, followed by reactive low blood glucose.

It's no wonder that daily drinking of sugary sodas has been linked to infertility in women. Even artificially sweetened drinks have been implicated in weight gain, increased blood glucose, and increased insulin.[9]

Elevated insulin is well known to interfere with the function of the ovaries, as explained in Chapter 9. Drink water instead of sugary sodas or diet sodas. Or use your good home water to make hot or iced tea.

CAFFEINE. Caffeine is a good slave but a bad master. When you use it only occasionally or in moderation, it provides a lift that many people enjoy. However, it affects the nervous system, and can cause anxiety and irritability.

 Caffeine, sometimes even in small amounts, can deprive you of a good night's sleep because it powerfully reduces the sleep hormone, melatonin.

Used to excess, caffeine depletes the body of B vitamins and raises blood glucose by overstimulating the adrenal glands. The latter effect triggers insulin release, ultimately causing hypoglycemia, fatigue, and the craving for more caffeine.

Caffeinated beverages are a factor in premenstrual syndrome (PMS), at least for some women.[10] In amounts exceeding 300 mg per day (about two to three cups of coffee), using caffeine relates to a delay in achieving pregnancy.[11] A higher incidence of miscarriage once pregnancy occurs has been found related to consumption of more than 200 mg of caffeine per day (about two cups of coffee).[12] Higher intakes increase these risks.

Coffee is the most familiar source of caffeine, but sodas, non-herbal teas, and chocolate also contain caffeine or related compounds which have similar effects. Table 6, "Caffeine Content of Selected Beverages" (below), contains a chart of the caffeine levels found in coffee, tea, and other beverages.

Caffeine affects blood vessel constriction, so if you are trying to cut back on a heavy-duty caffeine habit, it's better to reduce your caffeine consumption gradually— over a period of one or two weeks—to avoid withdrawal headaches.

TEA TIME

There is just something so special about serving and drinking tea. It's more than just the tea—it's the whistling kettle, the pretty teapot, the shiny tea tray, the coziness of relaxing with a warm, flavorful drink. It's the quick and easy welcome it offers to family and friends, in your kitchen or in another favorite room. It's so easy to prepare—and so healthful! Traditional black tea is not nearly as high in caffeine as is coffee, and many teas are particularly rich in phytonutrients and low in caffeine. Select green teas, white teas, or herbal teas. Sure, put in a little sugar or honey, if that's how you like it. It's fun to have a variety of teas in your home, so that you can offer your guests their choice.

TABLE 6
Caffeine Content of Selected Beverages

BEVERAGES, 8 OZ.	CAFFEINE CONTENT IN MILLIGRAMS (MG)
Coffee, drip	115-175
Coffee, brewed	80-135
Coffee, instant	65-100
Tea, iced	47
Tea, brewed (avg.)	60
Tea, instant	30
Tea, green	15
Hot cocoa	14
BEVERAGES, 12 OZ.	**CAFFEINE CONTENT IN MILLIGRAMS (MG)**
Mountain Dew	54
Diet Coke	45.6
Pepsi-Cola	37.5
Diet Pepsi	36
Coca-Cola Classic	34

(Source: www.wilstar.com/caffeine.htm; from National Soft Drink Association, U.S. Food and Drug Administration, Pepsi.)

8. BOOST YOUR ABILITY TO DIGEST YOUR FOOD

To nourish the body, food must be digested and absorbed. Digestion refers to two processes: First is the chewing, churning and mixing that converts a meal into a thick liquid within the stomach and small intestine. Second is the secretion of many enzymes from the saliva, stomach, pancreas, and intestinal wall, which break down the large food molecules into smaller molecules that can be absorbed. Absorption is the transport of the small food molecules across the intestinal wall and ultimately into the bloodstream. Once in the blood, these absorbed nutrients are quickly sent to every part of the body, from the brain to the big toe.

If the digestive processes work ideally, you feel good after eating, with no sense of acid reflux, stomach pain, gassiness, or bloating.

With healthy digestion, you have normal bowel movements, without either constipation or diarrhea. Your food nourishes you, energizing you until the next meal or snack without craving for more food.

If eating is an issue for you, and you suffer from any of the problems just mentioned, here are some strategies to improve your digestion.

Don't graze! Three meals and a couple of snacks are just fine, but constantly eating or drinking (milk, juice, etc.) puts undigested and digesting food together. And while "grazing" is often recommended to keep blood sugar levels up, it actually has the effect of keeping insulin levels up. While it is natural for insulin levels to rise with each meal or snack, constantly eating small portions of food can keep the insulin levels up too high for too long. High insulin is damaging to the ovaries and contributes to overweight. Let your digestive system rest between meals and snacks.

Sit down to eat. Don't eat and drive! Spend a little relaxation time after meals. The part of the nervous system that stimulates digestion (the parasympathetic division) is often nicknamed the "rest/digest" division. These two rhyming words really do go together!

Try an acid appetizer before a meal. Yes, the traditional pickle is an example of a food that "gets the juices flowing." That means digestive secretions in the stomach, not just your mouth watering.

Chew your food thoroughly. Taste it and enjoy it. Chewing breaks up large food particles, but it also stimulates salivation and stomach secretions.

Avoid too much water during meals, since it dilutes your digestive secretions.

Watch out for food that disagrees with you. Whether it's melons, peanuts, spicy salsa, wheat, eggs, or dairy, almost everyone is sensitive to one food or another. It's possible that the previous tips will help with food that bothers you, especially if you eat the food in small portions. Obviously, if you have a major allergy to a particular food, complete avoidance is the only answer.

Help your friendly intestinal bacteria help you with digestion. Foods that "seed" your intestines with friendly bacteria, such as yogurt, sauerkraut, or kimchi (a fermented Korean food) often help with digestive problems. Foods that "feed" your friendly bacteria, such as the soluble fiber of many plant foods, are also good for your overall digestion. Such foods include whole grains, fruits, onions, mushrooms, asparagus, artichoke, beans, and flaxseed oil.

Just taking supplements of friendly bacteria can put a fast stop to gassiness, diarrhea, and bad breath (Such supplements are discussed in Chapter 3).

If it's your stomach that's giving you trouble, and the previous strategies aren't helpful, try a supplement of mixed digestive enzymes with meals. These are easily available at health food shops and natural groceries.

9: MAKE YOUR MEALS TASTY AND SIMPLE

Nutritious, tasty, simple to prepare—these describe the ideal meal. So far the focus has been on better nutrition. However, if you emphasize the principle of improving the ingredients of your familiar, favorite dishes, you will already have one important element of good taste: familiarity. You naturally tend to like what you are used to, and the freshness, naturalness, and gentle cooking of nutritious foods will automatically add gourmet taste. Good food tastes good!

SIMPLY SWEET

Once you get rid of prepackaged foods with their sugary additives, you'll discover that natural foods are often quite sweet. Constant consumption of soft drinks, baked goods, desserts, candy, and artificial sweeteners stimulates rather than satisfies your sweet tooth. Conversely, when you cut down on sweet junk food, your sensitivity to sweet taste will noticeably improve. The sweetness of carrots, cabbage, whole wheat bread, meat, and even grapefruit will pleasantly surprise you. Eliminating added sugar also enables you to enjoy the actual taste of the food itself. Strawberries, apples, watermelons, blueberries, and other sweet fruits will taste like the treats they really are!

Simplicity is a major consideration since so many of us are so very busy. The rule of thumb of using a greater variety of foods is of real value here. Many of the convoluted, time-consuming recipes in cookbooks are only an attempt to create variety where it really doesn't exist. For example, it's easy to scrub and microwave a white potato. So why peel it, boil it, mash it, fry it, or au gratin it? Instead of depending on so many inconvenient ways to disguise the same old foods, offer real variety in your meats, grains, beans, fruits, and vegetables, and prepare them simply. Instead of that potato, why not brown rice, baked squash, sweet potato, quinoa, corn on the cob, or baked beans? Refer again to Tables 2 and 3 (pages 14 and 15) for some ideas for increasing variety.

BREAKFAST. Hot cereals are traditional breakfast foods. However, if you use cold cereal, make it a point to use whole-grain cereals, rather than the over-advertised junk foods that have replaced real grain foods. Rolled oats, granola, bran muffins, multi-grain pancakes and homemade waffles are all excellent foods. Whole wheat cereals are nutritious, but wheat is so commonly used as bread that it's an excellent idea to avoid it in breakfast grains to increase your variety of food. Instead, why not try a wheat-free organic breakfast granola, complete with oats, seeds, and nuts?

Whole fruits contain natural sugars, but they also offer freshness and fiber. Freshness and fiber are much reduced in bottled fruit juices. You can improve your nutrition by eating a delicious orange or tangerine instead of drinking orange juice, or purple grapes instead of grape juice, or a grapefruit instead of grapefruit juice. As a habit, prefer the whole fruit to the fruit juice, and you will add real zip to your breakfast!

A good source of protein and some fat, along with the fruits just mentioned, will enable your breakfast to give you a long, slow release of nutrients, keeping your blood sugar steady and keeping you energetic and alert until lunchtime. Eggs are a protein and fatty food that really do "stick to your ribs." Milk is another good protein food. Cottage cheese, hard cheese, and yogurt are also excellent sources of protein. Putting butter, peanut butter, or cashew butter on whole wheat toast slows the release of glucose from the toast. If you prefer meat for breakfast, try some of last night's leftovers, but avoid commercially processed meats such as bacon and sausage.

LUNCH. Lunch is great for sandwiches of whole grain bread packed with tuna salad, chicken salad, toasted cheese, natural peanut butter, leaf lettuce, tomatoes, sloppy joes, and so forth. Expand your lunch menu with soups, tacos, wraps, corn bread, yogurt, fruit, eggs, last night's leftovers, or perhaps another breakfast food such as multi-grain pancakes. Or microwave a sweet potato and eat it with butter as part of your lunch.

DINNER. If you serve a traditional American-style dinner, you probably prepare the evening meal around meat, potatoes, a vegetable, and a salad. This pattern gives you something to work with! Broaden your protein menu with ocean fish, tuna, pork, chicken, turkey, or other poultry. Use the "potato position" for brown rice, sweet potatoes, corn, peas, baked squash, beans, or whole grain pasta. Then cook up a couple of hefty servings of dark green or yellow vegetables—whatever is in season or on sale. Make your salad last but serve it first and make it big!

Casseroles, stews, soups, chili, chicken and rice, lasagna, and baked beans are nutritious and economical ways to increase variety and improve your nutrition. In reality, such foods combine two or three of the four basic dishes above. Your favorites can be improved by substituting better ingredients for poor ones (Table 3, page 14-15) and adding the vegetables at the last minute.

I do not serve dessert with dinner except on special occasions. This not only eliminates extra sugar, but it also simplifies dinner preparation considerably. On the other hand, if your family is accustomed to dessert, why not try some fruit?

YOUR SWEET TOOTH

A slice of cantaloupe or watermelon, apples sprinkled with cinnamon, sections of seedless oranges, or a dish of fresh or frozen pineapple, blueberries, cherries, or strawberries after a meal is a good way to satisfy your sweet tooth without disrupting your blood sugar or spending valuable time on preparation. For a pretty table, put your fruit in a dessert dish at each place setting.

Get the Sugar Out! by nutritionist Ann Louise Gittleman contains many other ideas for low-sugar desserts. (See "Further Reading.")

SNACKS. Children, pregnant and nursing mothers, and anyone who tends toward hypoglycemia (often characterized by fatigue or irritability which improves after eating, or migraine headaches in the morning or late afternoon) may find snacks just about a necessity. A combination of whole carbohydrates, protein, and fats makes the best snack. The carbohydrates get the blood sugar up in a short time, while the protein and fat slow the release of sugars into the blood. As a result the blood glucose remains neither too high nor too low over a long period of time.

Yogurt, peanut butter on bread, seed-nut-raisin trail mixes, granola cereal with milk, cheese and whole-grain crackers, toasted cheese sandwiches, or hard-boiled eggs on a salad make good snacks. Sugary foods, including sweet fruits, are the worst snack foods, because they cause wide swings in the blood glucose when they are eaten without other food. Mothers of toddlers who wake up frequently at night or who resist bedtime may find that a hearty protein-rich snack before bed solves the problem. A protein-rich bedtime snack may also help prevent morning headaches in some individuals.

10: MAKE GOOD CHOICES WHEN YOU EAT AWAY FROM HOME

Breaking all the rules occasionally at a fast food restaurant can be fun, but if you must eat lunch or another meal away from home regularly, eating out can make improved nutrition harder to achieve. The truth is, you can get excellent, delicious, highly nutritious meals at fine restaurants, but you will pay real money for their fresh, whole, gently-handled ingredients! Here are some suggestions for those who are away from home during the day.

Eat breakfast at home every day and make it substantial. Have French toast, homemade bread with peanut butter, whole grain granola with milk, or eggs and fruit. Or eat a breakfast that seems like lunch—sandwiches, soup, cottage cheese, or leftovers from last night. Avoid the coffee-and-donut breakfast, which is a recipe for blood sugar swings that drain your energy, disrupt your concentration, and rattle your nerves. Before you leave home, fill up your stainless steel water bottle with some ice cold water, unless you are lucky enough to have purified drinking water at your workplace or school.

Pack up some good food and take it along for lunch. If you have access to a microwave oven, plan on last night's casserole, chili, lasagna, stew, or spaghetti. Or pack whole-grain sandwiches or cold chicken to go. Fruits, salads, yogurt, hard-boiled eggs, or tuna salad are other possibilities.

Rely less on vending machines for snacks. Take a trip to the grocery store and find some snack items. Trail mixes of raisins, seeds, and nuts, or yogurt, whole-grain granola bars, natural cheese, whole grain crackers, baby carrots, celery, or fruits are all possibilities. Use vending machines for milk, yogurt, trail mixes, and other nutritious foods only.

Make good choices at fast food restaurants and cafeterias. Even fast food restaurants usually have salads available. Make digging into a vegetable salad a habit if you must eat out often at a fast food place or cafeteria. Choose meats that are not processed; for example, choose broiled fish, hamburger, chicken, or steak, rather than ham, hot dogs, bacon, or lunch meats. Can you get a baked potato? A bean burrito? Chili? A chef salad? Fresh fruits? Avoid the soft drinks, french fries, breaded chicken nuggets, breaded fish, processed cheese, and sweet desserts.

Make it a priority to eat the evening meal at home. There's no place like home for lots of things, including good nutrition. Eat dinner together as a family.

11: ENLIST YOUR FAMILY'S COOPERATION

Make no mistake about it—if your spouse or children rebel at your efforts to improve the family's nutrition, it's an uphill battle. For your spouse, the easiest way to gain his cooperation is by appealing to his taste buds. As the mother of nine children, I can offer some suggestions to encourage children to good nutritional habits and attitudes: First, keep junk food out of the house. Children can then be permitted to choose their own breakfasts, lunches, and snacks. A corollary to this is to limit screen time. There are better reasons than nutrition for doing so, but restricting the TV and computer will also prevent your children from being tantalized by the shameless advertising of worthless foods. As a significant side benefit, they will also get more exercise.

Next, encourage even the young children to participate in every phase of food preparation, from gardening to actual cooking. Then brag about it at dinner: "Lily picked the asparagus. Eva made the salad. Jonathan cooked the fish." The child who helps prepare the food is already prejudiced in its favor. I frequently set the table or act as "gofer" while my older helpers scrub vegetables, brown meat, or prepare cole slaw. When our children were younger, my husband and I also took the children shopping and let them select the fresh vegetables, seafood, and other items.

Actively teaching children about nutrition is an immense aid. Kids are impressed to find out that protein helps them grow big, or that vitamins keep them healthy. Of course, your own example is your best teaching aid; picky parents have pickier children! And to the extent that you as a parent avoid junk food, you will be pleased at how naturally your children follow your lead.

YOU WOULDN'T ALLOW THEM TO SMOKE...

Just as you teach your children about the dangers of smoking at an early age, teach them also not to drink sugary or diet beverages at all. Yes, your children may be slightly ahead of the crowd if they avoid soft drinks and boxed fruit juices, but many families, schools, and youth groups are now getting the message that these are prime culprits in the epidemic of childhood obesity, poor food choices, brain fog, and poor academic performance. What a help it is that bottled water is "cool" to carry!

BABIES. If you have not had children yet, you can plan beforehand to get future babies off to an excellent start in nutrition and save many problems later on. Sheila Kippley's *Breastfeeding and Natural Child Spacing* covers early solid feeding as well as the best nutrition: breastfeeding. I believe that my children's enthusiasm for salads, granola, vegetables, rice, fish, and yogurt is an outgrowth of their early feeding, which I learned from the first edition of this book. I never used baby food; in fact, I never even mashed my babies' foods, and I've never spoonfed them anything (other than yogurt, which is just too messy to qualify as a finger food).

Around the time my children were six months old and could sit up in the high chair with the family, I gradually introduced them to finger foods such as soft cooked carrots, asparagus, green beans, raw bananas, and tiny pieces of meat. Why spoon-feed a baby who loves to use his hands to put everything into his mouth? I've concluded that pureed baby foods spoil a child's taste for textured food such as salads and vegetables for years. The recognizable green beans and peas that inevitably appear in the diaper are probably nature's way of preventing the young child from obtaining too much nutrition from adult food at the expense of his mother's milk.

It's obvious that having babies sit at the table, watching Mom and Dad eat, whets their appetite for adult food. Togetherness at the table has a role in good nutrition! I have also noticed that babies who are permitted to feed themselves finger foods at the table are not nearly as prone to put small non-food objects into their mouths. Instead, they seem to graduate quickly from their fingers to a fork—not a spoon—just like they see Mom and Dad using.

THE FAMILY. Finally, strive for harmony at the dinner table. Such harmony has a value even beyond its role in family bonding. It's a real factor in good nutrition. Tension at the table, the American habit of eating in a rush, or other unpleasantness stimulates the "fight-or-flight" response. The fight-or-flight response interferes with digestive secretions and diverts the blood supply away from the digestive organs. Both digestion and absorption of a meal are decreased when the fight-or-flight response is activated. On a practical level, we have taught our children not to criticize food at the table, which spoils the meal for others and offends the cook! Instead, they may quietly pass up the occasional foods that they dislike, a practice that we have found goes a long way toward avoiding conflict at the dinner table.

MEALTIME

A gracious mealtime followed by a time of relaxation quiets the fight-or-flight nerves and encourages the "rest/digest" division of the nervous system, stimulating all aspects of the digestive and absorptive processes. Body and spirit are truly inseparable! The parents who set the tone of the dinner by inviting the Lord's presence, and then complimenting their children on their salad making, table setting, or pleasant manners, are helping to nourish both body and spirit.

12: USE THE "80-20" RULE

I've saved the best for last! This final guideline means that as you try for better nutrition, work toward a goal of 80 percent improvement. Having done that, don't worry about the imperfect 20 percent. It's simply not realistic to commit the time, effort, and expense to locating and preparing organically grown foods of prime freshness all the time. As you will see in Chapter 3, taking vitamin and mineral supplements helps to compensate for the inevitable inadequacies of the modern diet.

Completely avoiding all junk food all the time would restrict you from many memorable celebrations: cookouts with friends, birthday parties, weddings, Christmas. Sweets and treats are simply part of those good times! Your children are far more likely to accept your leadership in matters of nutrition if they understand that you are reasonable; that treats are not forbidden—but that they are *treats*.

SUMMARY — CHAPTER 1

TWELVE RULES FOR BETTER NUTRITION

1 Make protein the foundation of your meals.

2 Eat plenty of whole plant foods: grains, beans, nuts, vegetables, seeds, and fruits.

3 Choose healthful fats and oils.

4 Substitute more nutritious ingredients for less nutritious ingredients in your favorite recipes and dishes.

5 Eat a greater variety of foods (but avoid foods you are sensitive to).

6 Sharply limit your sugar intake.

7 Drink plenty of pure water instead of soft drinks and caffeinated beverages.

8 Boost your ability to digest your food.

9 Make your meals tasty and simple.

10 Make good choices when you eat away from home.

11 Enlist your family's cooperation.

12 Use the "80-20" rule.

ACTION PLAN: Try renumbering the above guidelines in your own order, ranking the ones that you need the most improvement on first, second, third, and so forth. For example, if you are drinking soda or have a heavy caffeine habit, guideline number 7 might be number 1 for you. If you also crave sugary treats, maybe number 6 is the rule that you would rank second. Or, if you are doing really well with your food choices, but often have digestive upsets, number 8 might be your number 1. No matter what, encourage yourself with the 80-20 rule!

OBTAINING & PREPARING NUTRITIOUS FOOD

2

Like a merchant fleet, she secures her provisions from afar. She rises while it is still night, and distributes food to her household.

— Proverbs 31:14-15

When nutritious ingredients have replaced refined foods in your home, it's easy to use them in the same recipes you have always used. And when your home contains no junk food, you can snack healthfully on whatever you choose from the kitchen. You will even do far less label-reading when you use whole natural foods, since they contain no added ingredients! The hurdle that many homemakers face, though, is to find out where to conveniently get the best foods they can afford.

This chapter addresses the issue of where to source healthy food, and then how to prepare it. It assumes you are as busy as you really are! It also includes reviews of two very useful cookbooks, either one of which will give you practical help in the matter of preparing good meals quickly and well.

OBTAINING NUTRITIOUS FOOD

If you are presently eating the worst of the American diet—processed meats, packaged mixes, frozen main dishes, boxed mac and cheese, and sweet grocery store baked goods—you can improve your nutrition immensely while still shopping at the same supermarket.

Besides your neighborhood grocery store, there are other sources of healthful foods which may offer better nutrition and sometimes lower prices. Following is a brief look at the nutritional possibilities of the supermarket as well as alternative food sources.

SUPERMARKETS

It's obvious that the explosion of interest in holistic nutrition has paid off well for the consumer at the grocery store. Many whole, natural foods are now stocked in entire sections. Organic brown rice, whole-grain pasta, beans, whole-wheat flour, granola, and natural peanut butter are readily available. The huge produce sections, with many organically-grown fruits and vegetables, make it easy to increase the assortment of fresh fruits and vegetables that you use. The variety of hormone-free poultry, quick-frozen ocean fish, eggs from free-range chickens, and tasty ethnic foods offered at most supermarkets is large and growing.

Even if a grocery store does not contain expanded sections of natural foods or produce, it can still remain the basic place to shop. Experienced nutrition-conscious homemakers favor the basics—produce, frozen vegetables, dairy items, meat, and fish—and bypass most of the processed foods.

Produce. In the produce department, it's easy to be overwhelmed by so many new and unfamiliar fruits and vegetables, so plan to browse a little someday soon. Challenge yourself to try just one new item each time you shop. Go ahead and bring home a kiwi or two. Or treat the family to a fresh pineapple. What about a bunch of fresh beets? Or some bright green Romaine lettuce or other leafy salad greens? Could you jazz up your salads with some red or yellow peppers? Those bright colors and spicy tastes are sure signs of foods rich in phytonutrients. What's on sale? Asparagus? Leeks? Artichokes? Yams? Acorn squash? Grapefruits? Watermelon? Cantaloupes? Cranberries? It's both nutritionally and economically sound to increase the variety of your fresh produce purchases by selecting whatever is in season or on sale.

Frozen Foods. Look around the frozen foods section for the frozen vegetables: green beans, broccoli, corn, peas, lima beans, and Oriental mixed vegetables. Bring home some frozen blueberries or frozen tropical fruits for a special treat. Prefer fresh to frozen, but frozen to canned. Avoid the frozen, prepackaged dinners or side dishes. With the right cookbook, as you will see, you will be soon making your own main dishes that are tastier, cheaper, and healthier in every way!

Dairy. In the dairy department, select natural yogurt and natural cheeses such as cottage cheese, cheddar cheese, or mozzarella cheese. Avoid processed "cheese foods." Choose butter instead of margarine. If you are attempting to overcome infertility or cycle irregularity, favor full-fat dairy products over no-fat ones. In some groceries, you may be able to get organically produced cows' milk, or goats' milk if you are allergic to cows' milk. Some grocery stores offer "DHA-containing" chicken eggs. DHA is the fatty acid that supports brain function and development, so reach for those!

Meats. In addition to beef and chicken, what other meats might you wish to try? Turkey? Lamb? Pork? Notice the labels—it's now possible to get meats that are labeled "hormone-free" and "antibiotic-free." Try to buy raw poultry that does not have flavored "juice" added to it. If you use meat on sandwiches, avoid the processed luncheon meats and make sandwiches from cold turkey, chicken or beef. Skip processed ham, bacon, hot dogs, and sausage also.

Fish. Basic, unbreaded fish fillets are healthier than the breaded, frozen kind. If you live inland, you may have trouble finding frozen fish that is not breaded or precooked, or the "fresh" fish flown in from afar is not very fresh at all! If that's the case, try stocking up on frozen fish fillets during Lent, when even stores that usually do not carry frozen perch, whiting, or whitefish fillets will have good buys on quick-frozen, unprocessed ocean fish.

FAST FISH

It's extremely fast and easy to cook raw fish. Defrost it and pat it dry. Season it on both sides (Old Bay 30% Less Sodium Seasoning is my favorite); dip both sides in corn meal. Pan fry at moderate heat in olive oil for a couple of minutes on each side. Top it with tartar sauce—crispy and delicious!

Look for **wild-caught** ocean fish instead of farm-raised fish. Fish do not make their own healthful fatty acids (abbreviated EPA and DHA); instead, they eat algae that contain the EPA and DHA. Farmed salmon, for example, are fed grains that alter their fatty acid content, detracting from the value of farmed salmon compared to wild-caught salmon. To avoid mercury-contaminated fish, check out the Natural Resources Defense Council's website: www.nrdc.org/stories/smart-seafood-buying-guide. They recommend American-caught fish, flash frozen, and stamped with the Marine Stewardship Council "Certified Sustainable Seafood" checkmark. As of this writing, haddock, flounder, sole, whiting, whitefish, and salmon are on the "least mercury" list. So are many other types of fish, including freshwater trout and marine invertebrates such as shrimp.

On The Shelves. In the center of the store, be sure to examine the ethnic foods section. Here you can find taco shells, dry beans, peas, and lentils for soup. How will you use them? Take a look at the wrapper; almost always you can find a recipe on it. I buy canned kidney beans and pinto beans for chili, and canned tomato sauce, which I use to make my own spaghetti, chili, or lasagna sauce. I use canned chunk light tuna occasionally (currently it is rated moderate for mercury content) for tuna noodle casserole or tuna patties. I also pick up commercially prepared condiments—ketchup, mayonnaise, tartar sauce, and mustard—from the shelves.

HEALTH FOOD SHOPS AND NATURAL GROCERIES

Health food shops and natural grocery stores are closely related. Health food shops are usually just miniature grocery stores that specialize in food supplements as well as organic and natural foods. Natural groceries, which are popping up all over, are generally larger than the traditional health food shops. They also emphasize organic and natural foods.

ORGANIC VERSUS NATURAL FOODS

It's helpful to understand these two terms before you purchase foods labeled as such. Certified "organic" refers to foods that are grown on mulched or manure-enriched fields without the use of chemical fertilizers, herbicides, or pesticides. With reference to animal products, it means that the animal was fed from such plant foods, and that no hormones or antibiotics were used. Importantly, certified organic foods do not include genetically modified foods (GM; GMO) or irradiated foods. "Natural" generally means unprocessed. "Natural" rice, for example, has not been refined after harvesting, but it has been grown using conventional farming methods and chemicals. Organic foods are the best, and their higher prices reflect the difference. They will contain more vitamins and minerals and less pesticide or herbicide residues than other foods.

Health food shops and natural groceries are more expensive than the large chain supermarkets, so they may appeal more to smaller families than to larger ones. But they are good places to get to know, because they carry several desirable items not found in most supermarkets. If you bake your own bread, in addition to organic flour, you can easily pick up baking yeast, sea salt, gluten, and nutritional yeast. You can find expeller-pressed canola oil, other expeller-pressed oils, and aluminum-free baking powder. You can get organic quinoa (a seed food cooked and used exactly like rice) and almond flour and whole-grain pasta. You will also find tasty breakfast cereals based on whole, organic grains.

Natural groceries and health food shops stock raw seeds and nuts. Some carry fresh-baked breads made with organic ingredients. Many feature locally-grown organic produce and DHA-rich eggs. Some may have organic milk. If you are hoping to buy top-quality bottled salad dressings, health food shops and natural groceries will have them. If you need gluten-free foods, or if you have allergies that restrict what you can eat, you will find these shops a real blessing. They most likely will have foods labeled just for you. Take a little time to look around, and ask the shopkeepers how to use unfamiliar items that interest you.

Health food shops are probably best known for their large selection of vitamins and minerals. In addition, they will have flax oil in capsules or bottles, as well as purified, good-tasting fish oil or krill oil to take as a supplement. Probiotics, friendly bacteria in capsules, can also be purchased at health food shops, as well as other healthy oils, herbs, and teas.

If you have access to a large natural grocery, you may be able to purchase fresh or frozen red meat, fish, and poultry. Look for their specials, and you may find prices equivalent to a typical meat shop.

If the nearest natural grocery or health food shop is inconveniently far away or too expensive for your budget, at least use it to purchase expeller-pressed salad oils, aluminum-free baking powder, sea salt, organic whole grain flours, and pasta.

FOOD CO-OPS

Food co-ops are member-owned natural groceries that are found in many communities. They can offer reduced prices to members as a result of direct bulk purchasing and no-frills shop keeping. These are excellent places to buy your organic grains, beans, flours, oil, honey, bran, nuts, peanut butter, breakfast cereals, and pasta.

Co-ops are wonderful for those who wish to eat nutritiously on a shoestring budget; if you are willing to work a few hours per month, you will get additional savings on your purchases. Chances are you will be able to bring your little ones to the shop as you work, as there is probably a corner space filled with toys to keep small hands occupied.

I get much of the nonperishable food for my family from our local food co-op. My monthly list includes the following, almost all of which is organically produced: whole wheat bread flour, wheat gluten, baking yeast, expeller-pressed salad oils, natural peanut butter, brown rice, granola cereal, other multi-grain cereals, oatmeal, bran, cornmeal, brown rice, quinoa, and pasta.

BUYING CLUBS

A buying club is another convenient way for cost-conscious homemakers to acquire natural or organic foods. It is especially practical if your family is large or if you have space to store nonperishable items, because most of the items are sold in fairly large quantities. A buying club is generally a small food co-op handled by a single family from their home. The member families order from the managing family a few days ahead of the monthly pick-up date, and on pick-up day they drive to the managing family's home to pick up and pay for their groceries. Pick-up day, in fact, is often a time to visit for a few minutes with friends who also belong to the buying club. To find the buying club nearest your home, try this website: www.coopdirectory.org.

FARMERS' MARKETS

Are you aware that many cities and towns feature wonderful farmers' markets where you can buy fresh produce brought in by nearby farmers? These markets are the next best thing to your own garden. The huge farmers' market in Milwaukee where I used to shop was filled with a huge variety of incredible bargains. We lived there as budget-conscious newlyweds, and my temptation was always to buy more than the two of us could possibly eat. We would visit the farmers' market on a Saturday morning, going home with brown bags filled with too much of everything.

These popular markets are usually open for a limited number of hours and days during the growing season only.

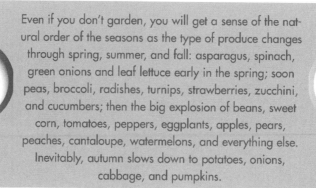

Even if you don't garden, you will get a sense of the natural order of the seasons as the type of produce changes through spring, summer, and fall: asparagus, spinach, green onions and leaf lettuce early in the spring; soon peas, broccoli, radishes, turnips, strawberries, zucchini, and cucumbers; then the big explosion of beans, sweet corn, tomatoes, peppers, eggplants, apples, pears, peaches, cantaloupe, watermelons, and everything else. Inevitably, autumn slows down to potatoes, onions, cabbage, and pumpkins.

Spend some time at your local farmers' market some Saturday morning. Shop carefully, and you will certainly find produce of gratifying freshness and vendors who are passionate about providing organically grown items. Make it a point to try something new every time. Ask the friendly vendors how they prepare, say, a rutabaga or a bunch of fresh kohlrabi.

The best thing about farmers' markets is that they are such fun to visit, especially if you would like to experience the old-time "down-home" way of getting to know the hard-working folks who grow your food. Not only are your purchases good for you, but they also support local family farmers and return money to the community.

COMMUNITY SUPPORTED AGRICULTURE
Community Supported Agriculture (CSA) is a rapidly-growing option that is a classic win-win for all involved. CSAs vary, but they can be summarized as groups of consumers who partner with a farmer to distribute the cost of production as well as the fruits of the soil among the members.

CSAs are good for the farm families, because they make a market and take financial pressure off the family farmers. They are good for the consumers, who have fresh, often organic, reasonably-priced produce, eggs, poultry, and red meat available in the natural timing of the seasons. They are good for the land, because organic farming practices enrich the soil. They are even good for production animals, which are permitted to graze to provide the recommended "pastured" meat that you may have heard about but have not been able to obtain. They are good for the community, because they create bonds between city folks and farm folks, and they recycle money within the community. They are good for the environment, because they cut the waste of trucking food from far away.

CSAs are eminently logical—why should Americans, who live in one of the most agriculturally blessed nations on earth, transport food across this huge nation? Isn't it more sensible to transport it across town?

Please look into the website www.localharvest.org to find out where there are local organic farms near you, and how to become a **shareholder** or **subscriber** in this type of cooperative venture.

PRIVATE FARMERS

Growing numbers of families own small amounts of land and are attempting to raise chemical-free vegetables, fruits, meat, eggs, honey, and dairy products for their own family as well as to sell for extra cash. If such an undertaking is out of the question for you, I can assure you that there are homesteaders around who would enjoy the extra cash of raising a free-ranging, antibiotic- and hormone-free lamb, goat, pig, or steer for you. No, you do not end up with a four-footed potential steak in your suburban garage! They take the animal to a custom butcher, and you literally pick up the pieces, all cut and wrapped according to your specifications. Rabbit, chicken, and other poultry are available in this way also.

Depending on the state that you live in, you may also be able to purchase raw cows' milk or raw goats' milk. For example, in some states you may legally own a share in a dairy herd, entitling you to the milk, which you may be able to pick up at a delivery point right in town.

GARDENING

Your own garden is good for the soul as well as the body, and it can be a wonderful family project, providing true quality time for dads, moms, and kids all at once.

Give yourself a couple of summers to get good at it, and please don't invest in a tiller or herbicides or even a spade until you read *Gardening Without Work* by the late Ruth Stout (See "Further Reading."). This book explains in a highly readable way the art of mulch gardening—using spoiled hay, straw, fall leaves, or grass clippings to prevent weeds, retain moisture, and fertilize the soil. It's the easy way to garden! Using a modified version of this method, we till our large garden only once every two or three years. We do use small amounts of conventional fertilizer and the low-toxicity plant product rotenone as a pesticide. You can learn more about mulch gardening by googling "Ruth Stout Gardening."

My suggestion for beginners is to plant whatever grows the best with the least care. Asparagus is on the top of my list. This hardy vegetable will produce for you the fourth year after planting, and will feed your family scrumptiously and effortlessly for years early each spring while you are just putting in the spinach seeds! High fencing for tall pole beans and edible pod peas (Sugar Snap, an incredible raw treat) will maximize your yields and minimize your bending. Nothing is easier to grow than sweet corn, and nothing compares with ripe corn picked as the water boils, or corn roasted on an outdoor grill. Beets, turnips, lettuce, onions, broccoli, Brussels sprouts, cabbage, cucumbers, peppers, and of course tomatoes are other easy-to-grow plants with high nutrient returns. If you have room outside your garden for some berry bushes, fruit trees, or grape vines, put some in. For example, one of the easiest fruits to grow is the Concord grape, which needs no spraying and thrives for years.

RAISING YOUR OWN EGGS, MEAT, AND MILK

Have you ever dreamed of homesteading on a few acres to feed your family yourself? If you already have the land to do so, why not give homesteading a try? If you are a young couple still not settled in your own home, I strongly encourage you to consider at least two or three acres zoned for agriculture. As a homesteader for the last thirty-five years, I would like to offer you just a little practical perspective.

First, fence in that garden we just talked about. In fact, fencing is first when it comes to livestock.

If you are just starting out with livestock, traditional dual-purpose chickens which are good for both meat and eggs are my first recommendation. They can be mail-ordered as day-old chicks. It is always a delightful day when we drive to the post office and pick up a chirping box of fluffy chicks. They are surprisingly easy to raise; often not a single tiny chick will die (if your brooding set-up is cat-proof!). If you can let your chickens free range, in about six months you will get delicious, nutritious eggs with deep orange yolks, and your homestead will be just about tick-free (but unfortunately it may also become flower-free!). Outsmarting local predators requires shelter, fencing, awareness, and an intelligent herd dog that has been taught to be part of the prevention, not part of the problem.

We value these traditional chicken breeds for their independence and willingness to forage for food, as well as for their good health, longevity, beauty, and ease of care. We have butchered our old hens and young "heavy layer" breed cockerels ourselves, but we find it more convenient to pay to have them butchered locally. By the way, old heavy-breed hens, about two or even three years old, make a most delectable chicken stew, complete with thick yellow broth.

We have also raised turkeys, ducks, and geese for a bit of variety on the homestead and at the table. No, you do not need a pond to raise ducks or geese! Geese, which live on grass, produce a dark meat that tastes much like beef. Roast goose makes a festive dinner. If you want to kick it up a notch, but on a small scale, a few dairy goats for milk and meat are my second recommendation. Again, good fencing is essential, and you will need the advice of others to get started.

But well-bred dairy goats, purchased at reasonable prices from experienced herdsmen who take pride in their high-quality does and bucks, are easy keepers. Champion dairy goats are bred for physical soundness, longevity, health, ease of milking, and ease of giving birth. A good goat will give a gallon of milk a day for several months. Goat milk is hypoallergenic to most people, and is a healthy raw food. It must be cooled rapidly to taste good, a technique my daughter has perfected using an electric ice cream maker with a metal sleeve that is cooled in the freezer. Goats are seasonal breeders, which means that they tend to kid in the spring, and thankfully are dry during the coldest months of winter. Like most homesteaders, we do not keep a buck, but rather take our goats to the best breeders we can find in our area. We butcher our goat wethers (young castrated males) ourselves, which saves a great deal of money, as custom butchering is about half of the overall cost of the meat.[1]

Our family has additionally raised sheep, rabbits, and even a pig. We have found spring lambs easy to raise, but we prefer to purchase them rather than breed sheep ourselves, though in the past we have kept ewes and a buck sheep. Lamb and goat meat, by the way, tastes very similar. A lamb or young goat wether can be home-butchered somewhere around 100-150 pounds, a manageable size.

Our family has never raised cattle, because of our preference for more variety and our inability to butcher so large an animal ourselves. All of our children have been enthusiastically interested in our small livestock, and we are glad that they know first-hand what goes into breeding and birthing, and into producing meat, milk, and eggs. I admit that I find livestock raising much more fun and satisfying than my original first love, gardening.

If homesteading is your dream, as it was ours when we were a young couple, I urge you to make it come true.

You can contact your local 4-H office where there are clubs for poultry, dairy and meat goats, sheep, cattle, rabbits, and hogs.

OBTAINING NUTRITIOUS FOOD

THE RIGHT COOKBOOK

The right cookbook could be the most important ingredient of all for preparing healthful meals. The ideal cookbook should use all natural ingredients; it should provide lots of options so that recipes can be adapted to your taste or pantry supplies; it should cover a wide variety of nutritious foods; it should contain mostly quick and easy recipes; and every single recipe must be delicious! Here are my recommendations; either or both of these will fill the bill:

Saving Dinner: The Menus, Recipes, and Shopping Lists to Bring Your Family Back to the Table, by Leanne Ely, is a cookbook that will jump-start you on your way to real, natural, tasty homemade dinners, and a great variety of them. (See "Further Reading.") This book not only offers very quick-to-cook dishes, but also gives you weekly menus and even shopping lists. It is set up by season, focusing your emphasis on fresh, natural, and thrifty ingredients. There are many nice touches—for example, the summer menus do not use the oven at all. The sidebars offer helpful tips on soaking beans, cutting squash, and marinating meat. It contains no dessert menus, but with all the tasty foods to start with and the spices for added flavor, you will not miss dessert. Some homemakers may wish to follow the menu plans closely, but for most others, just the recipes are more than enough to help you to bring the family back to the table. Leann Ely is also the author of several other cookbooks.

Whole Foods for the Whole Family, published by La Leche League International (see "Further Reading"), was written by and for busy mothers who wish to eat holistically while still "cooking American." It's somewhat more comprehensive than *Saving Dinner* and offers more instruction for those who have never had much experience in home cooking. It has many, many basic recipes, but it also has sections on making your own whole wheat bread, peanut butter, sprouts, yogurt, and even baby food. It explains how to cook brown rice, quinoa, dried peas, and beans. It features many meatless main dishes and many ethnic dishes, but it has a whole section on meat cookery—even several recipes for liver! There are also desserts that require very little added sugar and are loaded with nutrients. The book includes an appendix that lists recipes that are easy to make, easy to freeze, especially quick to prepare, and so forth. Browsing through it is a delight; you learn about basic nutrition, and it teaches you elementary kitchen skills that you despaired of ever learning. I love this book!

KITCHEN APPLIANCES

Once you have acquired nutritious whole food, whether from grocery or garden, you will be storing it, preparing it, and serving it. Many of the tools that are already in your kitchen are well-adapted to these tasks. Others that you may not use are also worth considering.

The refrigerator is basic, of course, and the bigger the better. Many natural, unprocessed foods must be refrigerated—for example, salad oils and peanut butter. You will need space for all your fresh produce. A deep freezer (or even two freezers) is especially useful for those who garden or raise their own meat. A microwave oven makes it easy to cook white potatoes, sweet potatoes, and other vegetables. It's great to reheat a plate of food quickly.

FOOD PROCESSOR

Nothing will help you increase your consumption of good food like a Cuisinart® food processor. It turns out huge amounts of green salads and cole slaw in seconds. It slices fresh beets, tomatoes, and stew vegetables such as carrots and celery. It chops onions, cold chicken for salad, and tuna for tuna patties. It grates potatoes for potato pancakes. It can be used to make peanut butter, mayonnaise, salad dressings, and natural pumpkin pie. It can chop mozzarella cheese or cheddar cheese into a fine topping. It grinds meat for those who butcher their own animals. I have also noticed that the smaller pieces that it produces seem to help young children really enjoy their salads.

A good food processor such as the Cuisinart® will repay you for years in big, fresh salads with minimal clean-up or maintenance. I use my medium-sized Cuisinart® just about every day, and have done so for as long as I have had one. I can recommend this brand heartily; my first one lasted for 17 years of almost daily use.

RICE COOKER

Goodness, what a convenience! You scoop out the rice with the measuring cup, rinse it three times, fill up the pan, which is marked so that you can easily determine the right amount of water, and push the button that says "Brown Rice." An hour or so later the rice is ready, and the cooker beeps. It doesn't matter if dinner is not yet ready, because the rice cooker automatically shifts to a warming mode. If you wish, you can use it at the same time to steam vegetables. We are eating organic brown rice quite a bit more since we have the rice cooker, and I am always amazed at how versatile rice is. And as a bonus, the rice cooker will also cook quinoa, a nutritious seed that can be substituted for just about any dish that calls for rice. Just make sure that your rice cooker's cooking pan is BPA-free (BPA is bisphenol-A, an organic substance that hardens plastics, but acts as a potential hormone disrupter).

The best thing about a rice cooker is that you can put the rice in and forget it.

BREADMAKER

A breadmaker is the most incredible little robot ever introduced into a kitchen. You drop in the ingredients, set the timer, and in three hours you take out a fresh, fragrant loaf of bread. There is very little clean-up, because the pan releases the bread with hardly a crumb left behind. You can set the breadmaker to have the bread ready any time: the next morning, before supper, or as you go out the door to take dinner to a friend. Most important, the breadmaker can make 100 percent whole-wheat bread with all natural ingredients and no artificial preservatives or *trans* fats.

Bread that can be perfectly sliced (just like store-bought bread) is essential if your family is going to use homemade bread daily. If it is crumbly or if it squashes as you try to slice it, it won't be good for sandwiches. That's why you will need to add gluten to 100 percent organic whole wheat bread, as is noted in the recipe below. I have not invested in one of the slicing templates that promise to enable you to slice the bread uniformly, because I have not had any difficulty with this. I do have a good serrated bread knife, though.

BAKING BREAD

If you don't have a recipe that suits your taste and nutritional goals, you will need to modify a recipe. A problem with breadmakers is that your friend's favorite recipe won't necessarily work well in your brand of breadmaker. You might try the basic whole wheat recipe for your own machine, and then adjust it for better nutrition. Or try mine (below) and alter it as needed. In general, bread that is too high and sinks in the middle needs less water, less honey, less gluten, less yeast, or more salt. Bread that is too heavy may need more water, honey, gluten, yeast (or another brand of yeast), or less salt. My recipe is based on an original one for whole wheat bread that came with my first breadmaker, but it has been modified beyond recognition. Don't give up on your ideal bread too soon—it may take half a dozen or more bad loaves before you create the perfect recipe.

Here is my one and only bread recipe, made for my Breadman breadmaker. I hope it will work well for your willing little kitchen servant.

MARILYN'S
Bread Recipe

Ingredients	You will need:
1-1/2 cup warm water	Breadmaker
3 1/2 cups hard organic whole wheat flour	**Yield:**
2 tablespoons gluten	1 two-pound loaf
2 teaspoons salt	
2 tablespoons butter	
1/4 to 1/3 cup honey	
2 teaspoons granular baking yeast	

Directions:

1. Drop ingredients in, set timer, and savor the fragrance of baking bread in your kitchen in a couple of hours.

2. When the buzzer sounds, remove the steaming loaf. Invite your husband to the kitchen table with you to enjoy a warm slice, covered with melted butter.

"Give us this day our daily bread." The Lord Himself taught us those words.

Once you have the perfect recipe, don't change it. In my home, all of the family members who make the bread have this recipe memorized, so that it is simple to start a delicious loaf of bread right before we go to bed. I also store the right-sized measuring cup or measuring spoon in each container of ingredients, so that it's hard to make a mistake.

YOGURT MAKER
Using a yogurt maker will save many dollars spent on yogurt and will produce better yogurt than you can buy. Several different brands of electric yogurt makers are available inexpensively through department stores. Some make one large batch of yogurt; others make it in individual one-cup servings. Many health food shops carry powdered yogurt starter, which ensures good tasting yogurt every time.

MAKING YOGURT IN A YOGURT MAKER

First, scald the right amount of milk in a saucepan to kill off bacteria. Then allow the milk to cool down to a temperature compatible for the friendly bacteria that will convert the milk to yogurt. If you are in a hurry, you can set the pan in a sink of cold water. Once the temperature has dropped enough (according to your yogurt thermometer), you stir in the yogurt starter. You place the mixture in the yogurt maker, plug it in, and in a few hours or overnight you remove the warm yogurt. Once it cools in the refrigerator, it's ready to eat with some jam, honey, or fruit as a sweetener. Homemade yogurt is thinner than the grocery store type. Don't be disappointed if that's how it turns out. Your yogurt maker will come with recipes to help you use more of this wonderfully nutritious food.

PRESSURE COOKER
I recently bought a two-gallon stainless steel Presto stove top pressure cooker. I am already in love with it! For example, I took some home-butchered meat and quickly cooked it and made Chinese curried lamb with wine sauce (actually goat kid meat).

On another busy afternoon I made a stew from start to finish—so fast. I guess some people love their crock pots to slow-cook a meal, starting in the morning, but I'm just the opposite: My pressure cooker is my fast cooker!

The Instapot is the electric version of the stove top pressure cooker, and you may like it even better. It multi-tasks as a crock pot, rice cooker, and yogurt maker, but the pressure cooking feature is the one that will help busy homemakers the most.

POPCORN POPPER

Our popcorn popper is used so frequently that it stays out on the counter, along with the rice cooker, breadmaker, and food processor. The air-popped popcorn avoids overheated oil, though it is not quite as crispy as the oil-popped variety. Popcorn topped with melted butter really does make a quick, easy, delicious, nutritious snack.

WATER PURIFICATION SYSTEM

Are you remodeling your kitchen? If so, why not install a reverse osmosis or solid carbon block water purification system? It will provide convenience and an improvement in your health, especially if you have city water or a shallow well. And what a great way to motivate yourself to kick the bad habit of drinking soft drinks!

If a reverse osmosis system or solid carbon block filter will not fit into your budget (or your kitchen), what about a filter for your kitchen tap? Look for a high-quality one that removes both organic and inorganic contaminants, and change it as often as specified by the manufacturer. Then, purchase good quality stainless steel water bottles for family members who work or go to school outside the home. That way, all of you can carry your "homemade" water with you, instead of buying plastic bottles of very expensive and not necessarily contaminant-free water.

POTS, PANS, AND BAKEWARE

Stainless steel pots with tight-fitting lids are ideal for basic cooking tasks such as steaming vegetables. Your teakettle is another staple item; it's there for all the tasty and healthful teas that you can enjoy with family or friends, or just for an afternoon pick-me-up. A really big stainless steel soup pot is useful if there are to be leftovers. Mine holds four gallons, and I love using it to make large amounts of stew or chicken and rice or spaghetti sauce for my large family. A big, covered stainless steel roasting pan is another essential item. Each Sunday before church, we put a roast in the oven— usually our own lamb, goat meat, duck, goose, or chicken, surrounded with potatoes, carrots, and onions. The roasting pan does the rest until we come home and make the gravy. Cookie sheets, muffin pans, and cake pans are nice to have for your homemade desserts and muffins, which are more nutritious and better-tasting than store-bought treats—plus you get the fun and family time of making them yourselves!

A non-stick frying pan will encourage you to cook more frequently at home, since it is so easy to use and so quick to clean. Frying pans with high-quality ceramic surfaces, even electric ones, are readily available. My son-in-law, an excellent and health-conscious cook, insists, though, that his properly seasoned cast iron frying pan is as easy to clean as any non-stick type.

A slow cooker (crock pot) is not only good for stews and soups that you start in the morning, but it's also wonderful to take to potluck dinners, full of whatever you'd like to serve hot. You can even make your own extra-thick yogurt with your crock pot, as my daughter Rosemary, the mother of a large family, does.

ROSEMARY'S EXTRA-THICK YOGURT IN A CROCK POT

Buying enough yogurt for a family of eleven was proving inconvenient, so I modified one of the many available crockpot yogurt recipes to make a probiotic-rich breakfast food for my family. The secret is the added capsule of probiotics; it makes the consistency thicker without any extra effort on my part. If I start this at 9 a.m., I put the finished yogurt in the refrigerator at 9 p.m., and we all enjoy it the next morning mixed with a spoonful of strawberry jam, frozen berries, and homemade granola.

ROSEMARY'S
Extra-Thick Yogurt in a Crock Pot

Ingredients	You will need:
1 gal. whole milk	1 gallon crockpot
16 oz. plain yogurt with live cultures	1 cooking thermometer
1 probiotic powder	

Directions

1. Fill a 1-gallon crockpot almost to the top with whole milk. Remember to leave a little room for the 16 oz of starter yogurt ("starter") that will be added later. Turn it on high and heat it to 180 degrees. I set the timer for 3 hours, and it is ready when the timer goes off.

2. When it has reached 180 degrees, turn off the crockpot and leave it to cool until the milk is at 120 degrees. I lift the crock out of the metal sleeve to allow quicker cooling, and set the timer for 2.5 hours; it is usually ready between 2.5 and 3 hours later.

3. When you start cooling the milk, set your starter yogurt out to come up to room temperature. I also set out the probiotic pill so I do not forget to add it later.

4. When the milk reaches 120 degrees, I break open a high-quality probiotic pill, and stir that thoroughly into the room-temperature starter yogurt. Then I stir this starter into the milk. The added probiotics make the final yogurt very thick and creamy. You can stir the probiotics directly into the milk, but the powder will float and only thicken up the top two inches, so I put it in the starter first to distribute it more evenly.

5. Wrap the crockpot in a big towel to maintain the temperature. Let it sit for 6-7 hours. Then, move it to the refrigerator to cool and set. I could strain and drain it to make Greek yogurt at this point--but never have bothered to do so, as we find it is thick enough. If I decide to make it thicker yet, I will probably will just add two probiotic pills instead of one.

6. Enjoy it with some tasty homemade granola, a spoonful of jam, and some berries!

CANISTERS, CONTAINERS, AND OTHER KITCHEN ODDS-N-ENDS

Extra canisters are important for your flours, brown rice, quinoa, beans, whole-grain pasta, herbal teas, and popcorn. Glass dishes with tight-fitting plastic lids are just what you need to keep your leftovers in top shape. A good bread knife and cutting board are essential equipment for breadmaking. A hand-held pepper mill filled with peppercorns will enable you to season your food like a gourmet cook. If you take lunch with you, invest in insulated containers to keep hot things hot and cold things cold.

DINNERWARE

Finally, may I suggest something not directly related to food preparation? You need a beautiful set of dinnerware. (Yes, even if you have young children.) A beautifully set table with a lovely tablecloth and centerpiece adds such graciousness to your meals. Better yet, it encourages you to prepare your best meals for your family as well as for your guests.

SUMMARY—CHAPTER 2

GOOD FOOD SOURCES

SUPERMARKETS: Still a great place to shop, and getting better.

HEALTH FOOD SHOPS AND NATURAL GROCERIES: Get acquainted with one near you.

FOOD CO-OPS: Economical, especially if you work in it a few hours per month.

BUYING CLUBS: Good for large, cost-conscious families.

FARMERS' MARKETS: Fresh and fun.

COMMUNITY SUPPORTED AGRICULTURE GROUPS: A win-win for all involved.

PRIVATE FARMERS: Find one nearby for organic meat and eggs.

GARDENING: Good for the soul, as well as for the body.

RAISING YOUR OWN EGGS, MEAT, AND MILK

If it's your dream, make it come true.

RECOMMENDED SUPPLIES

COOKBOOK: Not an appliance, but you need Leanne Ely's *Saving Dinner* or La Leche League's *Whole Foods for the Whole Family*.

REFRIGERATOR: Make it big and store your flour and oils in it also.

DEEP FREEZER: For frozen vegetables, fruits, homemade sauces, and meats.

FOOD PROCESSOR: Cuisinart® for salads and many other tasks.

RICE COOKER: Foolproof rice cooking and vegetable steaming.

BREADMAKER: If you have one, use it!

PRESSURE COOKER: The Instapot is most marvelous as a pressure cooker for stews, beans, or other fast cooking.

YOGURT MAKER: Provides high quality and less expensive yogurt.

POPCORN POPPER: Fun and nutritious snacks.

WATER PURIFICATION SYSTEM: A wonderful addition to a kitchen.

KITCHEN POTS AND PANS: Pots with tight-fitting lids; stainless steel soup pot and roasting pan; cookie sheets, muffin and cake pans, ceramic non-stick or cast iron frying pan.

CROCK POT: Great for so many things, even for making extra-thick yogurt.

CANISTERS: For all those grains, beans, rice, and flours.

STORAGE DISHES WITH TIGHT-FITTING LIDS: Keep your leftovers fresh.

DINNERWARE: For a beautifully set table, every day.

BASIC SUPPLEMENTS TO CONSIDER

3

God also said: See, I give you every seed-bearing plant on all the earth and every tree that has seed-bearing fruit on it to be your food.
— Genesis 1:29

Do you get discouraged by much of what you read or hear about modern food? Have you concluded that it's simply not possible to get top-quality nutrition out of the food you buy and prepare? Do you have food sensitivities—to milk, wheat, corn, fish, eggs, or other good foods—that limit what you are able to eat? Are you in a situation where it's difficult for you to make your own food at home? Are you concerned about sprays on plants used for food and the diet of animals used for food? Would you like to be in the best health possible before you get pregnant? Are you hoping to improve your chances of getting pregnant?

There is a way of compensating for the inadequacies of our modern diet and even for the toxins in the environment: taking vitamin, mineral, and essential fatty acid supplements.

I rank the prudent use of vitamin, mineral, and essential fatty acid supplements as a health practice second only to holistic food in the benefits it provides. The purpose of this chapter is to provide an overview of vitamin, mineral, essential fatty acids, and a few other supplements; to explain the rationale for taking them; and to recommend a plan of supplementation which is within the limits of safety, comprehensive enough to be beneficial, and flexible enough to be tailored to your individual needs. The chapter ends with several practical suggestions to help you get the most benefit from taking supplements.

DEFINING VITAMINS, MINERALS, AND ESSENTIAL FATTY ACIDS

Vitamins and minerals are called **micronutrients** because they are needed only in tiny amounts compared to the **macronutrients**: proteins, carbohydrates, and fats. In terms of how much you need, the two essential fatty acids fall somewhere in between the micronutrients and macronutrients. Nevertheless, in this book micronutrients refers to vitamins, minerals, and essential fatty acids, because these three classes of essential nutrients can be added to the diet in pill form; that is, as supplements.

Vitamins are complex, carbon-based molecules synthesized by other living creatures but necessary to human life and health. As such, they must be obtained in the diet. Vitamins are divided into fat-soluble and water-soluble types: vitamins A, D, E, and K are fat-soluble; the various B vitamins and vitamin C are water-soluble. Vitamins are absorbed from the intestines and ultimately enter the blood.

Cells receive vitamins from the blood and use them for a variety of essential functions. Some are used to liberate energy from food molecules, some assist in cell division, some prevent oxygen damage to cellular parts, some enable various cell structures to be synthesized, and some help to rid the body of toxins. Many perform these tasks by serving as **coenzymes**; that is, they enable the cells' enzymes to do their job of sparking the multitude of chemical reactions taking place within cells.

> **If you envision an enzyme as a razor, the thin strip of metal which does the actual cutting is like a vitamin which serves as a coenzyme. The enzyme cannot work without it.**

Minerals are simpler than vitamins. They occur in the non-biological world, though most dietary minerals come from plant and animal foods. Calcium, phosphorus, and magnesium are minerals used in relatively large amounts in our bodies, because they are major components of bone. Potassium, chloride, and sodium are also abundant in the body. The others that our bodies require are **trace minerals**, needed only in tiny amounts. Iron, zinc, copper, chromium, selenium, chromium, and iodine are examples of trace minerals. Minerals are absorbed from the intestines into the blood, but many are more difficult to absorb than are vitamins.

Some minerals, such as magnesium, zinc, and selenium, perform a large number of functions in many different cell types. Iron is a mineral well known for its role in red blood cells, where it carries oxygen, but it is also used by almost all other cells to liberate energy. Like the vitamins, many minerals serve as co-factors for various enzymes within cells. Without the mineral as co-factor, the related enzyme cannot perform its vital function of enabling cellular activity to proceed at its normal, rapid pace.

Essential fatty acids are relatively long, thin, carbon-based molecules which are termed "unsaturated" because they do not contain as much hydrogen as is chemically possible. There are only two essential fatty acids, linoleic acid, also called the "omega-6" essential fatty acid, and alpha-linolenic acid. Alpha-linolenic acid, also called the "omega-3" essential fatty acid, is the precursor molecule of **docosahexaenoic acid** (DHA) and **eicosapentaenoic acid** (EPA), which are longer, more complex, and more fragile fatty acids used abundantly in brain tissue and in the reproductive glands. Essential fatty acids are most abundant within the seeds of certain plants. Linoleic acid (omega-6) is found in most natural plant food oils, such as corn oil, soy oil, sunflower oil, sesame oil, and safflower oil. Because it is unsaturated, it is chemically reactive and is subject to damage from light, oxygen, and heat. Linoleic acid is easy to obtain through the diet, so it is not necessary to supplement it.

Alpha-linolenic acid (omega-3) is harder to get, and is less stable than its more plentiful relative. Small amounts are found in canola oil, soy oil, walnut oil, and pumpkin seed oil, but flax oil is by far the most plentiful source of it. People who eat expeller-pressed, unheated flax oil regularly on their salads can get alpha-linolenic acid in a natural food form. Or, high-quality flax oil can be obtained from a health food shop and taken by the teaspoon. It should be kept in the refrigerator and used within two or three weeks of opening, so do not purchase it in large bottles. As many people do not like the taste of flax oil, supplementing it in capsules is a simple way of obtaining alpha-linolenic acid, and I recommend this practice highly.

 In my consulting as a natural family planning teacher, I have found supplementing flax oil very helpful to many of the reproductive problems discussed in Part 2.

You can purchase fish oil, generally cod liver oil, as a source of EPA and DHA. It is possible to get fish oils that are certified free of toxic heavy metal, including mercury, cadmium, lead, and other contaminants. These oils can even be purchased with lemon flavor, making the old stereotype of terrible-tasting cod liver oil obsolete. Or, fish oil is available in capsule form. Fish liver oils, such as cod liver oil, also have modest amounts of vitamins A and D.

Krill oil is another excellent way to get EPA and DHA. In krill oil, these two omega-3 fatty acids are complexed in a way that makes them more easily absorbed and used (more "bioavailable").[1] Krill are marine invertebrates that are low on the food chain, which means that they do not concentrate and store toxins such as mercury to the same extent that large fish do. Krill oil is also rich in the powerful red antioxidant,

astaxanthin, which protects the EPA and DHA from oxidative damage. On the other hand, cod liver oil is a fish oil that contains both vitamin A and vitamin D, making for tradeoffs if you choose one or the other.

EPA and DHA are not strictly essential, however. Human beings can make EPA and DHA from the omega-3 alpha-linolenic acid, such as is plentiful in flax oil, if vitamins B3, B6, C, and the minerals magnesium and zinc are available in the diet. Should you supplement fish oil or krill oil in addition to flax oil? If you are supplementing flax oil as well as the vitamins and minerals, or if you eat fatty fish weekly, you may consider fish oil or krill oil optional.

> However, a review of many research articles confirms that supplementing the diet with fish oil is beneficial to a long list of reproductive problems, including menstrual pain, infertility, pregnancy problems such as gestational diabetes and pre-eclampsia, postpartum depression, menopausal problems, and osteoporosis.[2]

Fish oil supplements also have a very positive effect on the brain development of children born to mothers who took such supplements.[3] Krill oil has not been studied to the same extent, but it contains the same DHA and EPA. It does not contain vitamins A or D, however, as fish liver oils do.

SUPPLEMENTING PROBIOTICS

Supplements of probiotics are capsules or powders containing living "friendly" bacteria. All of us must have friendly bacteria in the intestines, not only to provide vitamin K, B vitamins, and other nutrients, but also to crowd out disease-causing bacteria and yeast organisms. Gut bacteria are being studied extensively, and more and more benefits of the right kinds of bacteria are being revealed.

But why would you need a probiotic supplement? First, antibiotics kill off many types of bacteria, including the beneficial bacteria of the gut. Second, poor food choices, especially sugar and refined carbohydrates, promote yeast organisms and harm the friendly bacteria. Yogurt has been a traditional food to restore the friendly bacteria. Raw sauerkraut and kimchi (Korean fermented cabbage) or other fermented foods can do the same. But many people, for one reason or another, don't eat such foods regularly. People with poor digestion, allergies, or autoimmune disease may benefit from probiotic supplements. Probiotic supplements are also helpful to women who are prone to vaginal yeast infections. And they can put a quick stop to diarrhea.

If you choose to supplement with probiotics, look for capsules that are especially coated to resist dissolving until the capsule enters the small intestine. Your brand should contain several varieties of bacteria, it should be well packaged to prevent loss of bacteria, and it should list a very large number of "CFU's" (colony forming units, meaning living bacteria), in the range of several billion per capsule.

WHY SUPPLEMENT?

Why should you take supplements? There are a number of reasons to do so.

SUPPLEMENT TO MEET INDIVIDUAL NUTRIENT NEEDS

Based simply on the wide genetic variation of humans and the definition of average, almost everyone is likely to have higher than average needs for one or more of the 50 or so essential nutrients. You may not absorb particular nutrients well from the digestive tract, a problem that increases with age—even while your need for calories is decreasing.

> Entire groups are known to have higher requirements for particular nutrients than even a balanced diet may provide: pregnant and nursing women, dieters, smokers, drinkers, the elderly, oral contraceptive users, those who exercise vigorously, those under stress, and those with acute or chronic illnesses.

Some therapeutic drugs deplete micronutrients; for example, some over-the-counter pain medications lower levels of vitamin C, folate, and iron. Eating refined sugar depletes the body of B vitamins and several minerals. Supplements help ensure that you are getting enough of all the nutrients that you, as a unique individual, need for your particular circumstances.

SUPPLEMENT TO HELP YOUR BODY GET RID OF TOXINS

Vitamins and minerals help the body to detoxify harmful substances formed within the cells through normal metabolism, as well as those taken into the body because of their presence in the environment. For example, folate (folic acid), vitamin B6, and vitamin B12 enable the body to reduce the levels of homocysteine, a harmful byproduct of the metabolism of certain amino acids. Vitamin A helps the body to detoxify contaminants such as dioxin and polychlorinated biphenols (PCBs). Vitamin C and selenium help protect against toxic heavy metals such as lead. Many vitamins and minerals are needed as part of enzyme systems that the liver uses to change various metabolic wastes, hormones, prescription drugs, and environmental toxins into forms that make them less potent and easier to excrete.

SUPPLEMENT TO BEEF UP YOUR ANTIOXIDANT DEFENSES

The oxygen that is so essential to every living cell in your body has its price: It creates dangerous **free radicals**, also called **reactive oxygen species**, within cells. What is amazing is that **oxidative stress**, the damage done by free radicals, has been found to underlie many, many disease states, from heart disease to male and female infertility.[4] Cells fortunately have many strategies to neutralize the potential harm that oxidative stress causes. For example, vitamins A, C, and E, as well as the minerals selenium and zinc, are well-known antioxidants that are essential nutrients. Many nonessential dietary nutrients also act as antioxidants, including those found in colorful fruits and vegetables. Some antioxidants are available as supplements because of their powerful antioxidant potential. One of these, a derivative of algae called **astaxanthin**, has been studied for its effect on male fertility.[5]

SUPPLEMENT TO MAKE UP FOR NUTRIENT DEFICIENCIES IN MODERN

FOODS When you consider typical American food, a balanced diet providing sufficient vitamins and minerals becomes more illusion than reality. When people eat only a few different kinds of food, the chance for adequate intake of each vitamin, mineral, and fatty acid diminishes. Even if you are eating abundant fruits, vegetables, and whole grains, many nutrients are lost when foods are harvested in an under- or over-ripe state or when they are stored, preserved, heated, peeled, juiced, or exposed to air. Vitamin E, for instance, is damaged by exposure to oxygen, heat, and light. Even raw fruits and vegetables are not as nutrient-rich as they might be, since most are grown on depleted soils replenished with only a few minerals, and cultivated year after year. The domestic crops themselves are hardly "natural"—many have been extensively bred for traits such as high yield, drought resistance, uniform size, or firm texture, but not for vitamin and mineral content. Vitamin and mineral supplements are a practical way of compensating for nutrient loss that occurs as a result of modern methods of producing, preserving, and preparing food.

When it comes to the essential fatty acids, nutritional researchers are concerned that the typical American diet supplies far less of the omega-3 alpha-linolenic acid, DHA, and EPA than is ideal. Flax oil supplements can supply omega-3 alpha-linolenic acid. Supplements of either fish oil or krill oil can compensate for the lack of DHA and EPA.[6]

SUPPLEMENT TO COMPENSATE FOR AN INADEQUATE DIET

How many people are actually eating a balanced diet on a daily basis? Even though there is considerable controversy regarding what a "balanced diet" really is, most nutritionists agree that large numbers of men, women, and children are not eating healthy foods daily. The huge numbers of fast food restaurants which line American roadways tell a dismal tale. The problem of recycling millions of aluminum beverage cans reflects a bigger problem with human nutrition. My own experience as a college instructor has driven this point home to me: many, many young adults simply do not eat anything close to the diet they know they should.

Supplementing vitamins, minerals, and essential fatty acids helps overcome the deficiencies of a hit-and-miss diet.

SUPPLEMENT TO IMPROVE HEALTH PROBLEMS

A prime reason to consider careful supplementation of vitamins, minerals, and essential fatty acids is to overcome specific health problems. Scientific literature contains numerous studies demonstrating the benefits of specific micronutrients on a variety of human illnesses. These studies are published in respected, peer-reviewed journals by medical doctors and other credentialed investigators; double-blind studies are well represented along with promising open studies. Some of the books recommended in the "Further Reading" section contain extensive citations of current research involving nutritional healing for many human diseases.

SUPPLEMENT TO IMPROVE YOUR FERTILITY

Dr. Jorge Chavarro, M.D., Sc.D., of the Harvard School of Public Health assisted with the large Nurses' Study and is the author of *The Fertility Diet*. During an interview with the Couple to Couple League he was asked if a woman was going to make one initial change to improve her fertility, what would it be? His answer: "There are of course some things that are more important than others. Certainly the first is to take a multivitamin that contains folic acid and also iron. That should be the starting point: a multivitamin that contains folic acid."[7] He has an entire chapter in *The Fertility Diet* dedicated to taking a "multivitamin/multimineral supplement." As you will see in Part 2, supplements of specific vitamins or minerals can improve fertility. As one example, vitamin C in doses of 750 mg has been used to overcome female infertility, and it has been shown to raise progesterone.[8]

As another example, other researchers investigating the role of nutrition in male fertility wrote the following as they discussed their study: "…[T]he referenced daily intake or recommended daily intake (RDI) for vitamin C is 60 mg per day…. Our study raises doubts about whether the current RDI may underestimate vitamin C requirements needed with regard to semen quality."[9]

SUPPLEMENT FOR OPTIMAL HEALTH

Sensible supplementation can help you toward the goal of optimal health. Optimal health refers to more than just the absence of disease. It refers to a state characterized by abundant energy, emotional stability, and the ability to participate vigorously in life's work and recreation. While optimal health is a subjective condition, improved energy level and sense of well-being are common reports among supplement users and undoubtedly contribute to their widespread and continuing popularity. Chances are great that you have already been taking supplements yourself, even before reading this book.

We are currently seeing immense growth of interest in the role of micronutrients in health and healing. This trend has been given quite a boost as the baby boom generation enters its mature years, demanding alternative information on how best to preserve vigorous good health and to prevent degenerative diseases. The real question is no longer whether to supplement, but how to do so effectively and safely. For an updated, extensively referenced discussion of the value of supplementation, refer to *The Supplement Pyramid* by Michael A. Smith, M.D. (See "Further Reading.")

BASIC SUPPLEMENTS TO CONSIDER

Table 7, "Basic Supplements to Consider" (page 60), is a general plan for supplementing the micronutrients effectively, comprehensively, and safely. In many cases the suggested amounts of the vitamins and minerals in this plan are substantially higher than the well-known Daily Values (DVs) that are part of food labels. DVs are formulated to cover the minimal nutrient needs of the majority of healthy individuals, and to prevent classic deficiency diseases such as scurvy, beriberi, pellagra, and rickets. They are not formulated for overcoming specific health problems, nor are they intended to represent optimal intake. For example, published studies of vitamins and minerals used to overcome physical disorders, such as PMS or male or female infertility, often involve nutrient levels considerably higher than the DVs.

Among nutritionally-oriented medical doctors who are actively involved in healing through nutritional alternatives, a consensus seems to have developed regarding the amounts of the various vitamins and minerals that are commonly supplemented. The amounts of supplements listed in Table 7 are in the general range suggested by clinically experienced, nutritionally-oriented physicians, including Guy Abraham, M.D., who used double-blind studies to establish the link between PMS and nutrition;[10] the late William G. Crook, M.D., who pioneered medical and nutritional treatment of yeast overgrowth;[11] Julian Whitaker, M.D., author and founder of the Whitaker Wellness Institute in Newport Beach, California;[12] Michael T. Murray, N.D., researcher and author of numerous books on natural medicine;[13] the late John Lee, M.D., who is so well known for his research on natural progesterone for women that it is easy to overlook his constant emphasis on better nutrition;[14] Dean Raffelock, D.C., and Robert Rountree, M.D., whose clinical experience with pregnant and postpartum women has led them to strongly recommend nutritional supplementation;[15] Jacob Teitelbaum, M.D., who has published extensively on the relationship between fibromyalgia and chronic fatigue syndrome and nutrition,[16] and Michael A. Smith, M.D., nutritional researcher and author.[17]

Far more critical than comparing supplement dosages to the rock-bottom DVs is relating them to their toxic levels. Footnotes have been added to Table 7 where research has indicated a potential for toxicity.

If you are contemplating pregnancy, you should discuss your vitamin and mineral supplements with a nutritionally-aware health care practitioner. However, I have made every effort to recommend only supplement amounts that are safe before and during pregnancy and breastfeeding.

GUIDELINES FOR SUPPLEMENT USE

The following guidelines are offered to enable you to reap the considerable benefits of nutritional supplements and to minimize the possible risks.

1) PROPER DIET IS A HIGHER HEALTH PRIORITY THAN SUPPLEMENTATION

Supplements cannot compensate for a sugar-laden diet, a diet full of *trans* fats, a low-fiber diet, or a low-protein diet. Whole plant foods are full of an astonishing array of health-promoting molecules called phytonutrients, which are not part of vitamin and mineral supplements.

2) SEEK REALISTIC NUTRITIONAL COUNSELING WHEN YOU SUPPLEMENT

If you are in ordinary good health, that may just mean an OK from your family doctor or gynecologist. However, if you suffer from a serious disorder such as diabetes, celiac disease, an autoimmune disease, or liver, kidney, or cardiovascular disease, make every effort to find a holistic physician who is aware of the specific benefits as well as the specific risks that supplements may hold for you. A nutritionally-oriented medical doctor, sometimes called an **integrative physician** or a **practitioner of functional medicine** or **complementary medicine** can test your blood thoroughly. He or she may be able to recommend supplements to improve your particular health problem, and can also address any potential for overdose.

3) STRIVE FOR BALANCE WHEN YOU SUPPLEMENT

High doses of some nutrients can cause increased requirements for others. The B vitamins deserve special attention in this regard. While "balanced" B complex supplements in the suggested amounts are readily available, tablets of the B vitamin folic acid of 1,000 micrograms (mcg; equal to 1.0 mg) or more are still obtainable by prescription only. In the higher potency B-complex vitamin supplements, such as the 50 or 100 mg/mcg amounts, folate, in the synthetic form known as folic acid, is too low for balance, and should be taken separately in 400 or 800 mcg tablets, which are widely available without prescription (see Table 7). Folic acid may mask vitamin B12 deficiency in strict vegetarians and those with gastrointestinal abnormalities, but it is one of the safest and most valuable vitamins to supplement.

Other nutrients which must be properly balanced include calcium and magnesium; to take the former without the latter is to invite magnesium deficiency. Copper and zinc must also be balanced with one another. Magnesium and vitamin B6 are both involved in similar cellular work. Vitamins B6, B12, and folate work together in the body to reduce the buildup of the toxic metabolite homocysteine. Vitamin A increases the need for vitamin E, and vitamin E's activity is enhanced by selenium. Calcium cannot be absorbed and used in the bone without adequate amounts of vitamin D, magnesium, manganese, zinc, and folate. The hard-to-get essential fatty acid alpha-linolenic acid, found abundantly in flax oil, cannot be converted to its active forms without vitamins B3, B6, C, and the minerals magnesium and zinc. Vitamin E is required to prevent the oxidation of the essential fatty acids.

Because of the interaction of nutrients and the need for balance, I strongly recommend that any program of supplementation include all of the essential nutrients listed in Table 7. Even if research indicates that only one micronutrient has reversed a physical problem that you are attempting to overcome, this principle of balanced supplementation still holds true.

4) ALWAYS TAKE SUPPLEMENTS ON A FULL STOMACH, PREFERABLY IN DIVIDED DOSES WITH BREAKFAST AND LUNCH

Taking micronutrient pills between meals can unnecessarily irritate your stomach or intestines, and may decrease the absorption of some nutrients, especially the fat-soluble ones. Some people find that taking supplements with their evening meal causes them to have too much energy to fall asleep at night. Take your vitamins with breakfast and lunch, when you will appreciate the energy boost later in the day.

5) BEGIN TAKING SUPPLEMENTS GRADUALLY

The most common side effect of taking vitamin and mineral supplements is an upset stomach. If you begin gradually and you do discover that they upset your stomach, you can back off and increase them even more slowly. It may take a couple of weeks to work up to what you want to take.

6) PREFER NATURAL VITAMINS TO SYNTHETIC VITAMINS

Vitamin E is a complex molecule that occurs in either a **right-handed** form or in a mirror image (**left-handed** form). Human cells prefer the right-handed molecule. Synthetic vitamin E is a mixture of both. Natural vitamin E, manufactured by living organisms, is the right-handed form, and is more usable to the body as such. On a vitamin bottle, natural vitamin E is listed as "*d*-alpha tocopherol," while synthetic vitamin E is labeled "*dl*-alpha tocopherol." (The "d" actually stands for the Latin word for "right," and the "l" in "dl" for the Latin word for "left.") Vitamin B12 in the natural form, methyl cobalamin, is now easily available in health food shops; prefer it to the synthetic cyanocobalamin. Most other vitamins are chemically the same whether derived from natural sources or synthetic. However, "natural" vitamins often include other molecules that occur together with the known vitamin and may enhance the cells' ability to use the actual vitamin efficiently. For example, vitamin C is often found together with complex molecules called **bioflavinoids**. "Natural" vitamins are also less likely to have food colorings or preservatives in them.

FOLIC ACID OR FOLATE?

The synthetic form of the B vitamin folate, **folic acid**, is probably the best-studied supplement in the world. Folic acid is well known for its role in preventing birth defects in the developing baby: spina bifida, anencephaly, heart defects and other congenital malformations. It has been studied as an aid to fertility and as a means to decrease the incidence of miscarriage. Folic acid supplementation has even decreased the incidence of Down syndrome. (See Chapter 12.) Folate is involved in healthy cell division, including the critical maturation of the ovum that is completed just hours before ovulation. (See "Introduction to Part 2.")

New research reveals that a substantial minority of people, anywhere from 10-40 percent, have a genetically inherited limitation in their ability to use folate and/or folic acid.[18] Having this genetic variation causes such individuals to need more folic acid. Alternatively, the natural vitamin in the form of methyl folate is now easily available. L-methyl folate (also called metafolin) leap-frogs the enzyme limitation. It is most often prescribed to women who have been genetically tested for the **methyl folate** genetic variation, but it is available without a prescription.

Since the excellent research on this important nutrient has been done using the synthetic folic acid, the effective amounts of natural folate are still not known. I suggest that if you use methyl folate, start slowly, but use the same amount of folate as the studies using folic acid have suggested.

7) USE TIMED-RELEASE VITAMINS TO HELP PREVENT LOSS OF THE SUPPLEMENT INTO THE URINE

Taking vitamins often results in bright yellow urine, revealing that the vitamins indeed have been absorbed out of the intestines and into the blood, and providing evidence that the kidneys are extremely efficient at removing excess from the blood. Timed-released vitamins slow the absorption of the nutrients into the blood, and prevent some of the inevitable urinary loss, though it is usual to have bright yellow urine if you supplement. Timed-release vitamins may also decrease digestive upset.

Instead of timed-release formulation, you may prefer a supplement labeled to take several of the capsules or pills daily. Taking them throughout the morning and afternoon with meals or snacks is another strategy to reduce urinary losses.

8) LOOK FOR "AMINO ACID CHELATES" TO ABSORB MINERALS MORE EFFECTIVELY
Minerals are more difficult to absorb than are vitamins. The **chelated** forms of minerals are more absorbable than other forms, because chelation means that the mineral has been bound to another molecule, often an amino acid, and "hitches a ride" across the intestinal wall along with the amino acid or other molecule. Not all minerals listed in a good multimineral supplement will be chelated, but at least the iron should be, as in this form it is less likely to destroy other nutrients. Health food shop brands of supplements are usually formulated with these considerations.

MAGNESIUM AND CALCIUM CONSIDERATIONS

Plain magnesium oxide can be quite laxative, as it is not well absorbed. While some magnesium oxide is usually well tolerated, look for magnesium as a **chelate**: magnesium aspartate, magnesium gluconate, or magnesium citrate. These forms are better absorbed and far less laxative than magnesium oxide alone. When it comes to calcium, calcium citrate is a highly absorbable form, as are calcium lactate, calcium gluconate, and calcium malate. Calcium carbonate, which is not a chelated form, is the least expensive form of calcium. However, it is not as absorbable as other forms of calcium.[19]

9) READ SUPPLEMENT LABELS CAREFULLY
Examine the list of vitamins and minerals, and then the actual amount of each. Ask for complete labels on prescription vitamins, especially typical prenatal vitamins, which are surprisingly low in potency. Pharmaceutical house multivitamins are closely tied to DVs and are generally less potent than the health food shop brands, so I suggest that you obtain as complete a multivitamin/multimineral supplement as possible from a health food shop or natural grocery. Even so, you will probably have to round out these supplements with additional folate or folic acid, vitamins C and E, and magnesium, according to your particular health goals.

10) BECOME AWARE!
Refer to the books listed in the "Further Reading" section to gain knowledge and confidence in the value and safety of supplements.

A NOTE ON VITAMIN BRANDS

For the convenience of the reader, this book recommends several brands of multivitamin/multiminerals: Optivite PMT and Androvite for Men, by Optimox Corp.; Professional Pre-Natal Formula, by LifeTime; and ProCycle PMS, by American ProLife Enterprise. Since the publication of the second edition of *Fertility, Cycles & Nutrition* in 1992, the Couple to Couple League has recommended these because of their relative completeness, modest cost, availability, and in particular the solid research behind Optivite and the similar ProCycle PMS. Also recommended is the proprietary herb/vitamin/mineral mix Fertility Blend, which contains the herb *Vitex agnus castus*. The listed contents of each of these are provided in Appendix A at the end of this book.

Flax oil, fish oil, krill oil, probiotics, digestive enzymes and a few other supplements such as astaxanthin and coenzyme Q10 are recommended without brand names, but in general you should look for these in natural groceries or health food shops that are committed to high-quality products. I have no financial interest at all in any brand that I recommend or any other supplement that I recommend, nor have I ever. Other brands with similar natural vitamins, chelated minerals, and potencies (amounts) may be equally helpful. In all cases, obtain the approval of your health care provider.

TABLE 7
Basic Supplements to Consider

VITAMINS	DAILY AMOUNT	COMMENTS
A (Retinyl palmitate)	5,000-20,000 IU	Use 8,000 IU maximum if pregnant or seeking pregnancy.[a]
B1	25-100 mg	
B2	25-100 mg	
B3 (Niacin)	25-100 mg	
B6 (Pyridoxine)	25-300 m	Over 500 mg/day has been associated with neuropathy. Taking with other B vitamins and magnesium reduces potential for toxicity. Tested for safety during pregnancy. Seek nutritional counseling for amounts over 300 mg.[b]
Pantothenic acid	25-100 mg	
Choline	25-100 mg	
Inositol	25-100 mg	
Para-amino benzoic acid (PABA)	25-100 mg	

Continued on the following page

VITAMINS	DAILY AMOUNT	COMMENTS
B12	25-2,000 mcg	Safe and recommended for pregnancy.[c]
Folic acid	400-4,000 mcg	Rarely, masks vitamin B12 deficiency; take B12 also. Safe and beneficial for pregnancy.[d]
C	1,000-3,000 mg	Chewing it may increase tooth decay.
D3 (Cholecalciferol)	400-1,000 IU	
E	400-800 IU	Prefer natural to synthetic.

MINERALS	DAILY AMOUNT	COMMENTS
Calcium	500-1,000 mg	Raises the need for magnesium.
Magnesium	500-1,000 mg	
Iron	0-30 mg	
Iodine	150 mcg	
Copper	2-3 mg	
Zinc	25-50 mg	
Manganese	10 mg	
Chromium	100-200 mcg	
Selenium	100-200 mcg	
Potassium	from diet	

ESSENTIAL FATTY ACIDS	DAILY AMOUNT	COMMENTS
Flax oil	5-10 1-g capsules (1-2 teaspoons)	Requires vitamin E.
Fish liver oil	5 1-g capsules (1 teaspoon)	Should be certified contaminant free. Optional if flax oil is supplemented. Requires vitamin E.

a Rothman, K., and Moore, L. "Teratogenicity of high vitamin A intake" (*NEJM* 1995, 333:1369-1373). Beta-carotene, which is not pre-formed vitamin A, can be taken in amounts far higher than the guideline given here.

b Shrim, A., Boskovic, R., Maltepe, C., et al. "Pregnancy outcome following use of large doses of vitamin B6 in the first trimester" (*J. Obstet. Gynecol.* 2006, 26: 749- 751); Guy Abraham, M.D., also reports this upper level safe and beneficial during pregnancy when used as part of a multivitamin/multimineral containing other B vitamins and magnesium: Beck, S., Abraham, G. "Optivite PMT and Gynovite Plus Total Dietary Programs for Premenstrual Syndrome and Menopause" (Optimox Corp., 1992, p. 27).

c Raffelock, D., Rountree, R., and Hopkins, V. *A Natural Guide to Pregnancy and Postpartum Health* (New York: Avery, 2002, p. 131). These authors recommend up to 5,000 mcg vitamin B12 per day.

d Wilson, R. "Pre-conceptual vitamin/folic acid supplementation 2007: The use of folic acid in combination with a multivitamin supplement for the prevention of neural tube defects and other congenital anomalies" (Joint SOGC-Motherisk Clinical Practice Guideline, *JOGC*, Dec., 2007, 1003–1013); Goh, Y., and Koren, G. "Folic acid in pregnancy and fetal outcomes" (*J. Obstet. & Gynaecol.* 2008, 28:3–13). Folic acid supplementation in amounts up to 5,000 mcg is recommended to prevent neural tube defects. This amount does not mask vitamin B12 deficiency.

SUMMARY — CHAPTER 3

Vitamin, mineral, and essential fatty acid supplements help overcome nutrient deficiencies that may result from an individual's higher than average requirements. They help to detoxify metabolic and environmental toxins. They also compensate for foods that are raised on depleted soils, bred for qualities other than high nutrition, cooked, or otherwise processed. They help to overcome the effects of the widespread habits of poor nutrition, such as eating at fast food restaurants and drinking carbonated beverages. Studies show that vitamins and minerals can prevent or overcome diseases. Supplements can help you to achieve optimal health.

Table 7 provides a plan for supplementing vitamins, minerals, and essential fatty acids. In order to supplement safely and effectively, the following guidelines should be used:

1 Proper diet is a higher health priority than supplementation.

2 Seek realistic nutritional counseling when you supplement.

3 Strive for balance when you supplement.

4 Always take supplements on a full stomach, preferably in divided doses with breakfast and lunch.

5 Begin taking supplements gradually.

6 Prefer natural vitamins to synthetic vitamins.

7 Use timed-release vitamins to help prevent loss of the supplement into the urine.

8 Look for "amino acid chelates" to absorb minerals more effectively.

9 Read supplement labels carefully.

10 Become aware! Refer to the books listed in the "Resources" section of this book to gain knowledge and confidence in the value of supplements.

11 This book recommends several brands of multivitamin/multimineral supplements: Optivite PMT, ProCycle PMS, Professional Pre-Natal Formula, Androvite for Men, and Fertility Blend. Other supplements are recommended without brand names: Flax oil, fish oil, krill oil, probiotics, digestive enzymes, astaxanthin, coenzyme Q10, and a few others.

INCREASING YOUR ENERGY & DECREASING YOUR STRESS

4

A merry heart doeth good like medicine.
— Proverbs 17:22
(KJV)

Good nutrition alone is a powerful force for overall glowing health and high energy. Yet nutrition alone can't do it all. Before we get started solving reproductive problems in Part 2, we need to look at the role of sleep, exercise, and stress in overall health. But how are these topics related to better cycles and better fertility? Over time, as I consulted with women on cycle irregularity, breastfeeding, or infertility, I gradually realized that many women who are seeking information about one problem—for example, long cycles, PCOS (polycystic ovary syndrome), or perimenopause changes—are actually dealing with fatigue and stress as well. These two topics do impact the cycle and fertility directly. Fatigue and anxiety are common symptoms of PMS, as well as common symptoms of the perimenopausal "change of life." They reduce sexual desire. They are involved in postpartum blues. Stress hormones, short term, can delay ovulation, creating an unusually long cycle. Stress hormones, long term, can contribute to PCOS. The stress hormone cortisol from the adrenal glands affects the function of other hormones, including progesterone and the thyroid hormones.

Stress and fatigue are closely intertwined. Fatigue causes stress, and stress causes fatigue. Oppositely, high energy and calm nerves go hand in hand. Strategies that naturally increase your energy tend to reduce stress, so let's start with increasing your energy.

INCREASING YOUR ENERGY

Have you ever considered what it is that makes you feel energetic? For example, if right now you are feeling bright and chipper, can you explain why? If, on the other hand, you are feeling wiped out, can you explain it to yourself?

Four major factors underlie the subjective feelings of high energy instead of fatigue: steady blood sugar levels, adequate sleep, the right amount of exercise, and manageable stress.

The first three actually are powerful stress reducers. Since the topic of blood sugar control is basic to the "Twelve Rules for Better Nutrition" and has already been discussed, we'll just summarize blood sugar control later and get started with sleep and exercise as the tools to manage stress.

ADEQUATE SLEEP: QUANTITY AND QUALITY

Enough sleep is at least as important as good nutrition as a basic component of overall health. It's number one for high energy. It's also number one to reduce stress.

Good quality sleep, and enough of it, causes the stress hormone cortisol to drop like a rock. Healthy sleep cycles regulate a number of lesser-known hormones that control growth, repair, and even appetite.

There's simply no substitute for enough sleep. But are you getting enough? Many women know that they are not. Others believe that six or seven hours of sleep is enough, but chances are that you need eight or nine hours, maybe more, to feel and do your best. This is particularly true if you are pregnant or breastfeeding, or if you are under stress. I've had women tell me that they are fatigued from morning to night, and then ask me if there is some nutritional way to increase their energy. Yet when I ask them how much sleep they get, they may reply that they go to bed at 11:00 p.m. and get up at 5:00 a.m.! As important as it is, improved nutrition simply cannot compensate.

There is a good chance that *when* you sleep makes a difference. For some people, seven hours of sleep at night and a one-hour nap is more restful than nine hours of sleep at night and no nap. For myself, I am convinced that eight hours of sleep from midnight to 8:00 a.m. does me more good than eight hours from 10:00 p.m. to 6:00 a.m. Other "night people" can understand this, while you "morning people" might find exactly the opposite is true.

SLEEPING WELL

For some women (and men also),
it's not that you don't have time to sleep;
it's that you don't sleep well.

Not sleeping well could mean that you don't fall asleep right away, or that you wake up during the night or early morning and can't get back to sleep. Most often it is anxious thoughts that are keeping you awake. It's a Catch-22: Sleep reduces stress, but stress can reduce the ability to sleep. There are ways to break this cycle, and it's helpful to think about the nature of sleep in order to plan a strategy to improve it.

SLEEP RESTS THE BRAIN
First, sleep is for the brain. The muscles can rest while you lie down while awake, but not the brain. Sleep rests and recharges the *conscious* areas of the brain. Even during sleep, the brain continues to control its automatic functions, such as regulating heart rate, digestive movements, and breathing. It's the higher centers of the brain that rest only during sleep. Think about why you need to lie down to sleep: There are large conscious areas near the surface of the brain that initiate movement and maintain posture. Those conscious areas for muscle control cannot rest unless you sleep; if you do fall asleep sitting up, you slump over! Closing your eyes cuts out input to the large brain areas for vision, and sleeping in a quiet room rests the brain areas that process what you hear. Sensory input from the skin is sent to conscious areas also, which is why a comfortable bed in a room that is neither too hot nor too cold favors sleep. Fortunately, it's fairly easy to lie down in a dark, quiet, comfortable room, reducing a large amount of work that the conscious brain areas perform.

The one conscious area of the brain that is not always so controllable is the "prefrontal region," right behind your forehead, where you think, plan, review—and worry! Many people who have trouble sleeping will say that it is anxiety or worry that keeps them up or wakes them up. Sometimes just recognizing this and learning to limit that anxious mental activity is a help. Doing so will help your sleep last longer and become more restful. There are physical, psychological, and spiritual ways to deal with such anxiety, as we will see.

FALLING ASLEEP AND STAYING ASLEEP
Recognizing that low blood glucose turns on the "fight-or-flight" (sympathetic nervous system) response is helpful. If you wake up in the middle of the night, especially with anxious thoughts that prevent you from getting back to sleep, low blood glucose may actually be the cause. A protein-rich snack with a little bit of carbohydrate right then may help you get back to sleep. Having such a snack before bedtime may prevent you from awakening like that in the first place. Oppositely, though, a large meal before bed may keep you awake.

For some individuals, mild exercise before bedtime may be helpful to sleeping better, but for others, exercise, especially if it is strenuous, is too invigorating and is best done earlier in the day.

Keep your room very dark—even pitch black if necessary—if you have trouble falling asleep or sleeping well. Why? When the lights go out, the sleep hormone melatonin is released from the pineal gland, which is buried deep in the brain. Conversely, when the lights go on, the pineal gland receives the message from your eyes, and your melatonin output drops. Though melatonin is a natural sleep aid, even dim light can reduce its production. You make less melatonin as you age, and it drops quite a bit during premenopause. This means a very dark room becomes more important to your sleep quality as you grow older. Consider room-darkening blinds and clocks without lighted displays. This topic is developed further in Chapter 10 under the heading "Sensitivity to Night Lighting," since melatonin is a powerful antioxidant that can improve fertility.

 Caffeine causes melatonin to drop sharply, and is a well-known sleep disruptor.

Cutting down on a caffeine habit, and making the afternoon the last time of the day for any caffeine can help you get a good night's sleep. If you prefer a nap and are able to take one in the afternoon, be careful of the caffeine. Your morning coffee may need to be the last coffee until after your nap!

You will feel better, think better, look better, and enjoy life more if you go through it in a rested state. You will be more cheerful. You will manage stress better. Your immune system will work better. You will be able to control your weight better. And you will be more productive if you spend the time you need sleeping, because it will increase your energy and mental focus during your waking time. Getting the sleep you need makes your waking time much, much more pleasant—for you and for those around you.

GET YOUR "VITAMIN ZZZZ'S!"

1) Plan time for enough sleep. Go to bed earlier, get up later, have a daily nap in the morning, afternoon or evening. Aim for a minimum of eight to nine hours of sleep per day.

2) Have a flexible schedule for both sleeping and eating. Many hormones have a daily cycle that is established by the sleeping and eating schedules. Your personal routine really does help your hormones get onto their own routine and enables them to do their job better.

3) Don't drink coffee or caffeinated tea or eat chocolate in the evening.

4) Avoid looking at screens for about an hour before bedtime. The backlighting on some screens can interfere with the production of the sleep hormone melatonin. And exciting or disturbing news or programs can raise your stress hormones.

5) Have a protein-rich snack before bedtime if you are prone to wake up during the night with anxious thoughts or just with hunger.

6) Make your room quiet and comfortable, with a soft-enough or firm-enough mattress, and a cool-enough or warm-enough temperature. Soft earplugs can help with noise, such as a spouse who snores.

7) Experiment to see whether mild exercise in the evening might help you sleep better, or oppositely, might disrupt your sleep.

8) Most supplements are energizing, and taking them with dinner can make you too alert to sleep. However, magnesium and calcium supplements are good sleep aids, and can be taken right at bedtime (about 500 mg of each).

9) Sleep in a very dark room. Melatonin, your natural sleep hormone, rises after thirty minutes in the dark. Even a little night lighting can reduce melatonin.

10) If anxious thoughts or worries keep you from falling asleep or wake you up, try the following:

Take time in bed to review your worries, then put them aside for sleep.

Keep a pencil and paper near your bed to write down things you don't want to forget.

Form the habit of sleeping without your smartphone nearby.

Do a bit of quiet, comforting reading, such as spiritual reading.

Say a little prayer. Prayer not only connects us with God, but it also reduces stress.

11) Consider whether your sleep disturbance is part of premenstrual syndrome (PMS) or painful periods. Both of these have been related to sleep disturbances,[1] and yet sleep is helpful for both. See chapters 6 and 7 for self care for PMS and painful periods.

12) If you can't sleep, a little reading in bed may help. However, resting quietly in bed in the dark with your eyes closed can partially compensate for lost sleep time. As one young mother said, "If I'm horizontal, I'm resting!"

13) If you have a baby or young children, have nighttime sleeping arrangements that make it easy to meet their needs. That often means having the young one nearby at night, so that your sleep is minimally disrupted.

14) Taking a nap is a great way to keep up on your sleep if you are getting up at night to care for a baby.

15) With your health-care professional's approval, instead of using prescription sleep medications, try using natural aids. Melatonin supplements of 0.3 to 3 mg taken about thirty minutes before bedtime may be helpful. The amino acid GABA (gamma amino butyric acid) is also helpful, in amounts of about 100 mg taken before bedtime. This over-the-counter amino acid is an inhibitory neurotransmitter that is not habit forming. If you are pregnant or breastfeeding, make sure that you have your doctor's OK.

THE RIGHT AMOUNT OF EXERCISE

What about exercise? Your need for exercise is not nearly as demanding as your need for sleep. There's a wide range of exercise that is healthy. Still, too much exercise can leave you exhausted, while not enough leaves you sluggish. The right amount is invigorating. Everyone has had the experience of too much physical exertion leaving you drained, even for the next day—spading and planting a garden on a hot day, over-enthusiastically undertaking a new exercise program, or driving around town running half a dozen errands. (Even though much of driving a vehicle is done automatically by habit, it requires a great deal of sensory and motor activity, and a high degree of alertness. The eyes keep the brain busy. No wonder it wears you out!)

The right amount of exercise contributes to your sense of well-being in a number of ways. Physically, regular moderate exercise is a powerful way of regulating blood sugar levels, which is a major factor in your energy level. Exercise is a satisfying and very natural release for the "fight or flight" stress response. Exercise burns calories and increases your metabolism even during rest, contributing to a healthy body weight. It is mood elevating, especially if done in the outdoors and with a friend. Outdoor exercise in bright sun light decreases melatonin, which apparently causes it to "bounce back" at night, helping you sleep. Exercise is fun—or at least, you should find a way of making it fun.

Nevertheless, a big caution to those who know that they should be getting more exercise is to start gradually.

Right from the start, your exercise program should be pleasant and invigorating.

You are not likely to stick with it if too much too soon overtires you. How much is the right start? About thirty minutes of ordinary walking is a good place to begin. If that's not fatiguing, then increase to brisker walking for up to an hour. Getting brisk exercise for at least half an hour most days of the week is a minimal goal.

If you are already involved in an exercise program, the side benefits should be increased energy, sound sleep, and better stress control. If you are finding that the opposite is true, ask yourself if you are trying to do too much for your level of fitness.

Some women need to cut back on the amount or intensity of daily exercise in order to gain the benefits of physical activity.

Sometimes young athletes must push themselves hard during their sport's season. A focus on excellent nutrition and plenty of sleep is the best way to cope with the physical demands of athletic competition.

Good nutrition, enough sleep, and the right amount of exercise not only increase your energy, but they are physical keys to our next topic—decreasing your stress.

DECREASING YOUR STRESS

The term "stress" can mean a number of different things, but most people understand what you mean when you say you are stressed. To feel overwhelmed, to feel like you are not coping, to feel overburdened by circumstances or responsibilities, to feel worried or anxious—all these can be summarized in the expression, "I'm stressed out." What causes stress? Financial worries, difficult children, tension between spouses, too much work and not enough time, concerns about aging or sick loved ones, and broken relationships are all examples of situations that cause emotional stress.

 Sleeplessness, inadequate or excessive exercise, low blood glucose, sickness, pain, or allergies also stress the body. No matter what the stress, emotional or physical, it is well established scientifically that the body reacts in the same way.

The stress hormones epinephrine and norepinephrine (adrenaline) are released during stress, causing the heart rate and blood pressure to rise. They affect the brain so that you feel nervous, anxious, afraid, irritated, or angry, depending on what is happening around you. The response to stress "revs up your engine," which sooner or later will cause you to crash in exhaustion. Stress and energy are related.

How do you deal with stress? The most common suggestion is to cut down on your activities in order to reduce stress or avoid stressful situations. Of course that's not always possible. For example, if you are caring for a chronically sick or high-needs child, you simply cannot decide not to do so any more. Perhaps your job is the stressful activity, but given the options, you feel you have no other satisfactory alternative. Maybe it's all the chauffeuring you do, but then again, you value the opportunities you are making for your children.

As most women have learned, talking about your stress is helpful. A sympathetic friend can be a real comfort when you feel down. When we adopted our seventh child from overseas, I felt anxious for a couple of months afterward, even though everything about the adoption and our baby's health and adjustment turned out better than we ever hoped. It really helped for listening friends to explain it for me, "You've just had a major life change. Look at all the unknowns you've been dealing with. No wonder you're stressed. Who wouldn't be?"

Prayer is a great consolation in stressful times. I love the prayer that Catholics say at each Mass: "...Protect us from all anxiety as we wait in joyful hope for the coming of our Savior, Jesus Christ." Christians believe that the Lord is the Prince of Peace, and the fruits of His Spirit include peace. Who has not had comfort in prayer?

Yet sometimes none of the above seems to help. You see that you ought to be happy and at peace, but even little things continually bother you. You see others coping better with bigger burdens than you are doing with smaller ones. You question yourself, your commitments, your relationships with others, and even your relationship with God. What is the missing link?

THE PHYSICAL ASPECTS OF STRESS

Human beings are not disembodied spirits, nor disembodied emotions. We are integrated physical, emotional, and spiritual beings. While it's common to recognize the emotional and even the spiritual aspects of stress, all too frequently the physical component is completely ignored. That physical component ultimately rests with two small hormonal glands, the adrenal glands.

GET ACQUAINTED WITH YOUR ADRENAL GLANDS
The adrenal glands do so much that everyone should be aware of them and what they do. They sit atop each kidney, above the waist near the back of the abdomen. Each adrenal gland is actually two separate glands, one inside the other. The inner adrenal medulla produces the fight-or-flight hormones epinephrine and norepinephrine (formerly called adrenaline). These hormones are the ones that cause the pounding heart and anxiety of stage fright, or the bad reaction you may experience when flashing lights and a siren zero in behind your car as you are cruising along! They cause the classic fight-or-flight reaction—increased heart rate, elevated blood pressure, anxiety or anger, and a flood of glucose into the blood.

The outer part of each adrenal gland is called the adrenal cortex. Each adrenal cortex produces a large number of steroid hormones. One of these hormones, aldosterone, is essential for life—it enables the kidneys to conserve the right amount of sodium for the body, and it causes the kidneys to secrete excess potassium. "Male" hormones, called androgens, are synthesized by the adrenal cortex; in women, the androgens contribute to sexual desire. The adrenal hormone cortisol raises the blood glucose by stimulating the liver to generate glucose. Cortisol and other hormones from the adrenal cortex stimulate and regulate the function of the immune system. Most importantly, adrenal cortical hormones respond to stress—cortisol rises sharply in response to stress. Healthy adrenal glands make the right amount of these hormones at the right time.

STAGES OF STRESS
The great Canadian researcher Hans Selye detailed the response of the adrenal glands to acute and chronic stress into three stages, together called the "general adaptation syndrome." The first, the stage of alarm, is the acute reaction to a sudden stress. An example of such a stress might be a nasty skid on an icy road. The sudden flood of fear or anxiety is caused by the adrenal medullae (plural) releasing the hormones epinephrine and norepinephrine, but cortisol is also released. When things get back to normal, this response soon subsides.

The second stage, the stage of resistance, occurs when a stress is prolonged. For example, if for a significant period of time you are uncertain about a loved one's life or health, you may experience prolonged stress. During this second stage, the adrenal cortices (plural) produce increased amounts of certain hormones, including cortisol. Blood sugar is increased, insulin rises to lower the blood glucose levels, and other hormonal changes occur. You may feel a sense of ongoing dread, worry, or brooding anger. Subjectively, you would probably say, "I feel stressed, but I'm still hanging in there."

The third stage, which may occur if stress is prolonged or severe, is the stage of exhaustion. The adrenals no longer can produce the hormones which enable the body to compensate, and the body is prone to fatigue, inflammation, and illness. Subjectively, the person at this stage would say, "I'm on the brink. I just can't deal with anything anymore."

HOW STRESS CONTRIBUTES TO WEIGHT GAIN

Chronic stress causes the prolonged secretion of cortisol, as in the stage of resistance. One of cortisol's many functions is to increase blood sugar levels by stimulating the liver to convert amino acids into glucose. High levels of cortisol elevate blood glucose so much that insulin levels increase to bring the blood glucose back down. When insulin is high, it is very efficient at ushering the blood glucose into the fat cells, where the glucose is converted into saturated fat. The stress of the low blood glucose that results stimulates more cortisol. Keeping blood sugar levels steady, as outlined in Chapter 1, is the key to stopping this cycle of stress.

There are several important conclusions from Dr. Selye's pioneering research. First, *physical stresses*, not just emotional stresses, can put the body into any of the three stages of stress.

The physical stresses of blood sugar swings, lack of sleep, excess exercise, allergies, acute or chronic pain, acute or chronic illness, toxins such as nicotine or even therapeutic drugs, or nutritional deficiencies can cause or contribute to the same stages of stress that emotional trauma can.

The late, great nutritionist, Adelle Davis, wrote that major stresses such as surgery or being in a bad car accident could put the body into the third stage, the stage of exhaustion, in a matter of hours. Yet Adelle Davis taught that if the adrenal glands were nourished well enough to meet their increased needs during times of stress, the third and perhaps even the other stages of the stress response could be avoided.[2] Let's look at ways to reduce stress by keeping the adrenal glands healthy.

STRATEGIES FOR BETTER ADRENAL GLAND FUNCTION

1) GET ENOUGH SLEEP, OR REST IN A DARK ROOM IF YOU SLEEP POORLY
Sleep rests the adrenals, allowing the stress hormones to decrease.

2) KEEP YOUR BLOOD GLUCOSE LEVELS STEADY BY EATING GOOD MEALS AND SNACKS REGULARLY
As outlined in Chapter 1, making every meal and every snack a combination of protein, whole carbohydrates, and natural fats is an excellent way to maintain steady blood glucose levels. When you do so, you prevent your adrenals from being stressed by a drop in blood glucose, so that they do not have to respond with their anxiety-producing, sleep-disrupting hormones, epinephrine and norepinephrine.

3) ANTICIPATE KNOWN IMPENDING STRESSES WITH IMPROVED NUTRITION
If you know that you will be studying for finals next month, for example, plan on improved nutrition aimed at adrenal health for a few days beforehand.

4) CONSIDER SUPPLEMENTS WHICH CAN MEET THE HIGHER NEEDS OF THE ADRENAL GLANDS DURING PERIODS OF EMOTIONAL OR PHYSICAL STRESS
The adrenal glands require vitamin A; B vitamins, especially pantothenic acid; vitamin C (more vitamin C is found in the adrenals than in any other body organ); essential fatty acids; vitamin E; and the minerals zinc and manganese. Use a high quality multivitamin/multimineral supplement, with vitamin C in the range of 1,000-3,000 mg per day. Add about 5 grams of flax oil and/or 1 teaspoon of fish oil daily. Additionally, vitamin B6 and the mineral magnesium are nerve calming and are well worth supplementing. Vitamin B12 (1,000 mcg/day) is beneficial to both energy and mood. Table 7 in Chapter 3 contains dose ranges for all these nutrients.

5) DO NOT RESTRICT SALT, UNLESS YOU ARE DIRECTED TO DO SO BY YOUR PHYSICIAN FOR OTHER REASONS.
A lack of salt in the diet can stress exhausted adrenal glands by forcing them to manufacture the hormone aldosterone, which signals the kidneys to retain salt.

6) AS ALWAYS, SEEK THE APPROVAL OF YOUR HEALTH CARE PROFESSIONAL BEFORE SUPPLEMENTING

BACK TO BLOOD SUGAR

The most underrated contributor to high energy levels is blood sugar control. The blood sugar glucose is a preferred fuel for many of the body cells. The brain's cells have no choice; they ordinarily use only glucose. They are dependent on a steady supply of glucose brought to them by the blood. If they get the glucose they need, they can perform their activities efficiently, as can the other body cells. What happens at the cellular level determines what happens to the whole person, physiologically speaking.

The key to high energy, then, is to get the glucose into the cells, particularly the brain cells. This depends first on blood glucose levels that are high enough to carry sufficient glucose. But it is overly simplistic to believe that high blood glucose levels alone ensure the brain's nutrition. For example, in untreated diabetes, the blood sugar levels are much too high, yet most of the body's cells are starving because without insulin, the glucose they need cannot enter. This is an example of a disease state, but in all cases, a number of vitamins and minerals, especially the B vitamins and magnesium, are needed to enable glucose to enter cells efficiently and to be used as a fuel to drive cellular processes.

When the brain gets and uses the glucose it needs, there are two side benefits. The first is increased mental alertness and ability to concentrate. I am surprised at how frequently and casually a woman will remark, as if it is a normal experience: "I can't think straight when I'm pregnant." Childbearing is a natural life experience which does not damage memory or concentration. What most likely has happened is that such a woman has not met the increased nutritional needs of pregnancy, especially for B vitamins, and is experiencing minor blood sugar drops that affect her mental function. Pregnancy is a time when blood sugar control is more difficult, but even then blood glucose drops can be prevented or corrected with careful nutrition.

The second benefit of stable blood sugar levels is calm nerves. If the blood glucose levels drop, the fight-or-flight hormones epinephrine and norepinephrine must be secreted to restore them. The side effects of nervousness, anxiety, irritability and so forth explain why some people (not you or me!) get grouchy when dinner is late. The role of stable blood glucose levels forms the closest link between energy and stress.

HOW THE BODY MAINTAINS BLOOD GLUCOSE LEVELS

Before reviewing practical ways of maintaining blood glucose levels, it's useful to understand that the body has two distinct metabolic states for blood sugar control.

The first occurs right after you eat. During this time, called the "absorptive state," you use the fuel provided by the recent meal to maintain your blood glucose levels. The hormone insulin from the pancreas is secreted; its role is to keep the blood sugar levels from rising too high. It does so by enabling glucose to move out of the blood and into the cells for their energy needs. Insulin promotes storage of excess glucose in the liver, where it can be released later. Within the fat cells, insulin promotes storage of excess fuel as fat. Interestingly, the brain does not require insulin to get its glucose.

The second state, the fasting or "postabsorptive" state, occurs after a meal is digested and absorbed. During this phase, you maintain your blood glucose levels by releasing fuel from its storage locations within the liver and fat cells. A number of hormones stimulate this. Glucagon, a second pancreatic hormone; cortisol from the adrenal glands; and, if necessary, epinephrine and norepinephrine from the adrenals all maintain blood glucose levels by stimulating the liver to release its stored fuel. Notice the glands involved: pancreas, adrenals, and liver.

When the postabsorptive processes function well, you feel energetic and alert between meals, and, as a beneficial side effect, weight control is easier since you do not need to boost your blood sugar levels with another snack or meal. If you wake up tired or experience afternoon slumps which are noticeably helped by eating dinner, most likely the postabsorptive processes are not working as well as they might. Migraine headaches at these times are yet another symptom of poor postabsorptive blood sugar maintenance.

PRACTICAL STRATEGIES FOR MAINTAINING BLOOD SUGAR LEVELS

Below is a list of practical ways to maintain adequate blood glucose levels around the clock. The underlying strategy is first to eat in such a way that your absorptive state is prolonged. I like to put it this way: When you eat, you want to your food to raise blood glucose levels, but only moderately so that your blood sugar "flies under the radar" of excessive insulin release, which would cause a reactive drop in your blood glucose levels. The second goal is to provide the body with the vitamins and minerals that make the postabsorptive processes more effective.

1) **EAT REGULARLY.** Avoid long periods of fasting. Don't skip breakfast. Even under the best of conditions, there is a limit to how long and how well your postabsorptive processes can maintain adequate blood sugar levels.

2) **AVOID SUGARS AND REFINED STARCHES ON AN EMPTY STOMACH**. A sudden load of carbohydrates (sugars and starches, which are quickly digested to sugars) will rapidly raise the blood glucose, boosting your energy temporarily. However, high blood glucose triggers insulin, which can overcorrect the high blood sugar and leave you with a fatigue-producing drop in blood glucose called "reactive hypoglycemia." Even healthy

foods, such as fruits and whole grain breads and cereal, can trigger reactive hypoglycemia if they are eaten by themselves.

3) MAKE EVERY MEAL AND EVERY SNACK A COMBINATION OF PROTEIN, CARBOHYDRATES (FRUITS, VEGETABLES, GRAINS), AND FATS. Carbohydrates alone raise blood glucose levels rapidly, as noted above. However, proteins and fats slow the digestive processes and the release of glucose into the blood. All three together create a long-lasting absorptive state with steady blood sugar levels. The old expression is that such a meal "sticks to your ribs." Eggs, toast with butter, and an orange for breakfast; cheese and crackers for a snack; and any typical dinner menu with meat or fish, vegetables and salad are examples of such combinations.

4) CAFFEINE IS A GOOD SLAVE BUT A BAD MASTER. It raises blood glucose, giving you a boost. But it causes a reactive drop in blood glucose and stresses the adrenals, creating a roller coaster of blood sugar fluctuations that make you crave sugar or more caffeine.

5) AVOID THE ARTIFICIAL SWEETENER ASPARTAME (NUTRASWEET) which causes the body to release insulin, decreasing blood glucose levels. On an empty stomach this is responsible for a major side effect of aspartame consumption: headaches. Avoid other artificial sweeteners as well.

6) TAKE SUPPLEMENTS THAT SUPPORT NORMAL POSTABSORPTIVE BLOOD GLUCOSE LEVELS.
These are listed in order of importance. (For specific amounts, see Table 7, Chapter 3):

Vitamin C is used in large amounts by the adrenal glands, especially under stress conditions.

B vitamins, including folate (folic acid). These enable the liver to release glucose during fasting and the brain to use glucose efficiently. The B vitamin pantothenic acid is especially valuable to the adrenal glands.

Magnesium enables the body to use certain B vitamins. Dr. Guy Abraham, who carried out double-blind studies relating nutrition to PMS, noted that if the body is deficient in B vitamins and magnesium, the brain cannot efficiently metabolize glucose, and even small drops in blood glucose affect the brain's function, making the individual feel like a large drop has occurred.[3] This could explain why you feel as if you have the symptoms of low blood glucose, even though tests may show that you do not.

Essential fatty acids are essential to all glands, including the liver, adrenal glands, and pancreas, each of which is involved in raising fasting blood glucose levels. Supplementing flax oil (five to ten 1 g capsules daily), fish oil (1 teaspoon daily or five 1 g capsules), or krill oil (1-2 grams) enables you to meet the need for these essential nutrients.

Vitamin E prevents destruction of essential fatty acids.

Zinc is necessary to adrenal function.

THE ADRENAL GLANDS AND REPRODUCTIVE PROBLEMS

PMS. Premenstrual syndrome (PMS) often manifests itself with the symptoms of anxiety. PMS which does not respond to nutrition aimed at improving ovarian function, or PMS-like symptoms that are not related to the menstrual cycle, may indicate that the adrenal glands are involved. The adrenal stress hormone cortisol interferes with progesterone, and low progesterone is related to PMS.

POLYCYSTIC OVARY SYNDROME (PCOS). When stress of any type is prolonged (stage of resistance), cortisol rises, causing blood glucose to rise. In response insulin rises to drive the blood glucose into the cells. The chronic high levels of insulin interfere with the ovaries, causing them to produce excess androgens and inhibiting normal cycles. The high insulin is responsible for the weight gain that usually occurs with PCOS.

MORNING SICKNESS. Low blood sugar levels and low blood pressure can both bring on nausea and vomiting in some pregnant women. Healthy adrenal glands help to increase blood sugar levels. The adrenal hormone aldosterone helps the body to conserve salt, which contributes to normal blood pressure. Attention to adrenal support can lessen morning sickness.

POSTPARTUM BLUES. Postpartum depression is related, at least in part, to adrenal function. During pregnancy, the placenta produces a hormone that stimulates the adrenals to produce large amounts of their hormones. The effects of this hormonal change are positive; for example, pregnant women show a decreased response to stress, which is thought to be adaptive.[4] Once the placenta is passed after childbirth, the adrenals must be activated by the woman's own hormones from her hypothalamus. Failure of her body to produce adrenal hormones can result in postpartum depression, as if in a stage of exhaustion. It may take several weeks to months for her adrenals to recover.[5]

Can nutrition improve the recovery of the adrenal glands after childbirth? As noted previously, these glands need vitamins, minerals, and essential fatty acids to do their job. The nutritional stress of pregnancy and the physical stress of childbirth can certainly contribute to adrenal burnout. *A Natural Guide to Pregnancy and Postpartum Health*, by Drs. Dean Raffelock and Robert Rountree, is an excellent book which deals specifically with nutrition for "pregnancy recovery," as they call it. I recommend it highly for anyone attempting to overcome stress-related mood problems. (See "Further Reading.")

A recent research review article has confirmed that low levels of omega-3 fatty acids, especially DHA (docosahexaenoic acid), contribute to postpartum and other depression. DHA is lost during pregnancy, and the authors suggest that supplementation with omega-3 fatty acids either during pregnancy or after birth should be considered.[6] Both fish oil and krill oil are sources of DHA, and flax oil contains the essential omega-3 fatty acid that can be converted to DHA in the body if vitamins and minerals are present. Chapter 3 offers more information on the topic of fatty acids.

MISCARRIAGE. Miscarriage is accompanied by a sense of loss, but all too often guilt also complicates the emotional response. I am frequently contacted after such a loss, and I counsel that adrenal burnout caused by blood loss as well as the emotional trauma may well be triggering the anxious feelings of guilt that so often illogically accompany miscarriage. A strong emotional support system comes first, but I also recommend the nutrition detailed in this chapter.

INFERTILITY. The stress of infertility can certainly be explained as an emotional stress. Paying attention to nutrition for adrenal support, as outlined above, makes it easier to take "one day at a time." On the other hand, don't let anyone try to convince you that you need only to "relax" to get pregnant. To suggest that an infertile couple "just relax" is an unkind and counterproductive counsel.

IS STRESSING OVER STRESS COUNTERPRODUCTIVE?

Most of us simply can't avoid daily stress, whether it is caring for a high-needs child or working at an unpleasant job. What we can do is to look at the physical aspects of stress. Understanding stress should convince us to eat better, allow more time for sleep, put a little more exercise into our life, and take supplements which support adrenal function. Dealing with stress is not counterproductive!

MENOPAUSE. As the hormones of fertility decline, the adrenal glands must produce their sex hormones to compensate. Healthy, well-nourished adrenals smooth the way to menopause and beyond.

For an interesting dietary approach to reducing the stress hormone cortisol, see *The Adrenal Reset Diet*, by Alan Christianson, NMD. (See "Further Reading.") It is particularly aimed at weight loss, but is useful to understand the adrenal glands and their need for good nutrition.

One day in late August I got my hair cut by a woman who kept saying she was having a terrible day. "I should be happy," she said. "My husband loves me and I have two wonderful sons. But I just feel so stressed lately! Especially today." It was a Monday, and she mentioned that the day before she had accompanied her two young sons on a Boy Scout hike into the woods. "My allergies just went crazy," she said. I explained that the adrenal glands respond to allergies by putting out stress hormones. Hers were probably exhausted by the exposure she had experienced hiking through a lush Indiana woodland in August. When your adrenal glands are exhausted, you feel like you can't cope. I went home and lent her a copy of a previous edition of this book, to encourage her to look into nutrition. You can build your adrenals back up.

ANOTHER "DIETARY" APPROACH TO STRESS

FAST AND FEAST IN LENT

Author unknown

Fast from judging others; feast on the Christ dwelling in them.

Fast from emphasis on differences; feast on the unity of life.

Fast from apparent darkness; feast on the reality of light.

Fast from thoughts of illness; feast on the healing power of God.

Fast from words that pollute; feast on phrases that purify.

Fast from discontent; feast on gratitude.

Fast from anger; feast on patience.

Fast from pessimism; feast on optimism.

Fast from worry; feast on divine order.

Fast from complaining; feast on appreciation.

Fast from negatives; feast on affirmatives.

Fast from unrelenting pressures; feast on unceasing prayer.

Fast from hostility; feast on non-resistance.

Fast from bitterness; feast on forgiveness.

Fast from self-concern; feast on compassion for others.

Fast from personal anxiety; feast on eternal truth.

Fast from discouragements; feast on hope.

Fast from facts that depress; feast on verities that uplift.

Fast from lethargy; feast on enthusiasm.

Fast from thoughts that weaken; feast on promises that inspire.

Fast from shadows of sorrow; feast on the sunlight of serenity.

Fast from idle gossip; feast on purposeful silence.

Fast from problems that overwhelm; feast on prayer that undergirds.

(*The Marist Messenger*, March 2003. Used with permission.)

SUMMARY—CHAPTER 4

1 The underlying causes of low energy and a sense of high stress are related, and the opposite is also true—high energy and calm nerves go hand in hand.

2 The factors that contribute to high energy are adequate sleep, the right amount of exercise, and blood glucose control.

3 Strategies for better sleep include arranging for time for enough sleep, sleeping in a dark room, avoiding caffeine in the evening, and solving worries before bedtime.

4 Strategies to stabilize blood glucose levels, including regular meals of protein, carbohydrates, and healthy natural fats, increase your energy and decrease your stress.

5 Vitamin, mineral, and essential fatty acid supplements, especially B vitamins, vitamin C, magnesium, and flax oil, fish oil, or krill oil, are useful to the adrenal glands, which manage stress.

6 Better adrenal health helps you cope with the stresses of PMS problems, morning sickness, postpartum blues, miscarriage, infertility, and menopausal changes.

CHECKLIST FOR PHYSICAL CAUSES OF ANXIETY

When you are bothered by feelings of anxiety or when worries come on, you probably already know the probable cause, whether it is a sick child, preparation for your wedding, or trouble with coworkers. But it is a good idea to ask yourself what physical factors may be making the level of anxiety or worry worse.

___ Lack of sleep

___ Low blood glucose

___ Skipping meals

___ Caffeine

___ Allergies acting up

___ Sickness or infection

___ Poor diet recently

___ Too much exercise

___ Eating too many sweets

___ Cooped up without enough exercise

___ Pain of a headache or some other pain

___ Medications

She had enough to
eat for a long time —
he and she and her
household. The jar of
flour did not go
empty, nor the jug
of oil run dry.
— 1 Kings 17:15-16

Q: How important is body weight to regular cycles and fertility?

There is a comfortable range of body weight that is good for fertility, and it varies from woman to woman. Your chart can help you out. If you are trying to conceive and your cycles are rather long, but you do ovulate and do have a normal luteal phase of (about 12-14 days), you may be a just few pounds underweight, or your body weight may be normal, but your body fat may be slightly too low. Ways to gain weight or body fat are discussed in Chapter 8, along with more information on the luteal phase of the cycle.

Oppositely, what if you are carrying a few extra pounds? If your cycles look "textbook," with more or less regular ovulation and normal length luteal phase, you are probably at a weight that works just fine for you.

Yet for some women, those few extra pounds may be producing enough extra estrogen that the luteal phase is short and the temperature and mucus patterns are hard to read. The effort to lose some of the extra pounds will pay off in many ways, most likely with better cycles. Chapter 9 covers PCOS, which most often occurs with overweight, and also has a section devoted to overweight without PCOS.

If you are overweight and trying to conceive, you may wish to bring your weight down toward average, even if your charts look fairly close to ideal. Normalizing body fat goes a long way toward decreasing elevated estrogen levels. When estrogen drops down, progesterone levels will often rise—an effect that is beneficial to fertility. When these two hormones are in the right balance, other hormones will tend to improve. When healthy, whole foods are used for gradual weight loss, insulin levels tend to drop, which again improves the reproductive hormones.

Q: I know that your book isn't really about dieting or weight loss, but since you're on this subject, do you have any suggestions for the best way to lose weight? I probably need to lose 20 pounds.

People are so individual when it comes to weight loss that the best approach is to try the weight loss program that seems to meet your needs best. Any diet plan that helps you avoid sugar and refined carbohydrates will help you out. That's why low carbohydrate diets work, and why the Mediterranean diet, which is quite different, also works. But equally as important, look for more than just a particular diet plan to help you lose weight. Here are some ideas that may help you.

Would you enjoy a support group? Weight Watchers is the traditional one, but many churches and Y's have groups that meet to encourage one another on weight loss.

Is exercise part of your life? Even if weight is not coming off fast (or at all), many of the health problems associated with overweight are very much improved by regular brisk exercise.

Is your weight gain stress related? An interesting book called *The Adrenal Reset Diet*, by Alan Christianson, N.M.D., proposes a pattern of eating that is aimed at lowering the stress hormone cortisol. The book explains exactly how cortisol raises blood sugar, which raises insulin, which drives blood sugar into the fat cells, where it is converted to fat. (See "Further Reading.")

What triggers your weight gain? Family parties, treats at work, travel with poor (or rich!) food choices and too little exercise—all such situations put temptation in front of you. Recognizing the situations that tempt you to overeat can help you avoid them or make alternative food choices.

Are you getting enough sleep? Tired people eat to stay awake. This is an overlooked factor, if only because lack of sleep is so common. Research has related inadequate sleep to weight gain in women.[1]

Are you someone who nibbles all day? Try extending the time between eating, so that you are only eating four or five times daily. Conversely, if you are someone who skips breakfast, eats a light lunch and then makes up for everything at dinner, you might try the same thing—four or five meals or snacks daily.

What is your family history like? Be reasonable with yourself, working within that genetic framework. Your ideal weight may be heavier than someone with different genes. Do you weigh yourself daily? It's much easier not to gain weight than to lose weight. Checking your weight often helps you get started on weight control before a big weight gain occurs.

Is craving for sweets and caffeine what drives your weight gain? If so, please read the next question and answer.

Finally, if weight loss is an ongoing struggle, you may profit from visiting a holistic medical doctor, often called a "functional" or "integrative" medical doctor.

Q: **I don't actually need to lose weight, but I know I eat way too much sugar. I don't really know where to start.**

Don't plan on giving the sugary foods up entirely; instead, plan on cutting down on them. A really good idea is to promise yourself that you will have treats only after a full meal, or only after a nutritious, protein-rich snack followed by a big glass of cold water. This will almost automatically reduce the amount of sugar that you eat or drink, and it will also limit the swings in blood sugar that create the craving for more. And don't underestimate the value of a salad with salad dressing, a handful of nuts, or a hard-boiled egg in satisfying your appetite and reducing those sugar cravings. Proteins and fats both slow down the digestive system, and give a sense of fullness that naturally curbs the cravings.

Keeping sweets out of sight or even out of the house or workplace is a great help, and limiting what you do eat to small portions is another strategy. Let's face it—most of us have a compulsion to finish the piece of food we start eating, so picking up one bite-sized piece of candy is better than trying to eat only one bite of a full-size candy bar.

Another way of dealing with sugar cravings is to use raw fruits, especially acidic raw fruits, to satisfy it. Along with the fruit sugar, you will get fiber and many other nutrients. The acid has the effect of slowing stomach emptying, which helps keep the blood sugar from rising too high. Just be careful that you don't overdo it, such as by eating a large bunch of sweet grapes on an empty stomach. But you can eat quite a few strawberries or blueberries or a large apple or orange or half a grapefruit without defeating your purpose.

For variety, try dark chocolate-covered almonds, peanuts, or cashews. They are crunchy, and also contain protein, natural fat, and fiber, and so are very filling. The slight bitterness of dark chocolate is reminiscent of coffee—and there is a little caffeine lift in it, too.

If it is "sugar water" you crave, meaning soda pop, why not go cold turkey, substituting unsweetened iced tea or ice water? Yes, it is breaking one habit and replacing it with a new one, but the fresh fruit or dark chocolate-covered nuts just mentioned can really help out. Dissolved sugar, as is in pop and sweetened juices, is the worst offender when it comes to blood sugar swings.

Eating a good diet is always a higher nutritional goal than taking supplements, but in this case starting general supplements a week or two before you begin to break your sugar habit will make it easier to change. This is true because certain micro-nutrients, notably the B vitamins and minerals, tend to regulate blood glucose levels. "Hypoglycemia" in Chapter 6 mentions specific nutrients which may help to reduce these cravings by improving blood glucose control. See also "Yeast Overgrowth/Gut Dysbiosis" in Chapter 10, since intense sugar cravings may relate to yeast problems.

An excellent book, *Beat Sugar Addiction Now!* by Dr. Jacob Teitelbaum, proposes four different causes for sugar cravings: fatigue, adrenal burnout, yeast overgrowth, and hormonal imbalances. He offers targeted solutions for each type. I have been particularly impressed with his suggestion to use 5-hydroxytrptophan (5-HTP) to overcome sugar cravings. While Dr. Teitelbaum suggests up to 300 mg per day, 100 or 200 mg may be helpful. Particularly if you take medication for depression, you absolutely must have your health care practitioner's approval before taking 5-HTP. (See Further Reading.")

Q: **For one week I tried increasing my family's whole grains by switching to oatmeal for breakfast instead of our usual boxed cereals. It gave my husband and me such bad gas that I don't think we'll ever try it again!**

This situation can happen to anyone who tries to make a major dietary change. Your digestive tract is accustomed to one type of food, and suddenly, it has to deal with something far different. A gradual change is the right answer as you move from refined foods to whole foods. It may also help to add good-quality yogurt to your diet, since yogurt contains healthy bacteria which can replace the gas-producing bacteria now thriving in your intestines. Better yet, get a probiotic supplement. Such supplements contain millions of "friendly" bacteria to crowd out the bad ones in your intestines. Just follow the directions on the bottle. Pharmacies also carry natural remedies for gas, such as "Beano," a source of enzymes which are helpful in preventing gas from any plant food, not just beans. Many people eat oatmeal without gas problems, and chances are you can, too.

Q: **Milk and milk products just don't agree with me. What should I do for calcium since I avoid milk products?**

It's not just the calcium; equally as important is the protein and natural fat in dairy products, especially if you are pregnant or breastfeeding. You can easily get calcium from supplement pills, but you must get your protein from your food. Each cup of milk or yogurt contains about 8 grams of protein, and an ounce of cheese contains about 7 grams. A three-ounce serving of lean meat or fish contains about 15 to 18 grams of protein. An egg contains about 6 grams of protein. A peanut butter sandwich made with two pieces of whole wheat bread and two tablespoons of peanut butter contains about 10 grams of protein. Therefore, a serving of meat or fish can replace the protein of two servings of dairy, or a large egg and a peanut butter sandwich can replace the protein of two servings of dairy food.

But back to calcium: The cole crops—cabbage, broccoli, cauliflower, brussels sprouts, and kohlrabi—and dark leafy greens are good sources of calcium, but it is still prudent to supplement calcium. Calcium supplements should also contain magnesium, preferably in an amount equal to or nearly equal to the calcium. Vitamin D3, along with magnesium and dietary fat, is necessary to assist with the absorption and use of calcium. (See Table 7 for amounts.)

It's worth mentioning that there are two basic reasons for the statement that "milk just does not agree with me." You may be lactose intolerant, which means that you do not produce enough of the digestive enzyme that breaks down lactose (also called milk sugar). If that is the case, you can purchase tablets of lactase, the enzyme that you are lacking. Products such as "Lactaid" will do the job. You take the tablets only when you eat a dairy food, such as milk or ice cream.

Milk allergies are the other likely possibility. A reaction to the protein in milk is not the same as lactose intolerance, and is best dealt with by avoiding milk to the extent that you need to. Or, if you are allergic to cows' milk but are not lactose intolerant, you may be able to use goats' milk instead. Some individuals who cannot tolerate pasteurized milk can enjoy raw milk, if they can obtain it.

Q: I would like to eat more beans, since they are a healthy food, but do you have any ideas how?

I bet you are eating more beans than you realize. Peanuts are actually a bean, so natural peanut butter qualifies. So do peas. Then there are chili beans, and beans in Mexican cuisine, baked beans, and lima beans. Though not beans, tree nuts are another important source of vegetable protein, so that snacking on all kinds of nuts is another way to emphasize vegetable protein. And one final point: if you are trying to eat more vegetable protein and less animal protein, if you are a typical American, you are likely eating animal protein far in excess of what you really need. Between milk, cheese, eggs, and meat, it is possible that just using moderation in the animal proteins will help get a healthy balance established between animal and plant proteins.

Q: Is Nutrasweet a safe substitute for sugar?

NutraSweet (aspartame) has caused a variety of adverse reactions in some individuals. Headaches, seizures, visual disturbances, dizziness, fatigue, depression, confusion, and memory loss are among the most common complaints. Dry mouth and intense thirst, creating a craving for more, is another common report. Women have reported heavy or scant menses and worsened PMS while using aspartame-containing products. These reproductive disturbances may occur because phenylalanine, which comprises about 50 percent of the aspartame molecule, stimulates the secretion of prolactin from the pituitary gland. Excess prolactin secretion is well known to affect the fertility cycle.[2]

Q: What about other sweeteners?

If you are planning to frequently use the new substitutes for sugar, my advice is short—don't. Small amounts may be acceptable, but how much can you get away with and still have optimum health? If you are only going to use a little, such as an occasional sweet drink, sweeten it with sugar or honey. Nutritionist Ann Louise Gittleman's *Get the Sugar Out!* explains the problems with the various artificial sweeteners, including aspartame (NutraSweet, Equal, Canderol) and the very similar sucralose (Splenda). She does recommend stevia, which is a sweet herb that can be used to sweeten drinks or foods.[3]

Q: I am concerned about the mercury and other contaminants in fish, as I am hoping to become pregnant.

The benefits of fish far outweigh the possible mercury issues. For example, a large study showed that pregnant women who consumed very little fish had a higher risk of their children having developmental problems compared to the children of women who ate more than the amount recommended by the government while they were pregnant. In effect, the study showed that the risk from the loss of the nutrients in fish (among them protein and DHA), was greater than the risk of harm from exposure to traces of contaminants.[4]

However, you can have it both ways. How? Eat fish with the lowest levels of contamination. The guidelines change, so check the website of the Natural Resources Defense Council: www.nrdc.org/stories/smart-seafood-buying-guide. Fish that my family enjoys include whitefish, whiting, and perch, which as of this writing are on the "least mercury" list. Canned chunk tuna, which we use once a month or so, is on the "moderate" list, to be eaten fewer than six times per month.

Q: I'm so frustrated by everything I read: if it's milk, it's got hormones. If it's fish, it's full of mercury. If it's eggs, it's cholesterol. If it's fruit, it's too sugary. Or if it's not too sugary, it's been sprayed. I even read that potatoes produce more "sugar shock" than candy.

Whoa! Don't let this kind of perfectionism discourage you from getting started with better nutrition. It's better to improve your diet to the extent you can than to skip the nutritious whole foods you mentioned because of these kinds of concerns. You may wish to reread Chapter 2, "Obtaining & Preparing Nutritious Food," which addresses at least some of your concerns. Taking vitamins, as recommended in Chapter 3, helps the body to compensate for the various inadequacies of the food we eat.

Rule 5 from Chapter 1, "Eat a greater variety of foods," is particularly helpful if you are concerned about unwanted additives or toxins that may be in foods that you buy. Not only will you get more vitamins and minerals, but you will also limit your exposure to what you are trying to avoid. How much variety? The late, great nutritionist, Adelle Davis, who wrote in the 1950s, suggested in her book *Let's Cook It Right*, that a homemaker should have thirty different menus for dinner.[5] You can see how following that old guideline would keep your consumption of tuna fish, for example, well within the recommended limits of safety discussed above.

Eggs are back on the healthy list, after several years of caution because of the high cholesterol content of their yolks. And while it is true that a plain cooked potato, by itself, really does increase blood glucose levels rapidly, who eats one all by itself? You have it as a side dish with meat, usually with butter, gravy, sour cream, or a cheese sauce. Protein and fatty foods significantly slow down the release of glucose from starchy foods like potatoes. Potatoes are also a good source of potassium, vitamin C, and iron.

Q: My food budget is stretched to the limit. Any suggestions on ways to change to all the good food you recommend without increasing what I am already spending?

Using food dollars prudently is a growing issue for everyone, not just those on the tightest budgets. I think everyone agrees that fast food is more expensive than home-cooked meals, especially if you factor in the soft drinks. In the supermarket, substituting basic whole food that you prepare at home instead of prepackaged items will definitely save you a few dollars. It's the fresh produce that increases your food bill the most as you try to eat more fresh fruits and vegetables.

Here are some ideas to help you make those dollars cover everything they should. First, the cheapest sources of protein are beans, eggs, milk, and chicken. Whole milk is a better buy than skim milk. In my hometown independent grocery store, even hormone- and antibiotic-free chicken is sold, usually on Mondays, at a reduced price, along with "reduced for quick sale" red meat. Might there be a store like that near you? Do you have room in your freezer if you find some really good buys?

Whole grain pasta is not much more expensive than the white variety, and tomato sauce to make your own meat sauce is another inexpensive, nutritious item. Brown rice is wonderfully nutritious. Look for a breadmaker on sale after Christmas, and then make your own bread. Making your own yogurt is yet another way to improve your nutrition at a much lower cost than store-bought. (See Chapter 3 for making homemade yogurt.)

Potatoes, onions, and cabbage are very good buys in the produce department, and usually other seasonal items are on sale. Meanwhile, your own garden can help out in a big way, especially if you freeze your beans, peas, broccoli, and sweet corn. Your local farmers' market is another place to find bargains, particularly at the very end of the day or of the week.

Unhealthy junk food and fast food can really waste food dollars. Instead, indulge in the family fun of making treats in your own kitchen. Peanut butter or oatmeal cookies, no-bake cookies, tapioca pudding made with plenty of eggs, homemade ice cream, or buttered popcorn are examples that give families entertainment as well as a treat.

Make a conscious effort to cut down on food waste to save dollars. Don't let that lettuce or celery in your vegetable crisper go bad. Rearrange your refrigerator and store leftovers right up on the top refrigerator shelf where you will see them immediately, and use them for breakfast or lunch the next day. Make French toast with day-old homemade bread, or make smaller loaves if you consistently have leftover bread. If it is something that is not the best as leftovers, such as fish fillets, ask your family members how many they would like before you start defrosting. A freezer will save you many food dollars, so be sure to have a signal light or some other means of being alerted in case it ever loses power.

Q: I would like for my teenage daughter to take ProCycle or Optivite for better periods. Can she take a full dose at her age? She is 15.

Your daughter's body weight is more important than her age. If she is 100 pounds or more, she can take the labeled dose. If she is less than 100 pounds, try a three fourths dose as a maximum. This guideline applies to girls who already started having periods or will probably soon start.

Q: I don't think I can afford supplements. Any thoughts about their expense?

Comprehensive multivitamin/multimineral supplements are more costly than one-a-day type vitamins. I personally feel that time is money; that is, the extra productive time I have because of the added energy they give me is well worth the monetary investment. But I took this question to a friend of mine, a divorced mother of three young children who works only part-time for their sake. She is on the tightest budget of anyone I know, but she always serves holistic food to her family. She replied:

"I buy health food store vitamins before I buy anything else. It's my highest priority for off-budget items. I can't afford to be sick, or miss work, or miss school. My kids and I hardly ever get sick any more. I would be sick four or so times a year before I took vitamins."

As the admen say, good nutrition doesn't cost, it pays. For many people, insurance and paid sick leave mask the true financial cost of poor nutrition.

Q: Would you please explain the difference between flax oil and fish oil? Should I choose one of these, or should I take both? And where does krill oil fit in?

The analogy I use to explain how flax oil and fish oil are alike and how they differ is this: Imagine that cake is essential to your body. There are two ways that you can get cake, because you cannot "make it from scratch." First, you can get a whole cake at a bakery. Or, you can get a cake mix and add water and butter and eggs. Then you can make the cake yourself. Fish oil, which contains the fatty acids EPA and DHA, is the whole cake; that is, it contains the finished products. EPA and DHA are long, highly unsaturated·fatty acids that our cells use for a number of vital processes. Flax oil is the cake mix. It contains an abundant amount of the hard-to-get alpha-linolenic acid, the "omega-3" essential fatty acid. If B vitamins and minerals (the water, butter, and eggs of the analogy) are available, the cells are able to convert alpha-linolenic acid into DHA and EPA.

Krill oil, to continue our analogy, would be like the whole cake, conveniently delivered to your door. It has the same EPA and DHA as fish oil, but the biochemical packaging makes them more easily available to the cells.

Besides the pre-made DHA and EPA, cod liver oil (but not all fish oils) contains modest amounts of vitamins A and D. It is available purified of contaminants, and in lemon or other flavors.

In addition to the hard-to-get alpha-linolenic acid, convertible to EPA and DHA, flax oil contains phytonutrients called lignans, which are weak estrogens that, at least in males, act as anti-estrogens. In women they may block the function of stronger estrogens, a beneficial function. High-lignan flax oil also serves as a prebiotic, nourishing healthy bacteria in the intestines.

My experience in consulting has shown that the use of flax oil has been very positive in virtually every aspect of female reproductive health, whether it is in overcoming infertility of unknown cause, lightening heavy menstrual periods, or reducing hot flashes or vaginal dryness.

Because of this consulting experience, I have a preference for flax oil over fish oil, but taking both is also an excellent practice. A teaspoon or two of flax oil (5-10 grams or five to ten 1 g capsules) and one teaspoon of fish oil (5 grams) are just fine if you want to get the overlapping benefits of both. Or, try krill oil instead of the fish oil. Just be sure to take vitamin E also, about 200-400 IU daily, as these unsaturated nutrients are vulnerable to oxidation, and vitamin E is a major antioxidant.

Q: I started taking flax oil, and I think it helped me get pregnant after irregular cycles and infertility. But it gave me a rash around the corners of my mouth. I would like to keep taking it, but is there any substitute for it that I might not be allergic to?

Yes, you can get pumpkin seed oil at health food shops. It has alpha-linolenic acid, though not in the same high amount as in flax oil. You will need more capsules to get the same amount of the alpha-linolenic acid. Ask the shopkeeper for a comparison of their brand of pumpkin seed oil with flax oil.

Q: Vitamins upset my stomach. Do you have any suggestions?

This is one of the most common reasons why people don't take vitamins. First, always take vitamins with a meal, and start very gradually with the lowest dose. Some people find that freezing their vitamins makes them go down more easily with less stomach upset. This may just help you to swallow the pills, or it may delay the dissolving of the vitamin long enough to make a difference.

WHY DO YOU GET STOMACH UPSETS?

Let's consider for a moment a possible cause of your sensitive stomach. Some people get upset stomachs because they have excess stomach acid, but others actually get upset stomachs because they don't produce enough acid to begin digesting their food. A little self-help trial to see which might explain your digestive upsets is to try the following: squeeze a fresh lemon into a glass of water, and have a few sips of it with food that causes your stomach to be upset. If it makes your stomach feel worse, you may be producing too much acid. There are many over-the-counter remedies for acid stomach.

If, to your surprise, drinking the lemon water makes you feel better, or does not bother you, it may be that you do not produce enough acid to activate digestive enzymes in your stomach. The acidic lemon juice may be helping out, so try having lemon juice in water with your meals. Some people with sensitive stomachs are also helped by digestive enzymes which can be purchased at health food shops or natural groceries.

Q: Ever since I started taking vitamins, minerals, and fish oil, I have been dreaming vividly practically every night. Is this a coincidence?

It's a sign of good mental function to remember dreams, and vitamin B6 and fish oil are probably the two nutrients that promote dreaming the most, though other B vitamins might be involved. If you do not care to "spend the night at the movies," as my husband puts it, take those supplements first thing in the morning. Cut down on the amount that you take if that doesn't work.

Q: What kind of vitamins should young children take?

Nursing babies and toddlers are fine with the vitamins they get through their mother's milk, assuming she uses supplements, including fish oil and/or flax oil. The quality of the mother's milk is improved by such supplements. For older children, health food shops have chewable vitamins, and vitamin C is especially helpful for their immune systems. However, make sure that your children brush their teeth immediately after taking chewable vitamin C, since it can promote tooth decay if left on the teeth. Avoid vitamins with food colorings in them.

When my kids were young, I had them take a half-teaspoon or a bit more of lemon-flavored cod liver oil daily to give them the EPA and DHA that are so important to their immune systems and brain function. They never had a problem with the taste, as it really is very mild tasting, and we started it at around two years of age. It's easy to purchase contaminant-free fish oil at health food shops, so look for this on the label. Our youngest child, who was adopted and was never breastfed, received a little fish oil daily in one of her bottles. It also helped with the problem of constipation, which is common in bottle-fed babies.

Dr. Julian Whitaker, founder of the Whitaker Wellness Institute in Newport Beach, California, recommends chewable vitamin pills for children beginning around age four. He suggests that the supplements include 125-250 mg of vitamin C, 25-50 IU of vitamin E, 2,000-4,000 IU of A and beta-carotene, 10-20 mcg selenium, 50-100 mg calcium, 200-400 IU vitamin D, 200-400 mcg folic acid, 5-10 mg B6, and 50-100 mg B12.

He additionally recommends supplemental DHA from fish oil.[6]

Once girls and boys are over 100 pounds, you can consider giving them an adult dose of a multivitamin/multimineral, or at least nearly an adult dose.

Q: I have four small children, and even though they are good kids, I feel constantly stressed out by the sheer amount of work around the house. Can nutrition make a difference?

The well-nourished person can perform a tremendous amount of work, day in and day out, without reaching wit's end. Cutting down on caffeine is the first step because it contributes to that anxious feeling. The mineral magnesium is probably the most noticeably nerve-calming nutrient, followed by the B vitamins, especially B6, vitamin C, zinc, and flax oil. Calcium supplemented without magnesium may cause nervousness and anxiety in some people, so be sure to supplement calcium with equal or almost equal amounts of magnesium. The nutritional strategies for keeping blood sugar up help to give you the energy to tackle the day's activities—see Chapter 1. Vitamin E may also boost your energy.

Many people would suggest that you hire household help for this common problem, but the price of one morning's help can buy you a month's supply of vitamins. I would choose the latter without hesitation, though I do not intend to diminish the role of diet, exercise, and adequate rest. The physical stress of multiple pregnancies, nursing, being on your feet constantly, and being on-call 24 hours a day—it's incomprehensible to me that anyone would advise women like you (or me) that they can function well without serious attention to the best nutritional support they can get.

Q: Are you implying that everyone ought to take vitamins in the amounts you suggest in table 7?

No. If you are completely satisfied with your health, your energy level, and your mental outlook, and you eat as healthfully as you reasonably can, you very likely do not need more than a basic vitamin/mineral supplement. My observation is that young adult men form the largest group in this category. This may explain why some women tell me that their husbands fail to understand the relationship between fatigue, moodiness, and nutrition—they simply have never experienced it.

Whether or not to take vitamins should not be an all-or-none decision. For example, those who are reasonably satisfied with their health, energy level, and moods may want to take a middle road by supplementing vitamins, minerals, and essential fatty acids at a low level as an "insurance policy." Others who have improved their health through diet and supplements may be able to maintain their good health through excellent diet and perhaps a low level of supplementation. In other words, taking food supplements (or not taking them) should relate to your perceived need, which changes with age, illness, pregnancy, stress level, and diet.

There are many good multivitamins available through health food shops and other outlets, and in the following sections of this book I mention four by name: Optivite, Androvite, ProCycle, and Professional Pre-Natal Formula. One of the reasons I recommend these is that the full dose for each is four to six tablets per day. This gives the users a great deal of flexibility in finding their own middle ground between high levels of supplements and none at all.

Q: I am trying to overcome infertility, so I am doing a lot of reading. Some books and websites recommend avoiding "hormone disrupters" like BPA and phthalates. How careful should I be to avoid hormone disrupters like these?

BPA is the abbreviation for **bisphenol A**, a chemical used in processing many types of plastic. It has been related to interference with estrogen, thyroid hormone, and testosterone. Because the awareness of its effects on hormones is growing, it's now easier to buy BPA-free kitchen items, such as cups, storage containers, and utensils. However, some of the new plastic replacements may be worse in terms of hormone disrupters, so glass, stainless steel, and ceramic items are better choices. Canned goods are usually put into cans lined with BPA, unless the label states "BPA-free." And checkout receipts are a source of BPA, which is more a problem for people who work as cashiers than for customers.

Phthalates are another class of chemicals that interfere with estrogen, testosterone, and thyroid hormone. Phthalates are in some plastics, in cosmetics, and in household cleaning agents. Air fresheners, fabric softeners, nail polish, perfume, shampoo, hair conditioners, hair spray, deodorants, and skin lotions are common sources of these chemicals, unless they are specifically labeled otherwise. Flexible plastics such as shower curtains and plastics used to package foods are another source of exposure.

What to do? First, always remember that the worst and most common hormone disrupter is the birth control pill, with its artificial estrogens and progesterones that interfere with natural hormones. Avoid the pill completely.

Second, apply the 80-20 rule to avoiding BPA, phthalates, and other such chemicals. That is, choose to avoid the worst offenders, such as perfumes, nail polish, and fragranced fabric softeners. Look for products that are labeled BPA- and phthalate-free. Such products are becoming more and more common as consumers like yourself become more aware.

Finally, don't become overly concerned with the effects of these chemicals. You can't avoid them entirely, but good nutrition and especially good supplements help your body to get rid of them.

Q: We are developing a different kind of eating problem in my family. Our teenage daughter has decided to eat a vegetarian diet which includes milk and eggs, but my husband still wants meat with our meals. So do I.

Meanwhile, my sister's family has gone gluten free. We are really having a problem making meals that everyone is happy with. It has even created a strain at family gatherings.

I would like to address only the social side of your problem, not any nutritional concerns, because an ovo-lacto-vegetarian diet can certainly be healthy, as can a gluten-free diet. But as people form "food tribes," they discover that one of the wonderful joys of good food, which is good fellowship, can get a bit complicated. Let me propose some guidelines, some for the cook, and some for the individual with a restricted diet for whatever reason—life or death food reactions, or as part of a philosophy such as concern for animals.

First, if you are the hostess/cook, can you offer an alternative for the family member or guest on the restricted diet? For years my husband has been sensitive to a variety of spices, and I have formed the habit of taking some of the food I am preparing out of the larger pot and putting it in a smaller pot and a serving dish for him. Before I freeze spicey meat-based sauces, I pull out some without spices and label it separately. There are times when I prepare a completely separate main dish for him, though usually it is something simple. I can say we are both good sports about this small extra effort.

As the hostess, you can also let your invited guests know what the menu will be, and see if it will be acceptable. If it is a guest with a highly restricted diet, often he or she will offer to bring a dish that works with their particular diet. By all means accept such an offer!

Second, if you are the family member or the guest with a restricted diet, can you help the cook by letting her know what you can and can't eat? If it is a matter of preference, can you make exceptions for the meal that you will be sharing? Or, it is a courtesy to offer to bring a dish that you can share with everyone, or at least that you can eat so that the cook can focus on the meal she has chosen to serve to the larger group.

PART 2
OVERCOMING REPRODUCTIVE PROBLEMS & CHALLENGES

As the title implies, the main purpose of this book is to offer suggestions on how to assist the natural fertility processes to function normally through self care, especially better nutrition. Therefore, Part 2 truly forms the core of this book. However, please keep three things in mind as you review the nutritional information that follows in the next eleven chapters.

First, a nutritious diet as described in Part 1 is always a higher priority than taking supplements for good nutrition. Second, when you look up a particular cycle problem, often only a small number of vitamin or mineral supplements are listed as potentially helpful. While these should be stressed, all of the vitamins, minerals, and essential fatty acids listed in Table 7 should be taken together to prevent imbalances as you supplement. Where a range of doses is given in Table 7, you can use the higher levels for micronutrients that are listed as helpful to your situation, but take lower levels of the others.

Finally, the suggestions that follow on these pages are not meant to replace the counsel of your health care provider. Nutrition and professional health care are by no means mutually exclusive, and happily, more and more doctors and other health professionals are deeply interested in the value of a good diet and nutritional supplements. A doctor's ability to diagnose, treat, and advise are great blessings. However, once a diagnosis is made, healing through nutrition should ordinarily be considered the first resort. If intervention through drugs or surgery becomes necessary, the value of continued excellent nutrition is even greater.

FEMALE REPRODUCTIVE BASICS

Whether you are reading this book to have more regular cycles, to overcome infertility, or to reduce your chance of a miscarriage, reviewing the basic events of the menstrual cycle will increase your understanding of how, why, and where nutrition can make a difference. What follows is a simplified summary of those events and their causes.

If you, however, are attempting to overcome infertility or repeated miscarriage, I especially encourage you to read the section entitled "Maturation of the Ovum: Egg Quality," which contains vital information that is unfamiliar to many women. The vocabulary in bold here will also be used in the chapters of Part 2.

PREOVULATION PHASE

During the first part of the menstrual cycle, as the menstrual flow is ending, the pituitary gland at the base of the brain secretes **follicle stimulating hormone (FSH)**. FSH stimulates a **follicle** (a tiny sac of cells containing an unfertilized ovum) in one of the two ovaries to begin to mature. As the follicle develops, it grows larger and secretes increasing amounts of estrogen. Estrogen causes the inner lining of the uterus, the **endometrium**, to thicken in preparation for a possible pregnancy. Estrogen also causes the cervix of the uterus to secrete a mucus discharge which is necessary for normal fertility and sperm migration. Depending on the quality of the mucus, natural family planning (NFP) providers refer to it as "less fertile" or "more fertile"; if it is absent the term "dry" is used.

OVULATION

When estrogen from the enlarging follicle rises to a critical point, it stimulates the pituitary gland to increase the secretion of a second hormone, **luteinizing hormone (LH)**. LH then stimulates more estrogen, and estrogen stimulates more LH, and therefore both hormones rise steeply for approximately two days. The spike of LH, called the LH surge, triggers ovulation. **Ovulation**, of course, is the release of the ovum from the follicle. That unfertilized ovum will be picked up by tiny "fingers" on the end of the fallopian tube, and microscopic hairs in the wall of the tube will move the ovum slowly toward the uterus.

The ovulated ovum will live only eight to twenty-four hours if it is not fertilized.

After that, it will die, and it is so very tiny that no remains of it will be observed. If conception is to occur, the ovum must be fertilized within those eight to twenty-four hours, an event that happens in the outer one third of the fallopian tube. Sperm must be able to swim "upstream" in order to fertilize the ovum.

POSTOVULATION PHASE

After ovulation, whether or not conception has occurred, the empty follicle gets a new look and a new name. It becomes yellowish and is called the **corpus luteum**, Latin for "yellow body." It secretes estrogen and especially progesterone, which prepares the endometrium for possible implantation of a newly conceived child.

Progesterone additionally causes the early, waking, "basal" temperature to rise slightly, a sign that can be observed and recorded on the NFP chart. The presence of progesterone, combined with decreased estrogen levels, also causes a distinctive change in the cervical mucus discharge. After approximately two weeks, if pregnancy has not occurred, the corpus luteum stops secreting progesterone, and the drop in this hormone causes the inner lining of the uterus to be shed in the process of menstruation.

Keep the term "corpus luteum" in mind because it is used frequently in scientific discussion of the fertility cycle. The postovulatory phase of the cycle is called the **luteal phase**, and inadequacy of the corpus luteum's ability to secrete progesterone is called **luteal phase deficiency**.

It's useful to realize that what happens before ovulation, during the preovulatory phase, sets the stage for the postovulatory time of the cycle. For example, if the follicle fails to develop properly before ovulation, it will become an inadequate corpus luteum after ovulation, and the result will be luteal phase deficiency.

ESTROGEN AND PROGESTERONE

While both estrogen and progesterone are necessary for healthy cycles and fertility, it is common for estrogen to be somewhat higher than ideal and for progesterone to be lower than ideal. This can result in a number of cycle irregularities, ranging from poor mucus patterns to PMS to infertility and even early miscarriage. Normal body weight, or rather, a normal amount of body fat, helps to keep estrogen in its lower, ideal range. Since high estrogen interferes with progesterone, progesterone tends to be higher if estrogen is lower. Some vitamin supplements have been shown to increase progesterone. These are vitamin B6[1], vitamin C[2], and folate[3].

The understanding of the normal fertility-menstrual cycle is at the very heart of NFP. Women who chart their mucus and temperature signs gain an extremely accurate awareness of where they are in their fertility cycles, and the benefits of this extend well beyond family planning. For example, if a woman is troubled by PMS, which is associated with the postovulatory (luteal phase), she will know from her fertility observations exactly when to expect PMS symptoms. Or, if a woman's thyroid function is low, her basal temperature will be abnormally low, even if blood tests fail to reveal it. If she is not ovulating, she will know, because she will not see the postovulatory temperature rise, even if she still has menstrual bleeding. (Such "cycles" without ovulation are called anovulatory cycles.) If her luteal phase is abnormally short she will easily see it on her chart, and will recognize it as luteal phase deficiency, even if her cycles are quite regular.

MATURATION OF THE OVUM (EGG QUALITY)

While many women who use NFP will find that much of the above information is simply a review, most women are not aware of the critical events that occur within the unfertilized ovum, especially during the *two days* before ovulation. If you are dealing with infertility even though you are ovulating, or if you are trying to avoid repeated miscarriage, or if you are interested in the possible prevention of certain birth defects, notably Down syndrome, please read on. If you are not concerned with these three topics, you may wish to skip the rest of this introduction.

The Life History of the Ovum

At ovulation, the unfertilized ovum contains only half as much genetic information as most other body cells. It is said to be **haploid**. In the human, that means it contains only 23 single chromosomes, whereas most other body cells contain 46 chromosomes in 23 pairs, and are called **diploid** cells. This is by design. When a haploid ovum is fertilized by a sperm, which is also haploid, the newly conceived human being will have the ordinary number of chromosomes, 46, and will begin to develop.

Meiosis: 46 to 23 Chromosomes

However, the millions of ova (plural of ovum) which develop in the ovaries of a baby girl long before she is born are all diploid cells, with 46 chromosomes. These diploid ova must become haploid cells before fertilization can occur. The time line for a diploid ovum to become a haploid ovum is one of the most remarkable physiological sequences in the human body. The process involves cell division by the diploid ova, and for reasons beyond the scope of this discussion, this cell division occurs in two separate events, called meiosis I and meiosis II. **Meiosis I** is the critical cell division that actually reduces an ovum from its diploid state (46 chromosomes) to its haploid state of 23 chromosomes. **Meiosis II** is the second cell division. It enables the ovum to eliminate extra copies of each chromosome which form normally as part of meiosis I.

Long before a baby girl is born, many of the ova in her ovaries die. The remaining ones begin meiosis I, but they are arrested in it. That is, the process is begun but is not completed until years later. When the girl reaches puberty, several follicles per month seemingly "wake up" and begin to respond to the hormones mentioned previously. Only one follicle per cycle (usually) takes the lead, and becomes the mature follicle that will burst open in ovulation. Some of the other follicles will continue to develop next month.

 But here's the key point: Within that single maturing follicle, the ovum is also maturing. How? By completing the all-important meiosis I, in which half of the genetic information is discarded. Amazingly, the ovum completes meiosis I during the two days just before ovulation. Truly a last-minute preparation for the big date!

Yet even more amazing is the fact that the final cell division, meiosis II, occurs only if the ovum is fertilized.

Ovulatory Causes of Infertility and Early Miscarriage

Why is this so vital? If the two cell divisions of meiosis occur normally, normal fertilization is likely and development can proceed. If, however, the meiosis I cell division is faulty, the unfertilized ovum will not end up with exactly 23 chromosomes.[4] If this occurs, the ovum is genetically imperfect. It may not be able to be fertilized at all, so that pregnancy cannot occur. In some cases such an ovum can be fertilized, but because of missing or extra chromosomes, development of the newly conceived child cannot proceed normally. The tiny child dies within a few days or weeks in what is sometimes called, unfortunately, a "blighted ovum" or "empty sac" pregnancy. Sometimes it is simply called an "early miscarriage," and is said to be caused by a "random genetic error." Despite the terminology, it is the loss of a child and often a great sorrow to the parents.

Down Syndrome

Very occasionally, when meiosis occurs abnormally before ovulation, the result is an unfertilized ovum with two number 21 chromosomes. Should this ovum be fertilized by a normal sperm, the newly conceived child will have three number 21 chromosomes.[5] This condition is Down syndrome, or trisomy 21, and unlike other similar genetic errors, it is mild enough that the baby, with extra love and extra care, can usually survive and grow and live to adulthood, despite some mental and physical disabilities.

What Does It Take for an Ovum to Complete Meiosis Correctly?

Answering this question has many implications, and new research is aimed at discovering the answers. If the ovum can complete meiosis I properly before ovulation, infertility of certain types will decrease. Early miscarriage without development of the child will decrease[6], and even the incidence of Down syndrome will decrease.[7]

It is known that the hormones FSH and LH stimulate the ovum to complete meiosis I. It is also known that folate (folic acid), vitamin B12, and zinc are involved in cell division. So are other B vitamins, notably vitamin B6, and the mineral magnesium, and the essential fatty acids. Vitamin C is necessary for folate function.

> **As the ova age within a woman's body, infertility, miscarriage, and the incidence of Down syndrome all increase. The ova are older, and they may not complete meiosis as well as younger ones did. Still, providing them with all of the nutrients that they need to undergo their cell division before ovulation occurs is the most fruitful way to overcome infertility and miscarriage related to the quality of the ova. Table 7 in Chapter 3 provides recommended amounts of these nutrients.**

Very new research is focusing on the understanding that the ovum uses a great deal of cellular energy to complete meiosis. As a result, coenzyme Q10 and **alpha lipoic acid** have been suggested as supplements for older women experiencing infertility, because these assist the cell with energy production.[8] The B vitamins are also involved with cellular energy production. Because energy production results in oxidative stress, the role of antioxidants such as vitamins C and E, zinc, and selenium is another topic of ongoing research.[9]

In obese women, the excess body fat may result in a disruption of the many hormones produced by adipose tissue, as body fat is technically called. Such imbalance "interferes with normal follicular development and oocyte maturation"[10].

More specific information on the topic of ovum maturation and egg quality is provided in Chapter 10, under the heading "Age-Related Infertility."

MALE REPRODUCTIVE BASICS

Unlike the woman's, a man's reproductive cells—the sperm—are produced in abundance beginning at puberty and continuing even into old age if a man remains healthy. This process occurs in the walls of the **seminiferous tubules**, which are the microscopic tubes coiled within each **testis** (plural is testes). There the sperm begin to form by meiosis, which is ongoing in the man.

SPERM PRODUCTION

Meiosis, the special cell division that only ovum and sperm can undergo, makes the sperm haploid (23 chromosomes in the human). As they mature, sperm lose cellular material so that their heads contain little more than the nucleus with its genetic material. The tip of the head forms an **acrosome**, which contains enzymes capable of digesting the covering material that surrounds an ovulated ovum. They develop a tail. They are the only self-propelled cells in the human species, and their ability to deliver their genetic material to the ovum depends on the whipping movement of their tails. Between the head and tail, a flexible midpiece contains tiny energy-producing units, the mitochondria.

Sperm production, though occurring at a very rapid pace in terms of numbers—perhaps one hundred million per da —is not particularly fast for each individual sperm. It takes two months for the sperm to develop from start to finish. Part of this time is spent outside the testes, in a coiled tube atop each testis called the **epididymis**. Both the testes and the epididymides (plural) must have a temperature lower than the core temperature of the body, or sperm production will not take place.

From the epididymis, the sperm enter the **vas deferens** (plural is vasa deferentia), the thin, muscular tube that enables the sperm to enter the pelvis. Immediately prior to ejaculation, the sperm are pushed through the two vasa deferentia. Each vas deferens enters the prostate gland, where it empties into the urethra. Three large glands, the two **seminal vesicles** and the **prostate gland**, secrete fluids into the urethra, forming the majority of the semen.

> **Both the production of sperm and the production of the hormone testosterone by the testes are stimulated by the hormones FSH and LH, the same hormones found in women.**

As you would probably guess, FSH and LH do not have a cyclic pattern of secretion as they do in women. As in women, excess body fat produces excess estrogen, which in obese men can reduce testosterone's effectiveness.

FERTILIZATION

Released by the millions into the female reproductive tract, the vast majority of the sperm cells soon die. Only a small minority are able to swim up into the fallopian tubes of the uterus. If an ovulated ovum is present, many sperm bury their heads into it; it is many times larger than the sperm cells. Together their acrosomes release enough enzymes to digest the covering. One sperm penetrates the ovum, and its nucleus soon fuses with the nucleus of the ovum.

> **Conception, or fertilization, has occurred, and the newly conceived human being has all the genetic information it will ever have, 23 chromosomes from the mother and 23 from the father.**

SPERM NUTRIENT NEEDS

The fast-dividing developing sperm cells need many nutrients to function efficiently. They require folate (folic acid), zinc, vitamin B12, and a number of other nutrients in order to provide for the constant, ongoing meiosis. They use B vitamins to generate energy. Selenium is necessary for the function of the midpiece. Vitamin C and E are essential antioxidants. Because of their small amount of cellular material, they are not able to neutralize the byproducts of their energy use efficiently, and must rely heavily on other antioxidants. The cell membrane and the acrosome must be relatively fluid, not stiff, so that the sperm can fuse to the ovum during conception. This requires, among other nutrients, the essential fatty acids. Meeting the nutritional needs of sperm production is the focus of overcoming male infertility.[11] (See Chapter 15 for more specific information on this topic.)

SUMMARY

In women, the fertility cycle begins with the preovulatory phase, in which estrogen is secreted by the follicle surrounding the ovum. Release of the ovum (ovulation) then occurs. The postovulatory or luteal phase follows, characterized by high levels of progesterone secreted by the corpus luteum.

The maturation of the ovum is a vital yet underappreciated factor in fertility.

In the two days right before ovulation, the ovum must undergo a key cell division called meiosis I. This requires several hormones, but it also requires a number of nutrients, including B vitamins, the minerals zinc and magnesium, and essential fatty acids. Nutrients that promote energy production, such as coenzyme Q10 and alpha lipoic acid are now being studied for their effect on female fertility. Antioxidants are also the topic of new research, since high energy production in cells, including the ovum, results in oxidative stress. Meeting the nutritional needs of the ovum as it prepares for ovulation is a key factor in fertility.

In men, sperm are produced at a high rate. Sperm need energy to move, and they need antioxidants to counteract their oxygen use. B vitamins, vitamin C, vitamin E, the mineral selenium, and essential fatty acids are among the nutrients needed for sperm production.

PREMENSTRUAL SYNDROME (PMS)

6

Her ways are pleasant ways, and all her paths are peace.
— Proverbs 3:17

Back when I was in my thirties, premenstrual syndrome (PMS) became a topic of great interest among women. Mood changes, fluid retention, craving for sweets—the premenstrual blues were talked about, written about, and researched. In fact, the first talk I ever gave at a Couple to Couple League convention was on nutritional self care strategies for PMS, and that presentation led to CCL's request that I write the first edition of this book. Now, however, with few exceptions, it's difficult to find new research or new books to help out with this all-too-common problem.

What has happened to research on PMS? I think the answer is this: The baby boom generation, who are in the midst of the change of life, are focused on menopause. Their concern with PMS, which affects women who have menstrual cycles, has declined. With half of all American women past menopause and many more soon to follow, the researchers have followed the demographics. Perimenopause, the transitional time before menopause, has replaced PMS as the hot topic when it comes to women's health concerns. But the truth is, the symptoms of perimenopause often include PMS. While it is true that PMS tends to become more severe as women approach menopause, it bothers many younger women as well, even teens.

The way that many medical doctors deal with PMS is to recommend the birth control pill. Yet for some women, the birth control pill can make PMS worse. If the PMS is so severe as to be classified as "premenstrual dysphoric disorder" (PMDD), the woman may also be prescribed anti-depressant medication. Fortunately, there are a number of natural self care solutions for PMS. The nutritionally-oriented research from the not-too-distant past is still very helpful for improving PMS.

No matter what your age, you can be optimistic that you can help yourself to overcome or improve PMS through better diet, specific vitamins and minerals, and other lifestyle improvements beyond nutrition.

DEFINING PMS

PMS is a actually a broad term, referring to a large group of symptoms which all have one thing in common—they occur mainly during the postovulatory (luteal) phase of the cycle, beginning two to three days to a week or so before the menstrual period begins. Severe PMS may start earlier and last into the next cycle, though most often it disappears when the menstrual period begins. PMS does not include menstrual cramps or heavy bleeding, topics which are discussed in Chapter 7. The symptoms of PMS can be classified into four categories, as summarized below in Table 8.

TABLE 8, SYMPTOMS OF PMS, FROM MOST TO LEAST COMMON*

PMT-A: ANXIETY	Characterized by anxiety, mood swings, irritability, and nervous tension
PMT-H: HYDRATION	Characterized by water retention, weight gain, swelling of the extremities, breast tenderness, and abdominal bloating
PMT-C: CRAVINGS	Characterized by cravings for sweets, cravings for carbohydrates, increased appetite; sometimes associated with headaches, fatigue, palpitations, and the "shakes"
PMT-D: DEPRESSION	Characterized by severe depression, forgetfulness, crying, confusion, and insomnia[1]

This classification was developed by Guy Abraham, M.D., who prefers the term "premenstrual tension" (PMT).

There are longer and more detailed lists of PMS symptoms, but most relate to the ones classified above. Premenstrual flare-up of acne is the only common symptom that doesn't easily fit into one of these four categories.[2] Women who are bothered by PMS usually experience more than one symptom, and their symptoms may change from cycle to cycle.

NUTRITION AND PMS

Gynecologist Guy Abraham, M.D., undertook pioneering studies on PMS and nutrition in the 1980s. His research is still truly remarkable for its holistic approach. He compared the daily diet of women who had PMS to the diet of women free from it. He observed the effect on PMS of consuming sugar and refined flour versus eating whole grains and vegetables. He considered the role of the healthy essential fatty acids versus the *trans* fats. Based on these studies, he developed a practical diet plan to improve the symptoms of PMS. At the same time, he researched the role of vitamins and minerals in PMS. Instead of recommending only one or two supplements, he formulated a complete multivitamin/multimineral for PMS, called Optivite PMT, and then tested it under double-blind conditions.

> Dr. Abraham's contributions to women's reproductive self care can hardly be overstated. Because his supplement recommendations tend to normalize the levels of estrogen and progesterone during the luteal phase, his PMS plan may also benefit women with short luteal phase, menstrual cramps, infertility, recurrent miscarriage, and endometriosis. For PMS as well as for these problems, the nutritional strategy detailed below is the practical self help that the Couple to Couple League has recommended since 1990, with much positive feedback from the many women who have implemented it.

PROPOSED CAUSES OF PMS

Here are some of the nutritionally-related causes of PMS, as originally proposed by Dr. Abraham. Understanding this research, though it is somewhat technical, is valuable because it helps you realize how and why nutrition makes a difference, not just in symptoms, but even more important, in the balance of estrogen, progesterone, and other hormones.

ABNORMAL LUTEAL FUNCTION (LUTEAL PHASE DEFICIENCY). Many women with PMS, especially those with anxiety and related symptoms (PMT-A), have estrogen levels that are too high and progesterone levels that are too low in the luteal phase of their cycles. This is a common hormonal imbalance, and is sometimes called **estrogen dominance**. Nutrition that tends to correct this imbalance by lowering estrogen and raising progesterone is beneficial to PMS, and it may also improve the other reproductive problems mentioned above.

B vitamins and diet play a role in regulating estrogen levels. If B vitamins are lacking, the liver cannot effectively inactivate estrogen, and estrogen rises.[3] Conversely, dietary fiber, which is the indigestible portion of whole plant foods, has the beneficial effect of reducing estrogen levels, apparently by "shielding" estrogens which are excreted in the bile from being reabsorbed back into the blood.[4]

Women without PMS were far more likely to take vitamin supplements regularly, especially B vitamins, and were found to eat twice as much dietary fiber compared to women troubled by PMS.[5]

Estrogen dominance can also be improved through nutritional means that raise progesterone. Excess estrogen itself decreases progesterone, so reducing elevated estrogen promotes better progesterone levels. Consumption of excess animal fats is implicated in PMS because these fats contain arachidonic acid, the dietary precursor of a harmful "local hormone," the prostaglandin PGF2α. This prostaglandin depresses the function of the corpus luteum, which produces the progesterone in the luteal phase.[6] Dr. Abraham found that women without PMS consume as much fat as those with PMS, but they use more vegetable fat, while women with PMS consume more animal fat.[7]

Naturally decreasing the hormone prolactin can help PMS. Prolactin, produced by the pituitary gland, is higher in some women with PMS than in women without it. High levels of prolactin decrease progesterone levels, contributing to estrogen dominance and PMT-A.[8] The hypothalamus controls prolactin primarily through inhibition, not stimulation, and prolactin will rise abnormally if it is not properly regulated. Vitamin B6 reduces prolactin levels by stimulating the production of dopamine, which decreases prolactin release.[9] Magnesium is also necessary for the synthesis of dopamine, and so can contribute to normal levels of prolactin. Zinc is another nutrient that suppresses elevated prolactin levels.[10]

Vitamin B6 (pyridoxine) supplements can elevate progesterone levels, which is key to overcoming abnormal luteal function.[11] This vitamin alone has significantly reduced the symptoms of PMS, especially anxiety, in double-blind studies.[12] Vitamin C, in a large, more recent study on infertility, has also increased progesterone levels significantly.[13] Dr. Abraham's complete diet and the supplement Optivite PMT, which includes large doses of both vitamin B6 and vitamin C, as well as magnesium and zinc, has lowered high luteal phase estrogen and raised low luteal phase progesterone to normal levels while reducing the symptoms of PMS.[14]

ABNORMAL FLUID RETENTION. The premenstrual fluid retention (PMT-H) that bothers many women with PMS is responsible for bloating, weight gain, and breast pain or tenderness. These symptoms relate in part to the hormone aldosterone, secreted by the adrenal glands, which sit atop each kidney. Aldosterone causes the kidneys to retain salt and water, and it is elevated during the luteal phase. Excess aldosterone secretion, which occurs in some women with PMS, increases loss of the mineral magnesium.[15] Magnesium works together with vitamin B6; both B6 and magnesium are necessary for the synthesis of dopamine, which in addition to lowering prolactin, also helps the kidneys to rid the body of salt and water.[16] That is, magnesium and vitamin B6 have a diuretic effect.

Intracellular magnesium levels have been found to be lower in women with PMS than in other women.[17] Women with PMS also consume more dairy products than do women without this disorder. High consumption of dairy products, with their unbalanced calcium to magnesium ratio of 10:1, inhibits the absorption of magnesium.[18] Reviews of experiments on the effect of magnesium supplements for PMS conclude that magnesium alone is beneficial for PMS.[19]

Moderate use of dairy products combined with plenty of green vegetables and whole grains naturally tends to balance calcium and magnesium.

Even when aldosterone levels are normal or low, high consumption of sugar, which is common in women with PMS, causes fluid retention within a day or two of a sugar binge.[20] Such sugar consumption depletes magnesium. And while excessive salt promotes fluid retention, adequate salt prevents over-secretion of aldosterone.[21]

HYPOGLYCEMIA. Women with PMS consume more sugar and refined carbohydrates than do others.[22] In addition to promoting fluid retention, sugar and refined carbohydrates trigger over-secretion of insulin. Insulin rapidly lowers the blood glucose, resulting in reactive hypoglycemia and symptoms such as craving for sweets, headaches, mood swings, and shakiness or faintness. (See Rule 6 in Chapter 1 for an explanation of the relationship between sugar consumption, insulin, and hypoglycemia.)

Insulin secretion is regulated with help from a beneficial local hormone, prostaglandin E1, so a deficiency of this prostaglandin may contribute to carbohydrate cravings (PMT-C). This prostaglandin is derived from linoleic acid, which is plentiful in many vegetable oils. However, for the dietary linoleic acid to be converted to the helpful prostaglandin E1, magnesium, vitamins B3, B6, and C, and zinc are all necessary. *Trans* fats, as in margarine, block this vital conversion. These damaging fats also favor the synthesis of the harmful prostaglandin F2α.[23] Conversely, alpha-linolenic acid, found abundantly in flax oil, is the precursor of the healthy "E3" series of prostaglandins, which increase the production of the beneficial prostaglandin E1, while blocking the production of the harmful F2α.[24]

Besides limiting sugary foods, both avoiding *trans* fats as well as taking in the healthy fats and oils, as explained in Rule 3 in Chapter 1, help to keep insulin levels normal. The undesirable insulin over-response to sugar can also be reduced by decreasing the ratio of calcium to magnesium. Dr. Abraham's preferred ratio of supplemental calcium to magnesium is 1:2, opposite the 2:1 ratio of these two minerals which is usually suggested by nutritional advisors.[25]

PMS DIETARY RECOMMENDATIONS

Dr. Abraham's nutritional recommendations integrate the above research into practical advice for women with PMS. He recommends plenty of vegetables, whole grains and beans, fish, and poultry, moderate use of dairy products, and limited red meat. Most important, refined sugar, *trans* fats, excess salt, as well as alcohol and caffeine, are to be restricted.[26] He suggests olive oil, safflower oil, and flaxseed oil to obtain the healthy monounsaturated fats and the two essential fatty acids.[27]

These recommendations, first published in 1983 and updated in 1990, are similar to the more recent dietary guidelines of *The Fertility Diet*, based on the Harvard School of Public Health's large Nurses' Health Study on ovulatory infertility in women. Both recommend whole plant foods, which are rich sources of magnesium, vitamins, and other minerals. Both have generous protein allowances, but encourage increased use of plant proteins. Both recommend healthful oils. Both emphatically discourage consumption of sugar, refined carbohydrates, and *trans* fats.

However, Dr. Abraham counsels limiting dairy products to two low-fat servings daily,[28] while *The Fertility Diet* recommends one to two servings of full-fat dairy products daily.

Based on the new research finding that use of full-fat dairy products improves fertility (and therefore hormonal balance), you may wish to use whole-fat dairy products rather than low-fat ones.

If you are able to obtain organic or raw milk, all the better.

That said, as you improve your diet to overcome PMS, use the "Twelve Guidelines for Better Nutrition" in Chapter 1. They are intentionally flexible, so tailor healthy food choices to your own needs and preferences. For example, you may find that extra protein in the form of meat or eggs, especially for breakfast, helps you to have more stable blood sugar and less sugar craving. On the other hand, your sister may find that high fiber snacks during the day do the same for her.

THE CAFFEINE CONNECTION. Dr. Abraham recommends limiting caffeine-containing beverages "because of their deleterious effects on breast cysts and mastalgia [breast pain]."[29]

Caffeine may cause benign breast cysts and breast pain to become worse.

There are conflicting studies on the effect of caffeine on PMS symptoms, but some studies have found a strong association between PMS and caffeine consumption.[30] Caffeine can make hypoglycemia worse, and many women find that it contributes to nervousness or anxiety. Dr. Abraham has noted that women with PMS seem to crave chocolate, which contains a caffeine-like substance—as well as high levels of magnesium![31] Author Jacob Teitelbaum, M.D., in fact, recommends moderate amounts of dark chocolate, up to a few ounces a day, for PMS.[32]

ASPARTAME (NUTRASWEET). Aspartame, the artificial sweetener chemical of Nutra-Sweet, contains 50 percent phenylalanine, an amino acid that stimulates the secretion of prolactin from the pituitary gland.[33] High prolactin levels are involved in luteal phase deficiency, which relates to PMS. Avoid aspartame, as well as other artificial sweeteners.

THE ORIGINAL PMS SUPPLEMENT: OPTIVITE PMT

OPTIVITE PMT, the multivitamin/multimineral supplement which Dr. Abraham formulated and tested, is an integral part of improving PMS. The full dose (six tablets), contains 300 mg of vitamin B6 along with substantial amounts of the other B vitamins and a high dose of vitamin C. It contains twice as much magnesium as calcium, and a significant amount of the mineral zinc. It should be taken all month long, not just during the luteal phase of the cycle. (See Appendix A for the complete contents of Optivite PMT.)

In an open study of Optivite, the most improvement was obtained among women with PMS when they took six to twelve tablets of Optivite daily for three or more cycles.[34] Results of three double-blind studies showed that three tablets daily of Optivite were ineffective against PMS, but six tablets per day were more effective than dietary improvement alone. "Once-a-day" type vitamins, used as a placebo, were useless for PMS.[35]

The multi-nutrient approach of Optivite, along with improved diet, is preferable to supplementing with any single nutrient. Even though vitamin B6 alone has been shown to reduce PMS,[36] the B vitamins work as a group, and are more effective if taken together. Vitamin B6 also depends on magnesium for its best function. Significantly, a recent study on infertility has shown that vitamin C (750 mg/day) raises progesterone while improving fertility.[37] Optivite contains 1,500 mg of vitamin C per full dose; undoubtedly this nutrient, which has been in Optivite since its original formulation, has been partially responsible for its positive effect on PMS and other reproductive problems.

> Optivite reduced the levels of estrogen and increased the levels of progesterone in women with PMS who had the high estrogen levels and low progesterone levels that are common with PMS.[38] Mainly because of this effect, I recommend Optivite not only for PMS, but also for self care of any other problem of estrogen dominance, including luteal phase deficiency, some types of infertility, endometriosis, and early miscarriage.

In over 100,000 women who have used Optivite for several years, no cases of vitamin or mineral toxicity have been reported.[39] While high doses of vitamin B6 alone can be toxic, Dr. Abraham credits this safety record to the balance of the micronutrients within the supplement. The other B vitamins and magnesium enable the body to process the B6 normally, decreasing the possibility of overdose. His advice for women to use the lowest effective dose is another probable reason for this safety record.[40] Nevertheless, you should discuss your vitamin and mineral supplements with your health care provider, and you should not exceed 300 mg of vitamin B6 per day. Instead, if six tablets of Optivite do not help your symptoms, increase magnesium to a total of 1,000 mg per day.[41]

My experience is that women with PMS begin to find relief, often within the first cycle of use, by taking six tablets of Optivite throughout the cycle along with an additional 500 mg of magnesium and three to six capsules of flax oil daily.

Optivite is available from the American Pro-Life Enterprise or from the Optimox Corporation. (See "Resources.") The package insert suggests up to six tablets per day plus 500 mg of additional magnesium. Since it is limited in folic acid (200 mcg), if you plan to become pregnant you should obtain additional folate (or folic acid) for balance (at least an additional 200 mcg/day, and as much as 4,000 mcg/day if it is suggested for other reproductive problems).

OTHER VITAMIN SUPPLEMENTS FOR PMS

PROCYCLE PMS. American Pro-Life Enterprise formulates ProCycle PMS, another excellent vitamin/mineral supplement specifically made for PMS. It is much like Optivite, with 300 mg of vitamin B6 and 1,500 mg of vitamin C per full dose. It contains more folic acid (800 mcg) than Optivite and twice as much vitamin D3, vitamin E, selenium, and chromium as Optivite. It contains 300 mg of magnesium compared to Optivite's 250 mg. Unlike Optivite, it contains no iron. This may seem like a disadvantage, but actually, many women are not anemic and do not need supplemental iron, and often it is the iron that causes stomach upset when you take a vitamin/mineral supplement. While Optivite is labeled for six tablets daily, ProCycle PMS is labeled for four tablets to achieve a full dose, making it more convenient to take. Appendix A lists the contents of ProCycle PMS; see "Resources" for ordering information.)

GENERAL SUPPLEMENTS. Instead of Optivite or ProCycle PMS, you may prefer to modify the general supplement program suggested in Table 7 (Chapter 3) for PMS. For example, Professional Pre-Natal Formula, which I recommend as a comprehensive supplement for women generally, can serve as your PMS multivitamin/multimineral, as long as you add 100-200 mg of additional vitamin B6. Professional Pre-Natal Formula is available through the American Pro-Life Enterprise. (Appendix A lists the contents of Professional Pre-Natal Formula.)

> In all cases, supplementing omega-3 fatty acids should be part of your strategy to overcome PMS. Try 5 one-gram capsules of flax oil to gain the valuable alpha-linolenic acid, and/or 1 teaspoon (5 grams) of fish oil. Or, you may wish to supplement instead with 1 gram of krill oil, which contains the omega-3 fatty acids in a more bioavailable form. Though krill oil is not nearly as well studied as fish oil, in a recent pilot study, when krill oil was given along with other nutrients, it was shown to be helpful for PMS, even in amounts less than 1 gram.[42]

OTHER OPTIONS FOR PMS

While improved diet, as outlined in Chapter 1, and Optivite PMT or ProCycle PMS, along with essential fatty acids, provide the most comprehensive self help for PMS, there are other approaches to PMS that may interest you. They are listed below, more or less in the order that I recommend them.

CHASTEBERRY EXTRACT. An old remedy for "female complaints" has been rediscovered and tested in a large, well-controlled scientific study for its effectiveness against PMS symptoms. It is chasteberry extract, also called "Vitex" (*Vitex agnus castus*).[43] Previous studies have also shown a positive effect of chasteberry extract on PMS,[44] including in women with known luteal phase deficiency.[45]

If you wish to try chasteberry to overcome PMS, I suggest that you use it as part of a product called Fertility Blend. This supplement contains chasteberry extract, but it also contains the antioxidants in green tea extract, and vitamin E (150 mg), folic acid (400 mcg), iron (9 mg in the preferred chelated form), magnesium (400 mg), and selenium (70 mcg). A study in 2006 examined the use of Fertility Blend for the achievement of pregnancy among infertile women. The researchers reported that chasteberry extract was safe and effective for use among women seeking pregnancy. Importantly, this study noted that chasteberry can increase progesterone levels and decrease prolactin levels.[46] Fertility Blend's complete contents are listed in Appendix A. (See "Resources.")

CALCIUM SUPPLEMENTS. Calcium is an essential nutrient which is best known for its bone-building effect. It is critical to nerve function as well, and it performs a variety of regulatory roles in the body. It cannot be absorbed without vitamin D, and the mineral magnesium enables it to work properly. Its levels fluctuate throughout the menstrual cycle.[47] (In fact, when I was a student in graduate school, I served as a subject in a study in which women took their basal temperatures daily, and then had their blood calcium levels measured before and after ovulation.) Women who get calcium and vitamin D from their diet are less likely to have PMS.[48] Even dietary vitamin D alone correlates with a lower incidence of PMS.[49]

Large studies have shown that calcium supplements alone, in the form of calcium carbonate or calcium gluconate, are effective against many symptoms of PMS.[50] However, I do not recommend calcium supplements alone as the remedy for PMS. You can obtain at least some of your calcium through use of dairy foods. If you do not use dairy products, supplements of calcium citrate, calcium malate, or other chelated forms of calcium, along with vitamin D3 and magnesium, may be most helpful. Try for total calcium (diet plus supplements) of about 1,000 mg per day. For example, since typical servings of dairy foods (milk, yogurt, cheese) average about 250 mg of calcium, if you have two servings of dairy products daily, supplement about 500 mg of calcium. A total of 500 to 1,000 mg of magnesium, ideally in a chelated form, can be supplemented to balance the calcium. Of course, it is prudent to improve your diet and to supplement comprehensively, as nutrients work together.

PROGESTERONE SKIN CREAM. If a serious attempt to improve your daily diet and vitamin, mineral, and essential fatty acid status is not effective after three months, you may wish to consider over-the-counter natural progesterone cream for PMS, in addition to continuing your improved nutrition.

The goal in using natural (**bio-identical**) progesterone cream is to raise progesterone to normal levels during the luteal phase of the cycle. The cream is rubbed onto thin skin, such as on the abdomen, neck, or inner arms. The suggested amounts to be used are noted on the product label. While progesterone is absorbed easily through the skin, the amount of it absorbed varies with the thickness of the skin, the skin temperature, and the blood flow to the skin.

If you choose to use progesterone cream, it is important to wait until a temperature rise of three days confirms that you have ovulated. Women who do not chart their temperatures may inadvertently use progesterone cream before ovulation and interfere with the cycle, as it is not natural for the ovaries to produce significant progesterone until after ovulation. Even though progesterone cream is a readily-available, nonprescription product, it is advisable to discuss its use with your physician, especially if you may become pregnant. If you have severe PMS, you may wish to try it immediately while you also implement better nutrition, but if you do so, aim to decrease the progesterone cream gradually as you improve your nutrition.

For detailed information on the use of progesterone skin cream, see the chapter on PMS in *What Your Doctor May Not Tell You about Premenopause* by the late John Lee, M.D., and colleagues. (See "Further Reading.")

BACK TO BASICS: NON-NUTRITIONAL ANTI-PMS STRATEGIES

CHARTING AS PART OF NFP. This suggestion really deserves to be at the top of the list.

> **Charting your symptoms—right on your NFP chart—lets you verify whether or not you have PMS and lets you know when to expect PMS.**

You can include notes on the type, severity, and duration of your symptoms, and you can track your progress as you implement self care. Using NFP may help you avoid PMS in another way; oral contraceptives worsen PMS in some women,[51] and PMS may become severe after a tubal ligation because the surgery damages the blood supply to the ovary, causing the ovary to function less well after the procedure is done.[52] Hysterectomy may also worsen PMS.

REGULAR OUTDOOR EXERCISE. Exercise is good for just about everything, and it is wonderful for improving the symptoms of PMS. It elevates your mood and gives you a physical outlet for stress. It helps you sleep better. Exercise that is done outdoors with plenty of natural sunlight is better yet, and there is even scientific evidence to support the common experience that bright light elevates your mood.[53] Who doesn't agree that there is nothing like a brisk walk on a beautiful day to make you feel great? Even walks in the bright snow may be helpful, but exercise in itself should be the goal, indoors or out, sunny or cloudy. Just don't overdo it, because too much increases your stress and is counterproductive. Start slowly if you are not accustomed to vigorous exercise.

REASONABLE BODY WEIGHT. Having your body weight at a comfortable level for you—not necessarily at some theoretical ideal weight—is helpful to preventing PMS,[54] and it tends to normalize the levels of estrogen. Especially if you are overweight, just a small decrease in weight may help you to feel better. See Chapters 5 and 9 for some recommendations for modest weight loss.

STRESS MANAGEMENT. Worrying about how to reduce stress can be a major stress! Here is some good news: Improved diet and supplementing vitamins and minerals helps decrease the hormonal response to stress, so that you "roll with the punches" better. That is, you reduce stress just by being well nourished, because poor nutrition is a physical stress. Exercise also reduces stress, provided you do something you enjoy at a level that does not leave you physically exhausted. See Chapter 4 for more information on stress.

ADEQUATE SLEEP. PMS can contribute to sleep disturbances, or sleep disturbances can contribute to PMS.[55] I am convinced that enough sleep is even more important than good diet, supplements, and exercise for decreasing stress. Putting good nutrition together with enough sleep may be all you need to decompress. When you sleep, the levels of the stress hormones cortisol and adrenaline drop, and that's beneficial to PMS. If more sleep means less work, or less chauffeuring, or fewer volunteer activities, try your best to say "no" to the extras that so many women try to fit into already full schedules. In addition, sleeping in a very dark room can increase your melatonin levels, contributing to better sleep and even raising your progesterone levels, as explained in Chapter 10 under the heading, "Sensitivity to Night Lighting."

OTHER POSSIBILITIES. If the guidelines given here are not helpful to you, consider factors other than PMS. Thyroid dysfunction, yeast overgrowth, and adrenal exhaustion are all possibilities to investigate, ideally with your physician's help. (See "Low Thyroid Function" and "Hyperthyroidism" in Chapter 8; "Yeast Overgrowth/Gut Dysbiosis" in Chapter 10; and Chapter 4, "Increasing Your Energy & Decreasing Your Stress.")

PMS DIET AND SUPPLEMENTS FOR OTHER CYCLE PROBLEMS

As noted in the opening paragraphs of this chapter, I recommend improved diet and Dr. Abraham's PMS supplement plan for several other female reproductive disorders, since it provides excellent overall nutrition and tends to normalize the levels of estrogen and progesterone. Some women have reported longer luteal phases, which are a sign of better progesterone levels, and others have noticed clearer mucus patterns. Some women believe that it has helped them to achieve a pregnancy after infertility or miscarriage.

The following anecdote illustrates several of these points.

A married couple who had never had children visited my husband and me to discuss their inability to conceive. They had taken our natural family planning classes as an engaged couple and had initially used the method to avoid a pregnancy. However, for over two years they had been trying to conceive, and the wife, whom I'll call Lana, was now 30. They had already undergone medical testing which confirmed that the husband's sperm count was normal and that Lana's fallopian tubes were unblocked.

I noticed that the postovulatory temperatures on Lana's charts were elevated for a shorter than normal number of days—evidence of possible luteal phase deficiency. "Does she have PMS?" I asked her husband. He nodded vigorously while she giggled. I explained the PMS nutritional plan to them, and we also discussed medical intervention as an immediate option, since the infertility had persisted for so long a time. Lana decided to take the recommended six tablets of Optivite and 500 mg of magnesium daily. Her day-to-day diet was already quite good, so she made no other changes.

"They helped everything!" Lana said of the vitamins. The supplements worked so well in reducing her PMS irritability that she and her husband jokingly called them her "nice" pills. The duration of her postovulatory temperatures increased by "at least two or three days." And she was pleasantly surprised to find that within a cycle or two, her painful menstrual cramps, which had been worsening for two years, also disappeared completely. Best of all, four months after she started the vitamins, she became pregnant. The baby, a girl, was born after a healthy pregnancy.

Incidentally, with her doctor's approval, Lana used six tablets of Optivite daily as her prenatal vitamin supplement, a practice approved by Dr. Abraham.[56] A recent study has confirmed that large doses of vitamin B6 during pregnancy, when it is often recommended to overcome nausea, do not harm the unborn child.[57] If you do use Optivite as a prenatal vitamin supplement, however, increase the folic acid (or folate) to a total of at least 400 mcg, and up to 4,000 mcg if you are an older mother or have had problems conceiving. ProCycle PMS (4 tablets) contains 800 mcg of folic acid, and is also safe for use during pregnancy with your doctor's approval.

Despite any confusion caused by the labeling, neither Optivite nor ProCycle PMS exceeds a safe limit of vitamin A. Each contains only 5,000 IU of true vitamin A (retinyl palmitate) per full dose; the other "vitamin A" is actually beta-carotene (7,500 IU), which has never been implicated in birth defects.

SUMMARY — CHAPTER 6

1 Premenstrual syndrome (PMS) refers to a group of troublesome symptoms (including anxiety, irritability, bloating, and breast tenderness) that may occur during the second half of the cycle in some women, ranging in age from the teen years to the perimeno-pause time.

2 One important cause of PMS is luteal phase deficiency, which means that estrogen is too high and progesterone is too low during the luteal phase of the cycle. This hormonal imbalance is often termed **estrogen dominance**.

3 Research by gynecologist Guy Abraham, M.D., showed that improved diet and vitamin/mineral supplements rich in vitamin B6, other B vitamins, vitamin C, zinc, and magnesium can improve the symptoms of PMS, even under double-blind conditions.

4 There are also other approaches to overcoming the symptoms of PMS, including supplements of the herb *Vitex agnus castus* (chasteberry), supplements of calcium, or use of progesterone skin cream.

5 Lifestyle improvements should be implemented to overcome PMS. These include charting symptoms, getting exercise, trying to achieve a more normal body weight if needed, reducing stress, and getting enough sleep.

6 The recommendations for PMS may also help to lengthen a short luteal phase, to overcome some types of infertility, to prevent recurrent miscarriage, endometriosis, and other problems related to estrogen dominance.

7 While no cases of vitamin B6 toxicity were reported in over 100,000 women using the PMS vitamin/mineral supplement Optivite for several years, it is prudent to discuss vitamin supplements with your health care practitioner. The vitamin A in the supplements suggested (Optivite, ProCycle PMS, and Professional Pre-Natal) does not exceed a safe dose for women who may become pregnant.

SHORTER, LIGHTER, & PAIN-FREE PERIODS

7

A woman afflicted with hemorrhages for twelve years, who was unable to be cured by anyone, came up behind him and touched the tassel on his cloak. Immediately her bleeding stopped.

—Luke 8:43-44

Some cycle problems are easier to solve than others. I have found that heavy and prolonged bleeding almost always can be improved with better nutrition. Cramps and menstrual pain will often improve once the menstrual period is lightened up, but there are also additional nutritional strategies aimed at decreasing menstrual pain. Because there is some relationship between heavy or long periods and menstrual pain, let's deal with heavy periods first.

HEAVY OR PROLONGED MENSES

The typical period lasts about five days, with two or three days of moderate flow and two or three days of light flow or spotting. If you are experiencing heavy or long periods and are in doubt as to whether or not it is normal, make sure your health professional is aware of your concern. If you have episodes of spotting or bleeding at times other than your expected period, let your health professional know. The vast majority of such episodes are explainable, especially with the information that you gain from your NFP charts, and in most cases your health professional will reassure you. Still, you need to know if fibroid tumors, endometriosis, low thyroid function, or some other condition is contributing to the problem. If heavy or prolonged bleeding has been ongoing, you should also ask for a test for anemia.

Even if your health professional assures you that you are in good health, why not try the nutritional measures outlined in this chapter to make your periods lighter and shorter as a matter of convenience? While up to a full week of menstrual bleeding or spotting is considered normal, a long or heavy period is not necessary to shed the lining of the uterus. Better nutrition can noticeably shorten the length of the menses as well as the amount of blood loss. As a side benefit, the better health of your mucus membranes can also make your mucus signs clearer and easier to read.

CAUSES OF HEAVY OR PROLONGED BLEEDING

Certain patterns of heavy or prolonged menses may indicate other problems, and charting can give you very good insight into what the underlying cause might be. If one of the following possibilities seems to fit, please also refer to the follow-up information, as noted.

ENDOMETRIOSIS. Severe menstrual pain is the foremost symptom of endometriosis, though prolonged or heavy bleeding may occur with it. Endometriosis is the final topic of this chapter, and that section offers specific self care options for you, but working closely with a compassionate physician who is an expert at helping you manage your endometriosis is essential.

COMING OFF THE PILL. Elevated levels of vitamin A, which are caused by oral contraceptive use, along with the synthetic hormones themselves, contribute to the very light bleeding typical of birth control pill users. Conversely, discontinuing the pill lowers vitamin A, sometimes resulting in heavy or prolonged periods. Refer to the section in Chapter 10, "Discontinuing Birth Control Pills," for a discussion of nutrition aimed at normal cycles following pill use.

LUTEAL PHASE DEFICIENCY. If your period starts with one to three days of light spotting while your temperatures are still elevated and then becomes a normal, full flow as your basal temperature drops; or if your period ends with a discharge which is brownish rather than the usual pink or honey color, suspect luteal phase deficiency. This term refers to a luteal (postovulatory) phase in which progesterone is too low. Often the premenstrual spotting, called **irregular shedding**, begins soon—too soon—after your temperature and mucus patterns have confirmed that you have ovulated. In addition to this chapter, see the section in Chapter 8 titled "Luteal Phase Deficiency."

BREAKTHROUGH BLEEDING (MID-CYCLE SPOTTING). In this pattern your temperature confirms that you have ovulated, but sometime around ovulation several days of spotting may occur. This may simply be from excess buildup of endometrium that is shed after the hormonal readjustment that follows ovulation. In addition to the nutritional information of this chapter, see Chapter 6, as the self care for PMS may also help breakthrough bleeding.

LOW THYROID FUNCTION. Low thyroid function is a common cause of heavy or prolonged menses. Suspect low thyroid function if your basal temperatures are low, in the range of 97.3 or below, during the preovulatory phase. You may or may not experience long cycle lengths. Your mucus pattern may be unclear with an ongoing less-fertile type mucus pattern. Even if you have had a test for your thyroid hormones that came back normal, you should still consider this possibility. See "Low Thyroid Function" in Chapter 8, in addition to the nutritional suggestions later in this chapter.

UNDERWEIGHT, LOW BODY FAT, AND/OR VIGOROUS ATHLETIC ACTIVITY. Along with heavy or long periods, you may have long cycles with a delay in ovulation, or you may have cycles followed by what appears to be periods, with your temperatures showing that you have not ovulated. If you are not charting, you may be puzzled to have some light and some heavy or prolonged periods which occur irregularly.

Your low body fat is the probable explanation. A marginal lack of body fat will cause a delay in ovulation at first, but as more body fat is lost, ovulation can cease altogether. Just a small gain in weight, perhaps three to five pounds, can improve the entire cycle. When the hormones that trigger ovulation kick in sooner, the endometrium repairs itself faster, meaning that the length of the period may shorten and lighten. When you gain enough weight, you are not likely to have long cycles with their unpredictable timing and bleeding pattern. If, on the other hand, more regular cycles cause heavier bleeding when before it was very light, try the nutritional strategies discussed below. Also refer to "Underweight or Inadequate Body Fat" in Chapter 8.

BODY FAT PRODUCES HORMONES

Body fat is an active tissue that produces several hormones. It is well known to produce estrogen, about one third of the estrogen in a young woman in her fertile years. It also produces the hormone **leptin**, which has a "permissive" role in the fertility cycle. That is, when body fat is adequate, enough leptin is produced to signal the hypothalamus that there is sufficient stored fat for a fertility cycle and potential pregnancy. Conversely, when body fat is inadequate, the levels of leptin are too low to signal the hypothalamus to secrete the hormones that launch the fertility cycle.

POLYCYSTIC OVARY SYNDROME (PCOS). If your fertility cycles are long, and you have prolonged or heavy episodes of bleeding at irregular intervals with or without the temperature rise that confirms ovulation, it may be PCOS that underlies your problem. In this case, your preovulatory temperature levels are usually normal (around 97.6°F.), and often your mucus pattern consists of on-and-off more-fertile mucus. If PCOS is contributing to heavy or prolonged bleeding, you may also tend to have abdominal weight gain and perhaps other signs of "male" hormones. See this topic in Chapter 9, as well as the information on basic nutrition for heavy or prolonged bleeding discussed later in this chapter.

FIBROID TUMORS. These abnormal but benign growths, which originate in the muscular layer of the uterus, are most likely to occur as you enter your late thirties or forties. Fibroids thrive on estrogen, so obesity is a risk factor, as well as the "estrogen dominance" pattern of hormones—high estrogen and low progesterone—that is common in the forties. Sometimes fibroid tumors cause no problems, but because they can interfere with the repair of the endometrium, they may contribute to heavy or prolonged bleeding at irregular times in the cycle. They frequently cause pain as well and can lead to the need for surgery. The basic nutritional information that is the focus of this chapter can help you to limit extra blood loss while you decide what course of action to take with the fibroids.

MISCARRIAGE. First, if you have experienced a miscarriage, I would like to express my sympathy for your loss. While I know that it is a difficult experience to deal with emotionally, it is important to care for yourself physically as well as emotionally as you recover. Bleeding after a miscarriage can be quite heavy and may be prolonged, depending on a number of factors. The nutrition suggested below can make the blood loss after a miscarriage considerably shorter and lighter, and nutrition for overcoming anemia can help you get your energy back sooner. It is likely that you will ovulate two to four weeks after the loss of your child, and if you avoid a pregnancy as you recover, you should expect a normal period about two weeks later.

Sometimes you may suspect that an early miscarriage has caused heavy or prolonged bleeding, but you may not be sure. Having a long cycle, even if followed by heavy bleeding, is not a sign of miscarriage in itself. In most cases it simply means that you have ovulated late—or maybe not at all—perhaps for one of the reasons listed above. On the other hand, if you have had at least 21 days of elevated temperatures without a period as part of your luteal phase, and then experience heavy or prolonged bleeding, particularly with unusual cramping, an early miscarriage unfortunately is the most likely cause.

CHILDBIRTH (POSTPARTUM LOCHIA)

After childbirth, your estrogen and progesterone levels drop and will remain quite low, especially if you are breastfeeding your baby, and considerable healing of the endometrium must take place. The nutrition suggested in this chapter will lighten and shorten the **lochia**, as the normal postpartum discharge is called. You will probably notice soon after the birth that when your baby latches on to nurse, you may have a brief increase in bleeding as the uterus contracts. That's good, because despite the slight increase in flow, the contraction of the uterus helps to limit the amount of blood loss overall. If you have had heavy postpartum bleeding in the past, I think you will be pleasantly surprised at the improvement that nutritional strategies make.

DIET FOR BETTER HEALING AND NORMAL BLOOD CLOTTING

Loss of much bright red blood that runs easily, as opposed to a discharge with mucus that lightens in color after three or four days, is a sign that the clotting and healing mechanisms are not working as well as they might. Proper clotting and the healing of the mucus membranes depends on sufficient amounts of many nutrients—vitamin A, B-complex vitamins, vitamin C, related phytochemicals called bioflavinoids, vitamin K, iron, and the essential fatty acids.[1] Vitamin E prevents destruction of the essential fatty acids. Calcium is necessary to proper blood clotting, and vitamin D is necessary for absorption of calcium. Zinc works along with vitamin A to maximize healing.

GOOD FOODS FOR BETTER HEALING AND NORMAL CLOTTING. Eggs are a good natural source of true vitamin A. Plenty of orange or yellow vegetables and fruits will provide beta-carotene, the precursor of vitamin A. Carrots, sweet potatoes, squash, and apricots are examples. Many whole plant and animal foods provide B-complex vitamins. Citrus fruits are the best source of vitamin C, and if you eat the white parts inside the rind, you will get bioflavinoids, which work together with vitamin C to promote tissue healing and stronger blood capillaries. Milk products, of course, provide abundant calcium, and the fat in whole milk products assists in the absorption of the fat-soluble vitamins A, D, E, and K. Raw pumpkin seeds and freshly ground flax seeds are the best food sources of the essential fatty acids. Organic, expeller-pressed canola oil provides some of both of the two essential fatty acids. Regular consumption of fish provides DHA and EPA, the active form of the essential fatty acids.

VITAMIN K SOURCE. Vitamin K is involved in the production of several clotting proteins. It is frequently assumed to be plentiful in the body since friendly bacteria within the large intestine synthesize it, and it is available in the diet if dark green leafy vegetables are eaten. However, antibiotics harm the intestinal bacteria, and typical Americans eat far too little of the vitamin K-rich foods. Emphasis on these foods and regular intake of bacteria-containing yogurt or supplements of friendly bacteria (probiotics) will help provide vitamin K, especially if nonessential antibiotics and aspirin, which deplete this vitamin, are avoided.

IRON FOR HEAVY BLEEDING. While you might think of iron only in terms of overcoming anemia, it actually helps to prevent heavy bleeding as well.[2] Good sources of iron are red meat, organic liver, blackstrap molasses, beans, eggs, and spinach.

SUPPLEMENTS FOR BETTER HEALING AND NORMAL BLOOD CLOTTING

MULTIVITAMINS/MULTIMINERALS. A multivitamin/multimineral supplement which supplies a balance of the vitamins and minerals mentioned in the preceding section is important to ensure that the endometrium has the raw materials it needs for rapid healing. Professional Pre-Natal Formula by LifeTime provides most of these specific nutrients in the amounts needed. It also provides the many nutrients, including iron, that are necessary to overcoming anemia, should blood loss be severe. (See "Resources.")

FLAX OIL. The two essential fatty acids (linoleic acid and alpha-linolenic acid) are neither vitamins nor minerals, so they are not found in vitamin/mineral supplements. Because alpha-linolenic acid is difficult to get in the Western diet—it is found in some seed oils, but is destroyed by exposure to light, heat, and oxygen—I strongly recommend that you supplement it. Flax oil contains a high percentage of alpha-linolenic acid. Three to ten 1g capsules daily makes a noticeable difference to a number of reproductive health problems, including heavy or prolonged bleeding.

If heavy bleeding is your only cycle concern, just taking three to five 1g capsules of flax oil starting two or three days before your period and continuing until your period ends is probably all you need.

However, vitamin E prevents destruction of the essential fatty acids, an example of why a comprehensive multivitamin/multimineral supplement is best.

FISH OIL. Instead of, or in addition to flax oil, you can use fish liver oil, which is rich in the fatty acids EPA and DHA. Fish oil is not essential; the healthy DHA and EPA can be made from the alpha-linolenic acid, as long as B vitamins, vitamin C, zinc, and magnesium are available. If you prefer fish oil, one or two teaspoons daily of good tasting, toxin-free, concentrated fish oil will provide what you need. Cod liver oil provides vitamin A and vitamin D, both beneficial to healing. Just be sure to get some vitamin E with it, about 400 IU daily.

VITAMIN A. Vitamin A can greatly reduce heavy or prolonged periods, especially if used in large amounts. If you are attempting to conceive, however, do not take more than 8,000 IU daily without consulting your doctor—at levels over 10,000 IU it has been associated with birth defects.[3] Reading labels can be confusing, though, as the listing "vitamin A" will be subdivided into retinyl palmitate or retinyl acetate, which are true vitamin A, and beta-carotene, which is not the same and has never been related to birth defects. Vitamin A is a necessary nutrient, and you should not fear healthy amounts of it, including the amounts found in fish oil supplements. If there is no chance of conception, 20,000-25,000 IU of true vitamin A daily is acceptable.

BIOFLAVINOIDS. The bioflavinoids, found abundantly in the white rind and sectional membranes of citrus fruits, strengthen capillary walls and therefore are useful to moderate the tendency to heavy bleeding. They are also available as supplements, and 1,000 mg tablets twice daily is the recommended dose.[4]

FAST ACTION FOR HEAVY BLEEDING

Sometimes heavy bleeding may catch you by surprise, whether it relates to your cycle, a miscarriage, or a postpartum problem. There are steps that you can take right away which are very helpful and fast acting. Capsules of chlorophyll, which is rich in vitamin K, work rapidly to reduce heavy bleeding, often within a couple of hours. They are available in health food shops in amounts of approximately 30 or 60 mg, and taking four or five capsules throughout the days of heavy flow is quite effective in reducing blood loss. Chlorophyll capsules only need to be taken shortly before and during the bleeding episode.

Chlorophyll in liquid form also rapidly controls postpartum bleeding, according to midwives familiar with its use. Like chlorophyll, cayenne pepper in tablets (also called capsicum) quickly slows any type of bleeding. Extra flax oil (ten 1 g capsules or 2 teaspoons) taken before and during the period will often lighten bleeding also, so much so that it may make chlorophyll or cayenne pepper unnecessary.

A SPECIAL CAUTION ABOUT MISCARRIAGE

I have spoken to several women who have lost frightening amounts of blood during an early miscarriage. In addition to the loss of their child, they have had to deal with the prolonged and unexpected physical weakness that such blood loss brings. The section above, "Fast Action for Heavy Bleeding," can moderate the bleeding caused by a miscarriage.

However, if you ever believe you are losing too much blood, especially with a miscarriage, make sure that you contact a doctor. Yet I know women who have phoned their doctor's office in the face of extremely heavy bleeding, only to be told to "wait and see." Such long-distance diagnosis of bleeding resulted in one friend of mine receiving several pints of blood after a harrowing ambulance run.

Better advice: Heavy bleeding and dangerously heavy bleeding cannot be diagnosed over the phone. You are the ultimate judge. If in doubt, go to a hospital emergency room.

DEALING WITH SEVERE BLOOD LOSS

The following anecdote illustrates how appropriate medical intervention and nutritional counseling enabled a young girl with severe **menorrhagia** (heavy menstrual bleeding) to recover from a frightening incident. Only twelve years old, this girl lost a large amount of blood during a heavy, prolonged period of which her parents were at first unaware. When they realized it, her hemoglobin was an extremely anemic 6.5 (normal is 12-16 mg/dl) and she was still bleeding. The attending gynecologist prescribed Provera (synthetic progesterone), but the little of it she did not vomit did no good.

At the parents' request, a transfusion of two pints of relatives' blood was arranged. It did not stop the bleeding, but it did bring her hemoglobin to an improved though still anemic 10. The gynecologist warned the parents that because of the severity of the situation, birth control pills were the probable next step, but he was willing to take a "wait-and-see" attitude for a short while.

The parents, concerned about the side effects of the Pill, turned to nutritional counseling. Cayenne pepper tablets (520 mg, five times daily) helped slow the bleeding significantly. The girl also began taking a balanced non-prescription multivitamin/multimineral which supplied 10,000 IU of true vitamin A, 75 mg/mcg of B-complex vitamins, 60 mg of chelated iron, and generous amounts of vitamin C, zinc, and the other micronutrients. The goal was to enable her body to produce its own clotting elements and more of its own hormones, and to overcome the anemia.

Her next period was very heavy but manageable. Two months later, she was no longer anemic and had a normal menses. Nine months later, her mother reported that she still tended toward heavy periods but was "definitely helped" by the cayenne pepper during her menses. Aside from the transfusion, her mother credits her daughter's faithfulness in taking the vitamins, cayenne pepper, and plenty of rest as the factors that enabled the girl to recover rapidly from this frightening incident.

Flax oil capsules are also helpful in cases like this, or in any case in which a woman is trying to heal from heavy bleeding or hemorrhage. In addition, chlorophyll capsules, which are a source of vitamin K, enable the levels of a key clotting protein, fibrinogen, to return to normal very rapidly.

OVERCOMING ANEMIA

If menorrhagia has been severe enough to cause anemia, as in the above anecdote, do not make the mistake of supplementing only iron to overcome it. The B vitamins, including folate (folic acid), B6, and B12, vitamins C and E, zinc, copper, and adequate protein are among the nutrients which are also necessary to produce new red blood cells. Good foods for overcoming anemia are liver, red meat, spinach, citrus fruits, and blackstrap molasses. Professional Pre-Natal Formula by Life Time is an excellent supplement for overcoming anemia. (See "Resources.") Also add three to five fish oil or flax oil capsules as part of your daily supplement.

PAINFUL PERIODS

Pain is a symptom of a problem; severe pain the more so. Menstrual cramps and pain may simply reflect common dietary or hormonal imbalances, or they may be a sign of endometriosis, uterine fibroids, infection, or other abnormalities. It is important to alert your health professional if your menstrual pain is worse than the moderate discomfort that is so common, especially among younger women who have never borne children. In most cases, the diagnosis will be **primary dysmenorrhea**—that is, pain during the period without any other problem such as endometriosis or fibroid tumors being involved. Primary dysmenorrhea is the main focus of the nutritional information that follows, though the chapter ends with a discussion of endometriosis.

CAUSES OF PAIN DURING MENSES

When painful menstruation occurs, it almost always is part of a period that follows ovulation, as opposed to an anovulatory cycle. The interplay of estrogen and progesterone, especially the drop in progesterone shortly before the period begins, is involved in the pain. The main culprits responsible for primary dysmenorrhea are inflammation-promoting prostaglandins, named PGF2α and PGE2, which are released from the endometrium during the menses. Not surprisingly, women with dysmenorrhea release many times more of these "bad" prostaglandins than do women without painful periods. These prostaglandins, which are actually found in the menstrual discharge, increase contractions of the uterus, decrease the blood supply to it, and increase inflammation. The result is pelvic pain that may feel crampy, achy, or congested. It is common for the ache to occur in the lower abdomen, or it can seem to originate from the lower back or from between the thighs. Some women experience nausea, vomiting, diarrhea, or headache along with their period.[5] Sleep disruption, with its own set of problems, is a common finding in women with period pain.[6] Can we solve this all-too-common cycle problem with nutrition?

Recent research provides us with a number of tested strategies to restore pain-free periods.

RISK FACTORS FOR DYSMENORRHEA

Girls who begin their periods at a younger-than-average age have a higher risk of dysmenorrhea. Having long or heavy periods is also a factor in painful periods. A new study indicates that obesity of the "apple" type, in which the body fat tends to be excess in the abdomen, is associated with painful menses, whereas more generally distributed overweight is not.[7] This suggests that polycystic ovary syndrome (PCOS), discussed in Chapter 9, may be an underlying cause of menstrual pain. Stress, smoking, and alcohol use are also risk factors.[8] Tubal ligation is a significant risk factor, because it may disrupt the blood flow to the ovaries, which in turn disrupts the balance of the ovarian hormones.[9]

DIET FOR PAINFUL PERIODS WITH HEAVY BLEEDING

Since heavy bleeding is a risk factor for painful menses, if you are having heavy periods along with pain, review the first part of this chapter and implement the nutritional strategies, especially the multivitamins and flax oil, to overcome the heavy bleeding. Doing so will very likely decrease your menstrual pain as well. Why? As it turns out, the same prostaglandins that cause menstrual pain are also involved in heavy bleeding.[10]

PMS NUTRITION FOR MENSTRUAL PAIN

Even though dysmenorrhea is not considered part of premenstrual syndrome (PMS), these two cycle problems share some common ground. In some cases, they may occur together. For example, dysmenorrhea is often thought to be a problem of teenage girls and young women that disappears after the birth of the first child, or gradually decreases with age. PMS, alternatively, is often considered to increase in incidence with age, up to the age of menopause.

However, while painful periods are common in adolescents, so is PMS. In one study of girls with dysmenorrhea, over 70 percent also had PMS.[11]

The understanding that inflammatory prostaglandins cause menstrual pain is another link between menstrual pain and PMS. This understanding has fueled interest in new nutritional research designed to reduce levels of the "bad" prostaglandins. Yet older nutritional research on PMS was also directed at reducing the very same prostaglandins, PGE2 and PGF2α. Newer research also provides interesting evidence that PMS mood symptoms occur at times when these inflammatory chemicals are high.[12]

This is not to overstate the relationship between PMS and dysmenorrhea, because there are significant differences. For example, while the **nonsteroidal anti-inflammatory drugs** (NSAIDs: aspirin, ibuprofen) are quite effective for menstrual pain, they are not helpful for PMS. Taken during the luteal phase, they may make PMS worse by blocking the production of helpful prostaglandins.[13]

Nevertheless, the PMS dietary plan in Chapter 6, which is interchangeable with the "Twelve Rules for Better Nutrition" in Chapter 1, is aimed at decreasing the inflammation-producing prostaglandins and stimulating the production of healthy prostaglandins. For this reason, you can use the PMS diet for menstrual pain that occurs without heavy bleeding. Do include dairy products in your self care to overcome period pain, as studies show that three to four servings of dairy foods daily reduce menstrual pain significantly.[14] If you do not use dairy products, calcium supplements may offer some of the same benefits (see below).

WATER FOR MENSTRUAL PAIN

What does the best drink of all—water—have to do with painful menses? The hormone **vasopressin**, also called the **antidiuretic hormone (ADH)**, is a factor in dysmenorrhea. Vasopressin, a hormone chemically related to the hormone of labor, oxytocin, stimulates contraction of smooth muscle, and when the smooth muscle of the uterus contracts excessively, you feel it as cramps. Medications have been used to decrease vasopressin in women with menstrual pain, who are known to overproduce this hormone.[15] However, there is a simple, natural, and effective way to decrease vasopressin—drink more water.

Drinking more water regularly, beginning about three days or so before you expect your period, reduces period pain in some women. You do not need huge amounts, but perhaps the eight glasses daily that many authorities recommend (but few women actually drink!).

SUPPLEMENTS FOR MENSTRUAL PAIN

FISH OIL. Fish oil, which is rich in the fatty acids EPA and DHA, has a strong anti-inflammatory effect. The "omega-3" fatty acid EPA is used by the cells to form beneficial "series-3" prostaglandins that block the production of inflammatory prostaglandins. Several studies confirm the value of fish oil for menstrual pain.[16] In a recent double-blind crossover study, just one capsule of fish oil daily, containing 180 mg of EPA and 120 mg of DHA, greatly reduced period pain, and reduced the use of ibuprofen by the subjects.[17] In another study, Catholic high school girls in Cincinnati, all with dysmenorrhea, were given fish oil in capsules (1080 mg of EPA and 720 mg of DHA, the amount in about two teaspoons of cod liver oil) or a placebo. During the study, which was carried out in single-blinded, cross-over fashion, the girls were instructed to take ibuprofen for pain as needed. On average, they took half as many ibuprofen pills for menstrual pain when they were using fish oil as compared to the placebo.[18]

In a study involving Danish women, fish oil, along with vitamin B12 (7.5 mcg/day), was used successfully to reduce menstrual pain. The authors noted that vitamin B12 strengthened the effect of the fish oil.[19]

 Natural fish oil (1-2 teaspoons daily), along with non-steroidal anti-inflammatory drugs if needed, is commonly used in Sweden by women with dysmenorrhea[20].

VITAMIN E. In addition to lightening the period, vitamin E is also helpful for reducing menstrual pain.[21] It is an antioxidant that protects the beneficial fatty acids from destruction, which promotes an anti-inflammatory effect. Try a total of 400 IU of natural vitamin E daily, along with the other recommendations here, to help with menstrual cramping and pain.

MAGNESIUM. Magnesium is a natural muscle relaxer, and is helpful to menstrual cramps.[22] About 500-1,000 mg/day is beneficial. However, pure magnesium oxide is far too laxative to take in this amount. Instead, use magnesium aspartate, magnesium citrate, or magnesium gluconate, which are chelated and are not nearly so laxative. Because magnesium is a natural sleep aid, taking it before bed may help you avoid the sleep disruption that period pain can cause.

CALCIUM. Like magnesium, calcium also enables muscle relaxation. Dairy products are the best source of calcium in the diet, and women who eat three to four servings of milk a day have been found to experience far less menstrual pain than women who do not eat dairy products.[23] If you cannot or do not use dairy products, be sure to supplement about 800 mg daily. Like magnesium, calcium is a natural sleep aid. Taking calcium supplements before bedtime promotes restful sleep.

VITAMIN D. This fat-soluble vitamin is essential to absorb calcium, and it has anti-inflammatory effects of its own. Many young women with severe menstrual pain have been found to have low levels of vitamin D, along with low levels of calcium, which are related to the vitamin D deficiency.[24] Extremely large single doses of vitamin D3 (300,000 IU), given once per month about five days before the menstrual period was expected, decreased dysmenorrhea very significantly.[25] However, for self care, huge doses of vitamin D certainly are not recommended; instead, try 400-2,000 IU daily, along with sufficient calcium and magnesium.

MULTIVITAMIN/MULTIMINERALS. Professional Pre-Natal Formula comes closest to "covering all the bases" for dysmenorrhea, but Optivite has also helped relieve menstrual pain, perhaps by increasing progesterone. (See "Resources.") Use either along with fish oil, or flax oil if you prefer. While flax oil has not been tested for dysmenorrhea, its omega-3 essential fatty acid can be converted to EPA and DHA if various vitamins and minerals are present.

 Flax oil is wonderfully helpful for lightening heavy periods that contribute to menstrual pain.

ENDOMETRIOSIS

Endometriosis is one of the most common causes of very severe pain during menstruation, pain during intercourse, generalized pelvic pain, and heavy or irregular bleeding. The disease apparently begins when endometrial tissue moves backward through the fallopian tubes during the menses and is deposited within the abdominal cavity. Living cells in this tissue can proliferate within the abdomen, and when these abnormal "implants" are stimulated by cyclic hormonal changes, they build up and then bleed, causing inflammation and intense pain. Yet such retrograde flow of endometrial tissue also occurs in women who do not have endometriosis. Because of this, researchers believe the disease also involves a dysfunction of the immune system as well as hormonal imbalances.

However, as much as the pain must be managed, it is the high rate of infertility that concerns many women with endometriosis, as about one third of women with the disease have fertility problems. If endometriosis is left untreated, infertility can be explained by scarring and inflammation from the endometrial implants. Yet the question remains: Why does infertility occur in women with milder degrees of the disease? Some possibilities may be problems with the endometrium that prevent implantation, ovarian hormone problems, ovulatory dysfunction (See Introduction to Part 2, "Maturation of the Ovum"), anti-sperm chemicals in the abdominal fluid, and luteal phase deficiency.[26] Resistance to the effects of progesterone because of inability of the receptors to respond to progesterone is one of several other areas of research.[27] An important new focus of research on endometriosis is "oxidative stress." [28] **Oxidative stress** refers to an imbalance between the natural production of reactive byproducts of oxygen usage within the cells and the ability of the cells to neutralize them.

LUTEAL PHASE DEFICIENCY AND ENDOMETRIOSIS

A strong link between luteal phase deficiency and endometriosis has been found by Dr. Thomas W. Hilgers, the founder of the Creighton Model of Natural Family Planning and the Paul VI Institute for the Study of Human Reproduction in Omaha, NE. He found that 54 percent of a group of 228 women with endometriosis had luteal phase deficiency.[29] Luteal phase deficiency refers to a hormonal imbalance characterized by low progesterone levels in the postovulatory (luteal) phase of the cycle. When a cycle is charted, it can be seen as a poor temperature rise and fewer than normal elevated temperatures following ovulation.

A study that compared women with endometriosis who were fertile to women with endometriosis who were infertile showed that the infertile group had low progesterone levels as well as elevated prolactin levels. The low progesterone seemed to be related to the elevated levels of the hormone prolactin; that is, high prolactin can affect the corpus luteum and decrease progesterone levels.[30] See "Luteal Phase Deficiency" in Chapter 8 for detailed information on this topic.

THE LINK BETWEEN PMS AND ENDOMETRIOSIS

Luteal phase deficiency may explain the high prevalence of endometriosis among women with PMS. As described in Chapter 6, abnormal luteal function is the most common cause of PMS. As long ago as the 1980's, Drs. Joel Hargrove and Guy Abraham found that half of 137 women with PMS who underwent exploratory surgery for menstrual pain and/or infertility also had endometriosis.[31] These researchers reported abnormal luteal function in women with endometriosis.[32] Dr. Hilgers has recently confirmed this finding, stating that "This group of patients [with endometriosis] also has a high incidence of premenstrual symptoms, making the underlying hormonal abnormality similar to that observed in women with premenstrual syndrome."[33]

PMS NUTRITIONAL STRATEGY FOR ENDOMETRIOSIS

Based on research that points to luteal phase deficiency as a cause of endometriosis, I recommend that you implement the complete PMS nutritional strategy, diet and supplements detailed in Chapter 6 as your basic nutritional self care for endometriosis.

This diet and supplement program has been shown to improve luteal function by decreasing estrogen and increasing progesterone levels, as referenced in Chapter 6. Progesterone secreted by the corpus luteum decreases contractions of the uterus, which may be one link between luteal function and endometriosis. I am not aware of any studies in which the PMS nutritional plan has overcome infertility specifically related to endometriosis. However, if you are experiencing difficulty in conceiving because of this disease, I encourage you to implement the complete PMS program vigorously. Be sure to include supplemental flax oil and fish oil in amounts suggested in Chapter 3 for their anti-inflammatory effect. I also recommend this nutritional plan to help prevent recurrence of the disease following surgery to remove the abnormal endometrial tissue.

CAN ENDOMETRIOSIS BE PREVENTED?

Until recently, very few studies have addressed this important question, though of course everyone agrees that prevention of a disease is preferable to having to cure it. Evaluation of the large Nurses' Health Study II found that the risk of endometriosis was significantly lower among women who consumed long chain omega-3 fatty acids (DHA and EPA) and was significantly higher among women who consumed *trans* fats.[34] A recent review of the literature confirmed this finding.[35] The Nurses' Health Study II also found that women with a high consumption of dairy foods had a lower risk of endometriosis, and that women with the highest levels of vitamin D in their blood had a lower risk of endometriosis also.[36] Blood levels of vitamin D have been found to be significantly lower in women with severe endometriosis compared to those without the disease or with mild endometriosis.

Here are my recommendations for young women who are concerned that they might be at risk for endometriosis, perhaps because a close relative has suffered with it.

1. Do not ignore severe menstrual pain. Yes, young girls are prone to period pain, but their concerns should not be ignored. Regardless of age, a health care professional, preferably a NaProTechnology practitioner, should be consulted if there is doubt as to how normal the level of pain is. (See "Resources" for more information about NaProTechnology physicians.)

2. A whole-foods diet rich in antioxidants, as described in Part 1 of

this book and emphasized again in Chapter 6, "Premenstrual Syndrome," is basic. Oxidative stress is known to occur in endometriosis.[37]

3. Conscientiously take multivitamins/multimineral supplements such as ProCycle PMS, Optivite PMT, Professional Pre-Natal Formula, or similar supplements that contain vitamin B6 (100-300 mg) and vitamin C (750-1,500 mg). Both of these vitamins can raise progesterone levels. In addition, a number of vitamins and minerals, including vitamin C, vitamin E, beta carotene, zinc, and selenium are in themselves antioxidants.

4. Take supplements of fish oil (5-10 g; 1-2 teaspoons) or krill oil (1-3 g). These contain the strongly anti-inflammatory DHA and EPA, the long chain omega-3 fatty acids found to reduce the risk of endometriosis.

5. Add supplements of magnesium and calcium. Both relax the muscle of the uterus, decreasing cramping and perhaps decreasing the backflow of the menses. Magnesium (500-1,000 mg per day) should be in the form of magnesium aspartate or magnesium citrate, not magnesium oxide, which is very laxative. Calcium supplements may not be necessary if dairy intake is high; if not, take 500-1,000 mg daily.

6. Take additional vitamin D3, up to 2,000 IU per day. Its anti-inflammatory properties make it a nutrient that may help prevent endometriosis. In addition, it is essential to absorb calcium.

7. An attempt to keep body weight near normal is important. Body fat contributes estrogen, and excess body fat raises estrogen. In turn, elevated levels of estrogen lower progesterone. Conversely, underweight can lead to low levels of progesterone. Normal progesterone levels relax the uterine muscle.

A large study has shown that comprehensive nutritional supplements were as effective as oral contraceptives or gonadotropin releasing hormone analogues (GnRH-a) in reducing the pain of women who had undergone surgery for severe endometriosis. (The latter drug, in particular, has significant side effects similar to severe menopausal symptoms.) In this study, the women were given vitamins A, B6, C, and E; the minerals calcium, magnesium, selenium, zinc, and iron; a mix of "friendly" bacterial supplements; and omega-3 and omega-6 fatty acids for six months. The authors noted that nutritional therapy can be used indefinitely, and the patients in the study not only reported less pain, but also significantly better overall health and vitality.[38] Obviously, if a woman with endometriosis is attempting to become pregnant or to use NFP, nutritional therapy offers additional benefits compared to drug therapies which suppress her own hormones. Though the amounts of the supplements were unspecified, all of them, except for the "friendly" bacterial supplements, have been part of Dr. Guy Abraham's PMS diet plan since the 1980s.

OTHER HELPS FOR ENDOMETRIOSIS

ENZYMES, HERBAL REMEDIES, AND HORMONAL SUPPLEMENTS. Susan Lark, M.D., a nutritionally-oriented women's medical doctor, recommends a comprehensive multivitamin/multimineral supplement, as well as supplements containing the omega-3 fatty acid, EPA, found in fish oil (600 mg EPA daily, the amount in approximately 1½–2 teaspoons of cod liver oil). In addition, however, Dr. Lark recommends taking the anti-inflammatory digestive enzymes bromelain (500 mg) and papain (200-300 mg) between meals. She also recommends the herb pycnogenol (60 mg/day).[39] Pycnogenol, which is available at many health food shops, has been shown to reduce menstrual and pelvic pain more effectively than medications that work through repressing the entire cycle.[40] If you are hoping to become pregnant, get your doctor's approval to use pycnogenol.

MELATONIN. A new, excellently-designed double-blind study has shown that supplements of melatonin, which is the "sleep" hormone secreted by the pineal gland in the brain, can decrease the severe menstrual pain caused by endometriosis. In this study, women were given 10 mg of melatonin before bedtime. Compared to controls receiving placebo pills, the women receiving the melatonin took 80 percent less pain medication. Within four weeks their reported period pain was significantly less. Their sleep also improved.[41]

That said, 10 mg/day of melatonin is a dose higher than the usual over-the-counter dose of 3 mg/day of melatonin. If you would like to try this approach, you should consult with your health professional if you choose to use more than 3 mg/day. If you might become pregnant, do not take melatonin without your health professional's approval.

YEAST OVERGROWTH. Candidiasis, also called yeast overgrowth, is discussed in Chapter 10. It has been linked to a number of reproductive problems, including endometriosis. *The Yeast Connection and Women's Health*, by the late William Crook, M.D., contains a chapter on this "connection." In this chapter he also notes the close association between PMS, menstrual cramps, and endometriosis.[42] (See "Further Reading.")

BEYOND SELF-CARE

If you have endometriosis, please make every effort to find a doctor who is an expert in this disease, and who is committed to doing his or her best to help you preserve your fertility if at all possible. NaProTechnology practitioners are medical doctors who are specifically trained to work in harmony the body's natural functions. They provide comprehensive diagnosis and treatment, including progesterone supplementation and surgery to remove the endometriosis implants. However, your own self care in the form of excellent nutrition can help with healing, reduce inflammation, reduce pain, and perhaps help prevent or overcome infertility. Continue self care diligently, even if you need surgery or other medical care.

The diet and supplements suggested in this chapter phenomenally helped a 24-year-old single woman with the worst dysmenorrhea I have ever encountered; in truth, I wonder if she actually had undiagnosed endometriosis. Her concerned older sister asked if she could bring her to me to discuss this problem. During our visit she described abdominal and back pain so wrenching she could hardly walk. She would be so ill that she spent three to five days in bed each month. I suggested that she consider Dr. Abraham's diet and nutritional supplements as explained in Chapter 6, including about 1,000 mg magnesium in a 2:1 ratio to calcium. She took the list of supplements and selected her own brands of vitamins from a health food shop. She felt "1,000 percent" better during her next period, and by the third cycle was "5,000 percent" better. Her sister and I chatted ten months later; she reported that the younger woman no longer misses any work, her PMS has also improved, and she is "5,000 percent better—at least!"

SUMMARY—CHAPTER 7

1 Heavy, prolonged, and painful menstrual bleeding are common problems that usually respond quite well to improved nutrition.

2 Underlying causes such as fibroid tumors, endometriosis, and low thyroid function should also be considered.

3 Diet and supplements aimed at improving the repair of the endometrium are helpful for prolonged or heavy bleeding, and less bleeding often reduces menstrual pain.

4 Besides improved diet and supplements, drinking more water, beginning two or three days before the period is expected, can help reduce menstrual cramping.

5 Menstrual pain has been helped by supplements of fish oil.

6 Since the same "bad" prostaglandins are involved in menstrual pain and PMS, the PMS nutritional plan described in Chapter 6 is helpful for dysmenorrhea.

7 Calcium, magnesium, vitamin D, and even supplements of melatonin have reduced dysmenorrhea.

8 New research into the causes of endometriosis has involved studies of supplements that decrease inflammation, including EPA and DHA in fish oil and vitamin D.

9 Nutrition directed at overcoming PMS and luteal phase deficiency is helpful to endometriosis, since women with endometriosis often experience both PMS and luteal phase deficiency.

10 Preventing endometriosis is preferable to needing to cure it. Eating an antioxidant-rich whole-foods diet, keeping body weight near normal, and taking a comprehensive multivitamin/multimineral and supplements of fish oil and vitamin D decrease the risk of endometriosis.

11 If self care does not reduce period pain, or if you suspect endometriosis, get medical help from a NaProTechnology physician.

FOUR COMMON CAUSES OF CYCLE IRREGULARITIES & FEMALE INFERTILITY

8

There is an appointed time for everything, and a time for every affair under the heavens.
—Ecclesiastes 3:1

It's amazing that the same information that allows couples to use natural family planning (NFP) to avoid becoming pregnant is extremely useful to couples who are hoping to become pregnant, but are having difficulty doing so. Why is this? In both cases, the NFP chart reveals the potentially fertile time. Couples who wish to postpone a pregnancy avoid relations during the fertile time, while couples having difficulty conceiving identify the fertile time and then specifically use that time in order to increase their chances of conceiving.

Trying to make your cycle more regular is helpful, whether you are postponing a pregnancy or are actively trying to conceive. If you are using NFP in order to avoid conceiving, a more regular cycle makes it easier to identify the potentially fertile versus infertile times, and therefore it often shortens the time of abstinence. This is true even though high effectiveness can be achieved despite irregular cycles, since modern NFP relies on ongoing signs of fertility and infertility. If you are trying to increase your chances of becoming pregnant, a more regular cycle is often a healthier, more fertile cycle with more frequent ovulations. Improving cycle irregularities with better nutrition is a basic self-help tool for those experiencing infertility.

If you are hoping to increase your fertility through self care, improved nutrition may help you to conceive, as it has for other couples in the studies cited in this chapter. However, even if your focus on nutrition does not help you directly, you will be in much better physical condition to respond to hormonal or medical therapy, if that's what it takes to help you to achieve your desire for a baby.

FERTILITY AND INFERTILITY: A CONTINUUM

Your fertility depends on complex interactions among several hormones which stimulate ovulation and maintain the cycle afterwards. As a review, please reread the information on the normal fertility-menstrual cycle which appears at the beginning of Part 2. It's also useful to realize that female fertility is not an "all-or-nothing" occurrence. Instead, there is continuum between normal high fertility, cycle irregularities, and complete infertility. This is not to imply that irregular cycles generally indicate infertility, although in some women some types of recurring cycle irregularities do signal decreased fertility.

Cycle irregularity differs from infertility by a matter of degree, as sprinkles differ from a rainstorm. That's why the same nutritional guidelines apply to fertile women with troublesome cycle characteristics as to women having difficulty in conceiving.

THE CONTINUUM OF FERTILITY: BREASTFEEDING. The experience of a typical nursing mother—as she gradually changes from complete infertility to normal fertility—can help you understand irregular cycles versus unexplained infertility in non-nursing women.

When the hormones of ovulation—FSH and LH—are consistently low, which is normal in a nursing mother with complete absence of periods (**amenorrhea**), follicle and ovum development doesn't occur and the endometrium doesn't develop. The result is that neither ovulation nor menstruation occurs. As such a mother begins to produce more of the reproductive hormones, cervical mucus appears and the endometrium develops. If the nursing mother does not ovulate, eventually the endometrium will be shed anyway, causing spotting or a full, sometimes prolonged episode of bleeding. Such a "period" without previous ovulation indicates that an infertile, **anovulatory cycle** has occurred. It's common for a breastfeeding mother to have one or several such anovulatory cycles and periods.

As the hormones of breastfeeding gradually decrease, increased FSH and LH may stimulate an ovarian follicle to develop to some extent, and an immature ovum, probably incapable of fertilization, may be ovulated. If so, a basal temperature shift occurs, although it might be less than the usual shift of 0.4°F. Since the levels of FSH and LH in the preovulatory phase set the stage for the function of the corpus luteum after ovulation, progesterone in the luteal (postovulatory) phase may be reduced. A sympto-thermal chart, on which the signs of fertility are recorded, will show this with a luteal phase which is quite a bit shorter than the normal twelve to sixteen days of elevated basal temperatures. Pregnancy is less likely to occur if the duration of elevated temperatures in the luteal phase is less than nine to twelve days. Spotting may also occur before the actual period begins, while the temperatures are still elevated. Such **irregular shedding** may be yet another manifestation of low progesterone. The entire pattern at this stage of the nursing mother's return to fertility often includes an extended patch of "more fertile" mucus before ovulation, as well as a delay in ovulation that may cause a long cycle.

Finally, in this example of the continuum of fertility, the cycle of the nursing mother returns to its familiar norms, and she may continue to nurse for many months while having fertile ovulatory cycles, and she may even conceive again while doing so.

THE CONTINUUM OF FERTILITY: WEIGHT LOSS OR EXCESS EXERCISE.

Another example of the continuum between fertility and infertility is the change that takes place in a woman who exercises vigorously, but does not eat enough food to maintain her body fat. If she would eat enough calories for the exercise and to maintain body fat, she could expect to have normal, regular cycles. However, if she loses too much body fat, she may at first experience a delay in ovulation, resulting in a long cycle. Or, she may seem to have no change in her overall cycle length, but charting will reveal that she is ovulating later in the cycle than before, and that she has developed a short luteal phase, which indicates low progesterone. If she continues to exercise vigorously and to lose more body fat, she may experience anovulatory cycles. That is, she may have a period, but she is not ovulating. If she loses more body fat, she will go into complete amenorrhea (no ovulations or periods).[1] Such a pattern is quite reversible if she can consume sufficient calories, or if she cuts down on the amount of strenuous exercise.

THE CONTINUUM OF FERTILITY: PERIMENOPAUSE.
Yet another example of this continuum occurs as women approach menopause. During this time, the menstrual cycles often become shorter, with short preovulatory phases along with short luteal phases. As more time passes, though, longer cycles with delayed ovulation become common. The last few episodes of bleeding are likely to follow anovulatory cycles, and by definition menopause is followed by complete—and permanent—amenorrhea.

There are a number of different causes of cycle irregularity in women. Sometimes the cause is not known for certain, but often the NFP chart provides excellent clues as to what is actually occurring. What follows are cycle irregularities that can be seen by charting, along with strategies to improve them. Even though you may never be absolutely certain of the cause of your cycle irregularity or infertility, you can take heart from the fact that nutrition by itself often improves cycle irregularity—and sometimes leads to long-awaited pregnancies.

LUTEAL PHASE DEFICIENCY

CHARTED SIGNS OF LUTEAL PHASE DEFICIENCY, also called "luteal phase defect" or "luteal phase inadequacy"

Short luteal phase (fewer than nine to twelve days of elevated postovulatory temperatures, or fewer than nine days of post-peak mucus days[2])
Premenstrual spotting
Postmenstrual brown bleeding or spotting
Poor temperature rise after ovulation
Extended mucus
Poor mucus quality or hard-to-interpret mucus
Amenorrhea
Early miscarriage
Infertility

In some women, the periods occur at quite regular intervals, and the entire cycle is short or normal in length, mainly due to the short luteal phase. In other women the entire cycle may be prolonged and sometimes irregular, as ovulation is delayed. In either case, when the cycle is charted it is obvious that the postovulatory phase is short. PMS often occurs with this pattern.

While it's possible for any woman to have a short luteal phase cycle occasionally, more often such cycles recur month after month. The hormone levels of the previous cycle set the stage for the next cycle, so that one cycle is intimately connected to the next. If your pattern of short luteal phase is occurring regularly, there are steps you can take to improve it.

Improving the short luteal phase will increase the postovulatory infertile time for couples avoiding a pregnancy, reducing abstinence, and it will increase the chance of conception for couples attempting to overcome infertility.

UNDERLYING CAUSES OF SHORT LUTEAL PHASE

Luteal phase deficiency results from low levels of progesterone during the postovulatory phase of the cycle.

The **corpus luteum**, which produces the progesterone after the ovum is released from the follicle, doesn't do its job as well or as long as it should. Since progesterone is the cause of the basal body temperature elevation during this time, low levels of progesterone cause the poor upward shift of temperatures and the short luteal phase. Progesterone distinctly affects the characteristics of the mucus, explaining why poor mucus patterns result. Progesterone causes growth in the thickness of the endometrium and prevents menstruation. When it is too low, spotting may occur before the full period begins, and dark red or brown spotting may follow or end the period.

What causes progesterone to be too low? Or more specifically, what causes the corpus luteum to secrete inadequate amounts of this hormone? One possibility is high levels of estrogen, caused by poor diet or by overweight. High estrogen levels decrease progesterone. "Bad" local hormones, called prostaglandins, are another cause, since they interfere with the function of the corpus luteum. High levels of the hormone prolactin may also be involved.[3] It is known that in breastfeeding women, high prolactin, which is normal while nursing, inhibits the FSH and LH and therefore inhibits the development of the follicle and corpus luteum. Sometimes prolactin is high in non-breastfeeding women, and it can do the same thing.

Low thyroid function can also underlie short luteal phase.

If you are experiencing very low preovulatory temperatures, in the range of 97.3°F or below, please refer to "Low Thyroid Function" later in this chapter. Vigorous exercise that causes you to lose body fat can also cause short luteal phases, and the topic "Underweight or Inadequate Body Fat" in this chapter is intended to help you get started on the goal of restoring normal cycles. Of course, if you are currently breastfeeding a baby, short luteal phases are a completely normal part of the transition from infertility to fertility, as explained in the introductory example of this chapter.

INFERTILITY AND RECURRENT MISCARRIAGE

Luteal phase deficiency results in an increased risk of infertility and miscarriage.[4] Many researchers attribute this to the poor development of the endometrium, which results in poor implantation of the embryo if conception occurs.

What happens before ovulation affects the luteal phase, and also affects fertility even before the time of implantation. If the follicle does not develop well before ovulation, the corpus luteum will also be inadequate, and will produce inadequate progesterone.[5] But equally important, immediately before ovulation, the unfertilized ovum must complete the critical cell division called meiosis I, as explained in the Introduction to Part 2. The same hormones responsible for development of the follicle and its secretion of estrogen before ovulation—FSH and LH—are also responsible for stimulating the cell division of the ovum, which is called the **maturation** of the ovum. If the hormonal stimulation early in the cycle is insufficient to cause the all-important meiosis I to occur properly, then the ovum will not be genetically normal. Most often it will not be able to be fertilized, so that conception cannot occur. If conception does occur with such an abnormal ovum, the newly conceived child cannot develop properly, and an early miscarriage will result.[6]

NUTRITION FOR LUTEAL PHASE DEFICIENCY

Can nutrition help you to overcome a short luteal phase and its related manifestations? The nutritional research says "yes!"

OVERALL DIET. Most of the underlying causes of luteal phase deficiency are also involved in premenstrual syndrome (PMS), which has been related to poor luteal function. The nutritional plan developed by Dr. Guy Abraham and explained in Chapter 6 is intended to correct these problems and to raise progesterone. For this reason, the overall nutritional strategy for improving luteal phase deficiency is to implement the PMS dietary guidelines of Chapter 6. The dietary recommendations of the PMS diet plan are very similar to "Twelve Rules for Better Nutrition" in Chapter 1, and can be used interchangeably. However, in addition you will most likely need to supplement vitamins and minerals to improve luteal phase deficiency.

VITAMIN B6. Vitamin B6 alone (200-600 mg/day) has lowered prolactin levels and restored regular cycles to women with the severe overproduction of prolactin that causes both amenorrhea and **galactorrhea** (milk in the breasts of non-nursing women).[7] Elevated prolactin levels can cause short luteal phase.

In a truly remarkable study, vitamin B6, a critical nutrient for PMS sufferers, was given in 100-800 mg/day doses to fourteen women who had normal menstrual cycles but also had PMS and infertility of eighteen months to seven years' duration. Ten of the fourteen had never borne a child, while the other four were experiencing secondary infertility. Twelve of the women conceived, eleven within six months of the vitamin B6 therapy. In this study, prolactin levels were not found to change, but progesterone levels were significantly increased in several of the women, indicating that the vitamin B6 had improved their luteal function.[8]

Please note that these amounts of vitamin B6 are not recommended by themselves. Instead, B6 should be taken in amounts not exceeding 300 mg daily, and along with other B vitamins and magnesium, as explained in Chapter 6. Vitamins and minerals work together.

VITAMIN C. Another important study has shown that vitamin C can increase progesterone levels to normal in some women with luteal phase deficiency, enabling some of them to conceive. Japanese researchers hypothesized that oxidative stress decreases the activity of the corpus luteum and causes it to secrete insufficient progesterone. They provided the antioxidant vitamin C or a placebo pill to 150 women with carefully diagnosed luteal phase deficiency as well as infertility. Of the women who took vitamin C (750 mg daily), 53 percent had a significant increase in their mid-luteal phase progesterone, from an average of 7.51 to 13.27 ng/ml (greater than 10 ng/ml was considered normal). Of the women taking vitamin C, 25 percent conceived within six months. Of the placebo group, 22 percent had improvement in their progesterone level spontaneously, and 11 percent conceived. The miscarriage rate was 16 percent in those taking vitamin C and 20 percent in those taking the placebo (though this difference was not statistically significant).[9]

It is worthwhile to note that in this study the vitamin C was discontinued as soon as pregnancy was confirmed, which I believe was an unfortunate aspect of the experimental design. I suspect that the miscarriage rate would have been significantly lower if the vitamin C, which is safe and beneficial during pregnancy, had been continued. The women in the study had previously experienced low levels of progesterone that were normalized by the supplementation of vitamin C, and continued vitamin C very likely would have continued to support their progesterone levels.

OPTIVITE PMT. The PMS nutritional supplement Optivite PMT, developed by Dr. Guy Abraham and recommended in Chapter 6, contains several nutrients (vitamin B6, magnesium, and zinc) that help to reduce prolactin. In reality, the supplement is designed to overcome the luteal phase inadequacy that may contribute to PMS.[10] Optivite's 300 mg of B6 and 1,500 mg of vitamin C are most likely responsible for the finding that Optivite, plus dietary improvement, has restored low luteal phase progesterone and high luteal phase estrogen to normal levels.[11] Mucus and temperature patterns returned to normal within three to six months in some women who followed Abraham's PMS nutritional plan along with exercise and stress reduction.[12]

Improvement in the length of the luteal phase as well as improved mucus patterns have often been reported to the Couple to Couple League by women who have taken Optivite. For example, a 27-year-old woman submitted three sympto-thermal charts (shown on page 144) to Couple to Couple League showing an improvement in her luteal phase from nine days to twelve days after taking Optivite for two months. Her ovulation also occurred earlier, from Day 30 to Day 17, during the second month of taking Optivite.[13] Such a change significantly reduces the days of abstinence in couples who are avoiding a pregnancy.

PROCYCLE PMS is a supplement which is very similar to Optivite, but contains no iron and is formulated for only four tablets daily. You may prefer to use it instead. (See Appendix A for complete contents of Optivite PMT and ProCycle PMS.)

From Chart 1 to Chart 3, this woman's cycle length reduced from 39 days to 30 days; the length of Phase 2 (the fertile time) reduced from 27 days to 14 days; and the luteal phase increased from 9 to 12 days.

FERTILITY BLEND. A nutritional supplement called Fertility Blend has also improved the rate of conception in women with infertility, while significantly raising the mid-luteal phase levels of progesterone in women with low progesterone before treatment. Fertility Blend contains green tea, which has antioxidant capabilities higher than that of vitamin C. It also contains the herb *Vitex agnus castus*, or chasteberry extract, which previous studies have shown to increase progesterone levels.[14] In addition, it contains the antioxidant vitamin E, folic acid, magnesium, selenium, and zinc, as well as other nutrients. (See Appendix A.) Of fifty-three infertile women taking Fertility Blend in a double-blind study, 26 percent conceived within three months, compared to 10 percent of women taking the placebo. Also of interest to NFP users was the effect on charted basal body temperature:

Women taking Fertility Blend in non-conception cycles averaged two more days per cycle of temperatures over 98.6°F compared to controls.[15]

A double-blind study using chasteberry extract alone produced similar results; 20 mg daily of *Vitex agnus castus* extract given to fifty-two women with luteal phase deficiency due to elevated levels of prolactin resulted in a reduction of their prolactin levels. Levels of progesterone returned to normal, as did the length of the luteal phase.[16]

SUMMARY OF RECOMMENDATIONS FOR LUTEAL PHASE DEFICIENCY.
Improve your diet as recommended in Part 1 of this book. Review Chapter 6, "Premenstrual Syndrome (PMS)," even if you do not have PMS. PMS has been related to luteal phase deficiency, and the details of diet and vitamins, minerals, and essential fatty acids for PMS have been studied, and are also helpful for luteal phase problems.

With your health care practitioner's approval, supplement Optivite PMT, ProCycle PMS, or Fertility Blend, along with flax oil and/or fish oil in the amounts recommended in Table 7 (Chapter 3). Chapter 6 compares Optivite PMT to ProCycle PMS, and also explains that any other brand of vitamin and mineral supplements can be used instead, as long as the amounts of the nutrients are similar.

Low thyroid function, strenuous exercise, underweight, or overweight can result in poor luteal phases.

See the sections in this chapter, "Low Thyroid Function," and "Underweight or Inadequate Body Fat" for a discussion of the first three topics. See Chapter 9's section, "Overweight Without PCOS" if you are experiencing short luteal phases which might be related to overweight. Finally, if you are hoping to achieve pregnancy at an older age, or if you have had recurrent miscarriages, see the section on "Age-Related Infertility" in Chapter 10, or "Repeated Miscarriage & Birth Defects" in Chapter 12.

LOW THYROID FUNCTION

CHARTED SIGNS OF LOW THYROID FUNCTION

Unusually low basal temperatures (preovulatory temperatures around 97.3 °F. and lower)

Heavy menses

Prolonged menses

Delayed ovulation

Long or very long cycles

Prolonged less fertile mucus

Short luteal phase

Anovulatory cycles

Unexplained infertility

Miscarriage

In addition, low thyroid function can also cause or contribute to reproductive problems not seen on the chart, notably:

Low sexual desire (low libido)

PMS

Painful periods

Galactorrhea (milk in the breasts of non-nursing women)

Low thyroid function can also be responsible for a number of non-reproductive problems—anxiety, mental confusion, intolerance to cold, weight gain, dry skin, hair loss, and ongoing fatigue.

If you have suffered from some of the reproductive symptoms of low thyroid function listed above, there is a good chance that your physician has already tested your thyroid hormones. It's well known that thyroid dysfunction can cause problems with a woman's cycle and fertility.

For reasons that are not always clear, however, low thyroid function may not be detected by blood tests for the various thyroid hormones. This problem of diagnosis has led to the term "subclinical hypothyroidism." Or, you may have had a diagnosis of hypothyroidism and are taking thyroid medication, yet you are still experiencing cycle irregularities. Insufficient thyroid hormone replacement could be involved.

THYROID HORMONES

The thyroid gland, situated like a small bow tie right at the base of the neck, secretes several hormones. The two most important ones are abbreviated "T4" for thyroxine and "T3" for tri-iodothyronine. Thyroid hormones contain iodine; T4 refers to the hormone with four iodines, and T3 contains three attached iodines. About four-fifths of the hormone secreted into the blood is T4; the rest is T3. However, T4 is much less active than T3, so all body cells themselves must convert the T4 into T3, a process that depends on several vitamins and minerals and on the intestinal bacteria. The thyroid hormones affect virtually all cells in the body by stimulating their various activities, which explains why low thyroid function can have such seemingly unrelated symptoms as hair loss, infertility, and mental confusion.

THYROID FUNCTION AND THE CYCLE. The major effects on the menstrual cycle and fertility occur because thyroid hormones affect or are affected by several other hormones, including estrogen, progesterone, prolactin, and cortisol. Low thyroid hormone can indirectly cause elevated prolactin, which in turn can be responsible for short luteal phase, long cycles, absence of cycles, infertility, and galactorrhea.[17] Low thyroid hormone levels can cause low estrogen and low progesterone, which may contribute to infertility.[18] Thyroid hormones enable body cells to use more fuel and to produce more heat.

When thyroid function is low, the basal body temperature is often lower than normal.

That is also the link between easy weight gain and hypothyroidism; without normal thyroid function, the cells burn their fuel more slowly than normal. Thyroid hormones also affect blood clotting; low levels decrease the production of coagulation factors needed by the blood, explaining at least in part the heavy menses that often occur with low thyroid function.[19]

BREAST SELF-EXAM FOR GALACTORRHEA (MILK IN THE BREASTS OF NON-NURSING WOMEN)

Even a very small amount of milk in your breasts can indicate high prolactin, which in turn may be related to low thyroid function. One natural family planning client of mine, who was infertile for several years after having had two children, was surprised to find out during a gynecological exam that she had milk in her breasts. It was just a small amount, but it was an important clue as to her infertility, which she was able to overcome. To check for milk in your breasts, perform a breast self-exam, carefully expressing each breast from the edge to the nipple, using both hands. Even a small amount of fluid should be reported to your physician, though galactorrhea is usually a sign of correctable hormone imbalances.

UNDERLYING CAUSES OF LOW THYROID FUNCTION

A number of factors may cause thyroid function to be abnormally low, resulting in either subclinical or full-blown hypothyroidism. Nutritional deficiencies can prevent the thyroid gland from doing its job. Iodine is well known to be essential for the production of thyroid hormones, but a number of other vitamins, minerals, and the essential fatty acids are also necessary for the production and activation of thyroid hormones.

One of the most common causes of hypothyroidism is **Hashimoto's thyroiditis**, an autoimmune disease in which one's own antibodies disrupt normal thyroid function. In some women, the thyroid gland may temporarily malfunction for a time after a woman gives birth, but it often corrects itself within a few months. Sometimes, though, persistent hypothyroidism begins after childbirth. (See Chapter 11's section on "Postpartum Thyroiditis" for more information.) Removal of the thyroid gland due to elevated thyroid function or thyroid cancer also produces hypothyroidism, which must be treated medically.

> **Low thyroid function can occur due to insufficient medical replacement of thyroid hormone, or replacement with T4 alone, instead of a mix of T4 and T3, as is more natural.**

Hormones from other glands also affect thyroid function. Normal levels of progesterone from the corpus luteum stimulate the thyroid. Progesterone enables the body's cells to bind T3, so that the cells can respond to thyroid hormone. Progesterone also decreases the production of a blood protein called thyroxine-binding globulin, an effect that increases the availability of thyroid hormone to the cells. Conversely, high estrogen levels block the function of thyroid hormones within the body cells.[20] The adrenal hormone cortisol, which rises during prolonged stress, also blocks the function of the thyroid hormones within the body's cells.[21]

NUTRITION FOR LOW THYROID FUNCTION

Improving the diet generally, as described in Chapter 1, is helpful to the entire body, and it is basic to glandular health. Ocean fish is one food to emphasize for thyroid function, since it is a source of iodine as well as omega-3 fatty acids. However, when it comes to low thyroid function, certain foods should be avoided or eaten in moderation.

FOODS THAT INTERFERE WITH THYROID FUNCTION. *Trans* fats found in processed foods such as shortening, margarine and fast foods, especially pastries, interfere with normal cellular function and should be avoided by everyone.

Unfermented soy foods eaten in significant quantities have anti-thyroid properties that can affect thyroid function.[22] Avoid soy milk, soy powder, tofu, and so forth as part of your self care for low thyroid function. (Intake of foods which contain soy oil, such as salad dressings, need not be restricted.)

Very high consumption of certain raw vegetables and fruits can also have anti-thyroid effects. These include cabbage, Brussels sprouts, broccoli, kale, radishes, turnips, spinach, mustard greens, peanuts, peaches, and pears. Please do not avoid these healthy foods entirely; if they are cooked, the potentially anti-thyroid enzymes are destroyed. According to thyroid patient advocate Mary Shomon, people who have had their thyroid gland removed and who are receiving thyroid replacement hormones do not need to be concerned at all, but even those who are dealing with low thyroid function can eat these vegetable and fruits, raw or cooked, in ordinary moderation.[23]

Finally, if you are fighting low thyroid function, you may wish to drink purified water. Both fluoridated and chlorinated water can interfere with the thyroid gland's use of iodine.[24]

SUPPLEMENTS FOR LOW THYROID FUNCTION. Adding iodized salt (not plain sea salt) to the diet has improved cycle irregularity and irregular mucus patterns in women who were using little or no iodized salt.[25] If you prefer not to consume extra salt, you can get iodine from a multivitamin/multimineral or from tablets of kelp, a type of seaweed (150–225 mcg of iodine is a typical daily dose). Besides iodine, the B vitamins and vitamins C and E aid thyroid function. True vitamin A from fish oil also helps the thyroid gland. (Some people with low thyroid function cannot turn beta-carotene, the precursor of vitamin A, into true vitamin A.) Recent research has implicated vitamin D deficiency to autoimmune diseases, including Hashimoto's thyroiditis.[26] The essential fatty acids found in flax oil stimulate all glands, including the thyroid gland, and the omega-3 fatty acids of fish oil have anti-inflammatory properties.

The mineral selenium is especially important to thyroid function, in part because it enables the conversion of T4 into the active form, T3. Selenium has important antioxidant and anti-inflammatory effects that have been studied recently.

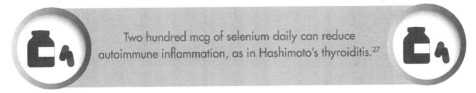

Two hundred mcg of selenium daily can reduce autoimmune inflammation, as in Hashimoto's thyroiditis.[27]

Smaller daily doses (80 mcg/day) have also been studied, but take a longer time (12 months) to reduce thyroid antibodies than the higher dose (200 mcg; 3 months).[28]

Zinc also assists in the conversion of T4 to T3, and should be included in your comprehensive multivitamin/multimineral (25-50 mg/day).

Making sure that you support your intestinal bacteria is yet another, perhaps surprising, way to support your thyroid function.

Intestinal bacteria help with the essential function of converting the inactive T4 form of thyroid hormone into the active T3 form.[29] Healthy gut bacteria decrease overall inflammation. Since inflammation is involved with all autoimmune disease, including autoimmune thyroid disease, it makes sense to eat plenty of foods which feed the intestinal bacteria, or supplement with a high-quality probiotic. See "Supplementing Probiotics" in Chapter 3 for more information.

I usually recommend Professional Pre-Natal Formula, ProCycle, or even Androvite for Men along with flax oil (five to ten 1 g capsules daily) when I see very low temperatures as well as poor mucus patterns and poor temperature rises on a chart.[30] (See "Resources.") I have seen women's basal temperatures gradually rise to normal, over a period of about two to three weeks, when they supplement as recommended here. I have also had the interesting experience of seeing the reverse—women with low basal temperatures and poor chart patterns whose charts improved substantially once they took a supplement like Professional Pre-Natal Formula, only to gradually revert back to poor patterns and low temperatures after they discontinued it.

As vital as iodine is to thyroid function, new research shows that *excess* iodine may be involved in autoimmune thyroid disease, including Hashimoto's thyroiditis. It may surprise you to find out that the excess iodine contributes to low thyroid function.

Lack of iodine worldwide, historically a cause of hypothyroid goiter, has been greatly reduced due to iodine fortification of salt with iodine. But surprisingly, new studies show that autoimmune thyroiditis has increased at the same time. Chronic high iodine intake is associated with an increased frequency of autoimmune thyroiditis. According to the author of one such study, "…The best approach would be adherence to a narrow iodine intake interval so that a given population may achieve prevention of iodine deficiency disease and minimalization of the risk of autoimmune thyroid disease."[31]

It's my opinion that excess iodine intake is from iodized salt used in restaurant food. Surely you have noticed how salty restaurant food is compared to your home-cooked food. That salty food is almost certainly salted with iodized salt. With the great increase in eating out—just look at the fast food places and sit-down restaurants along any American highway—it's no wonder that excess iodine intake can occur. The answer? The best nutrition comes from the food you prepare at home, where you can control the ingredients in your food.

Additionally, supplements of selenium (200 mcg) per day in a controlled study resulted in an average of 50 percent drop in anti-thyroid antibodies, which cause the autoimmune attack on the thyroid. The thyroid gland has the largest concentration of selenium in the body, and selenium has potent anti-inflammatory and anti-oxidative properties.[32]

OTHER SELF CARE

Moderate exercise done in cool weather, or cool-temperature activities such as swimming, may stimulate the thyroid gland, as it naturally responds to cold temperatures by increasing its hormonal output.

Oppositely, however, the stress of excessive exercise accompanied by loss of body fat may contribute to a **hypometabolic state** which includes lowered levels of progesterone.[33]

The late Rose Frisch, Ph.D., who studied Harvard University women athletes throughout her long career, observed the effect of excessive exercise on body temperature. She wrote that "the baseline temperature measurement of most of the well-trained athletes amazed us right from the start. Their evening temperatures ranged around 96.5°F. Practically no one had an evening temperature of 98.6°F."[34] While women do not need to have evening temperatures as high as 98.6°F., evening temperatures of 96.5°F. are certainly indicative of low thyroid function.

This effect may well be related to high levels of the stress hormone cortisol, which interferes with thyroid function. Excessive exercise is a stress that can take its toll on the thyroid. Besides engaging in moderate exercise only, other effective ways of lowering your stress hormones include eating a good diet, taking supplements of essential nutrients, and, maybe most important of all, getting enough sleep. Doing so is not just good for your moods and energy; it's good for your thyroid gland, too. (See Chapter 4, "Increasing Your Energy & Decreasing Your Stress.")

MEDICAL TREATMENT

Nutrition and other self care by themselves can improve the symptoms listed above. However, in some cases thyroid hormone replacement may be necessary. If so, you should be aware that there are more and more doctors who are willing to prescribe natural **Armour** thyroid replacement, because it contains the active T3 form as well as the less active T4 hormone. L-thyroxine (Synthroid, Levoxyl, Levothroid) contains the T4 hormone only. About 25 percent of people with subclinical hypothyroidism are actually taking T4 therapy alone, according to a recent review article.[35]

DIAGNOSING LOW THYROID FUNCTION. During my early years as an NFP teacher, I was often puzzled that women with several of the cycle problems listed above, such as very low basal temperatures, would test normal for blood levels of thyroid hormones. That puzzle was solved for me when I discovered the book *Hypothyroidism: The Unsuspected Illness*, by the late Broda Barnes, M.D. Dr. Barnes was a young physician before World War II. Like other physicians back then, he used physical findings such as heavy bleeding, infertility, and so forth to diagnosis low thyroid function, along with a clinical determination of basal metabolic rate, the oxygen consumption test. He treated patients diagnosed with low thyroid function with natural thyroid hormone, and found that it was effective in helping such women overcome heavy periods, repeated miscarriage, and infertility. When blood tests for thyroid hormone became available in the 1940's, these laboratory blood tests replaced the diagnosis based on the patient's symptoms and physical examination—but many fewer women were diagnosed with hypothyroidism, even if they still had clinical symptoms of it, or even if they had been on thyroid replacement and had been doing well with it.[36]

Instead of relying on blood tests that he considered inaccurate, Dr. Broda Barnes developed the **Barnes basal temperature test** for thyroid function. He studied the relationship between the underarm basal temperature and the "gold standard" oxygen consumption test, and found that the easy-to-take basal temperature correlated very well with the cumbersome but reliable oxygen consumption test. He considered basal temperatures below 97.8°F. a possible sign of low thyroid function. For menstruating women, he used preovulatory temperatures taken on Days 2 or 3 of the cycle; for other women, men, or children, any day's temperature was usable.[37] His book states that the underarm basal temperature is about the same as the oral basal temperature.[38]

I have looked at many NFP charts over the years, and on one point I disagree with the work of Dr. Barnes. While he states that basal temperatures below 97.8°F may indicate low thyroid function, I have seen many, many charts with preovulatory temperatures in the range of 97.3–97.7°F that seem otherwise completely normal, and the women were experiencing good health. This discrepancy may actually have to do with Dr. Barnes' protocol of using temperatures during Days 2–3 of the cycle, whereas I always consider the six low temperatures right before ovulation occurs and the temperatures rise.

When temperatures during the preovulatory time hover around 97.3°F and below, low thyroid function should certainly be considered if the chart shows other irregularities or if infertility is an issue. If you are not ovulating, any three or four basal temperatures in a row can give you the same information. Self-care to improve thyroid function, as described above, should be the first step, and should be tried for about three months.

WHY AREN'T THYROID TESTS COMPLETELY RELIABLE? There are several theories to explain why tests for thyroid function are not always accurate. First, the thyroid hormone in the blood is overwhelmingly the inactive T4 hormone, which must be converted in the tissues to the active form, T3. Direct testing of the active T3 hormone in each cell is not possible. The conversion of T4 to T3 depends on a number of nutrients, including the mineral selenium. Second, the standards for "normal" thyroid function may be too broad, even though the range for "normal" has been narrowed in the last few years. Third, high levels of estrogen can block thyroid function within the body cells, as can high levels of stress hormones.

DIFFICULTY IN DIAGNOSIS OF HYPOTHYROIDISM: ONE WOMAN'S EXPERIENCE

A woman I'll call Jane was very much helped by Dr. Barnes' research regarding the value of the basal temperature chart, other charted information, her own persistence, and the assistance of an open-minded medical doctor. When she contacted me, her preovulatory temperatures were as low as 96.3°F. Her temperature shift was poor, with only nine elevated temperatures in the luteal phase before the next menses. (Twelve to sixteen elevated temperatures are normal for the luteal phase.) She had brown bleeding at the end of the menstrual period, and then a pattern of less-fertile "tacky" mucus that began immediately and never changed to stretchy, more-fertile mucus.

Jane was in her mid-30's at the time and had four young children, none of them breastfeeding. She made some other notes on her charts, especially about the painful periods. She felt generally unwell, and was avoiding a pregnancy. Because of the chart problems—this was her monthly pattern—the abstinence phase was prolonged. She said she had low libido and bad PMS.

When I reviewed Jane's charts, I felt sure that the problem was low thyroid function, and suggested that she get her thyroid hormones tested. Jane did see her family doctor, who performed standard thyroid tests at her request. All came back normal. I encouraged her to seek further testing. She followed up by seeing a hormone specialist who performed new tests. All were normal. When Jane asked this doctor about a lump she found growing on the front of her neck, the specialist was not at all concerned about it.

Jane persisted and made an appointment with a second specialist. When she met him, he had her test results from the previous doctors in his hand, and he said as he walked into the consultation room: "I'm not going to redo these tests. You've already been tested twice. I'm going to put you on [an anti-anxiety medication]. Ninety percent of the patients who come here are anxious." When Jane called his attention to the lump on her neck, he completely changed. She left with an appointment for a biopsy of her thyroid gland and the fear that it might be cancer.

At this point Jane decided to use the services of a more holistic medical doctor in another town. This doctor took her history, reviewed her NFP charts and her previous medical tests, and concluded that she had low thyroid function. He recommended that she first have the abnormal growth on her thyroid evaluated and removed by a surgeon. She did so; it turned out to be a benign hypothyroid goiter.

Afterwards, the nutritionally-aware doctor prescribed supplements similar to those in this book to see if he could help her improve her thyroid function. (Jane had already tried the nutrition recommended in a previous edition of my book very conscientiously, but to no avail.) When nutrition failed to make a difference, the doctor started Jane on the natural Armour thyroid hormone. He very gradually increased her dose over a period of months.

A year later, Jane was so pleased with her improvement that she surprised me by mailing me a recent NFP chart. While her preovulatory temperatures were still low compared to most women's charts, they were noticeably higher than they had been. More significantly, her luteal phase, which had been only nine days long, was lengthened to twelve days, which is within the normal range. Her period was shorter and lighter, and her mucus pattern was very much improved and was completely normal. The time of abstinence the new chart required was far less than for her previous charts when her hypothyroidism was undiagnosed and untreated.

SUMMARY OF SELF-CARE FOR LOW THYROID FUNCTION. If your chart or symptoms fit those listed at the beginning of this section, make sure that you first improve your diet, and then begin taking a comprehensive multivitamin/multimineral, along with flax oil and/or fish oil. If you are very athletic, reduce your workouts until your cycles and health improve. Instead, try milder exercise in cool weather, or consider swimming to allow your body to experience lower temperatures, which may stimulate your thyroid function. If you are not able to resolve your symptoms, seek the assistance of a nutritionally-oriented health professional.

For overall information on thyroid dysfunction, refer to *The Thyroid Hormone Breakthrough* by Mary Shomon, which exhorts women to fight for accurate diagnosis and effective treatment for thyroid and related hormonal dysfunction. For a comprehensive view of autoimmune thyroid dysfunction (Hashimoto's thyroiditis) and self care to improve it, see *Hashimoto's Thyroiditis: Lifestyle Interventions for Finding and Treating the Root Cause*, by Isabella Wentz, PharmD. (See "Further Reading.")

HYPERTHYROIDISM (ABNORMALLY HIGH THYROID FUNCTION)

CHARTED SIGNS OF HYPERTHYROIDISM

Unusually high basal temperatures (preovulatory basal temperatures averaging 98.4°F and above)

Light menses

Short cycles

Short luteal phase

Irregular cycles

Lack of cycles

Infertility

In addition, hyperthyroidism may cause milk in the breasts of non-nursing women (galactorrhea).

Hyperthyroidism can also cause many effects not related to the cycle: intolerance to heat, excess perspiration, anxiety or irritability, a feeling of being "wired," fatigue, rapid heart rate, unexplained weight loss.[39]

This problem is the reverse of low thyroid function, but it can also contribute to cycle irregularity and infertility.

Hyperthyroidism is not nearly as common as low thyroid function.

The cause may be an autoimmune disease called Graves' disease that "tricks" the thyroid gland into producing excess hormone. Excess thyroid medication prescribed to treat hypothyroidism (low thyroid function) is another possible cause of hyperthyroidism.[40] Milk in the breasts may occur with hyperthyroidism because the imbalance in the control of the thyroid hormones elevates the hormone prolactin, which is responsible for milk production.

If you suspect that hyperthyroidism may be the cause of your cycle irregularities or infertility, you should first seek accurate medical diagnosis. You should also look into the possibility of iodine overdose. Kelp tablets, multiminerals, excess iodized salt, and ocean fish are sources of iodine that should be considered. Hyperthyroidism increases the need for all nutrients because it raises the body's energy expenditure, so excellent nutrition as outlined in Part 1 of this book is a basic part of recovering your health.

However, nutritional improvement alone cannot correct hyperthyroidism, and medical intervention may be necessary.

Treating hyperthyroidism may involve removing all or part of the gland, or prescription medications which interfere with its ability to produce excess hormones. Unfortunately, such treatments usually result in hypothyroidism, which becomes the long-term situation that must be managed medically. Mary Shomon, the author of *The Thyroid Hormone Breakthrough*, has also written *Living Well with Graves' Disease or Hyperthyroidism*. (See "Further Reading.")

UNDERWEIGHT OR INADEQUATE BODY FAT

CHARTED SIGNS OF UNDERWEIGHT OR LOW BODY FAT

Long cycles

Scant cervical mucus

Delayed ovulation

Short luteal phase

Anovulatory cycles (periods which occur, often irregularly, without ovulation during the "cycle")

Complete amenorrhea (absence of periods and therefore absence of ovulation)

Miscarriage

Infertility

If your basal body temperatures are low (preovulatory temperatures averaging 97.3°F or less), please also read "Low Thyroid Function." If your basal body temperatures are abnormally high (preovulatory temperatures averaging about 98.4°F), see "Hyperthyroidism" in addition to this topic.

UNDERLYING CAUSES OF UNDERWEIGHT-RELATED CYCLE IRREGULARITIES

According to the pioneering studies of the late Harvard researcher Rose E. Frisch, Ph.D., your body fat must contribute at least 22 percent to your total body weight if you are to have normal menstrual cycles.[41] It was Dr. Frisch who first amazed the world of human physiology by reporting that among slender women, losing or gaining as little as three to five pounds could cause the menstrual cycle to completely stop or to return again.[42]

Body fat profoundly affects female fertility. First and foremost, fatty tissue is an important source of estrogen. It converts androgens (male hormones) to estrogen, and during a woman's fertile years it provides about one third of her total estrogen. Second, lean women make a less potent form of estrogen than do women with more body fat, and the less potent estrogen has less ability to stimulate the various reproductive functions. Third, thin women have higher than average amounts of a blood protein—sex hormone-binding globulin—which binds estrogen; therefore, they have less free estrogen available for stimulation of the reproductive organs.[43]

Finally, in excessively lean women, the part of the brain that controls the pituitary gland, the hypothalamus, does not properly stimulate the fertility hormones FSH and LH. Normally the hypothalamus secretes a hormone, GnRH, in pulses every ninety minutes or so. GnRH stimulates FSH and LH. When the body lacks sufficient fat, the hypothalamus no longer secretes GnRH in the normal pattern. In response, FSH and LH levels drop and are secreted in patterns similar to that of pre-adolescent girls. The hormone leptin, produced by the fat cells, stimulates the normal release of GnRH. A lack of body fat results in a lack of leptin, and so the GnRH secretion drops.[44] For these and for other reasons still being investigated, being too lean adversely affects your cycles.

CAUSES OF LOW BODY FAT

 Cycle irregularities and infertility are more related to low body fat than to low body weight.

Understanding why your body fat is low is the first step to making the adjustments necessary to restore your cycle regularity or your fertility. Your low body fat could just be part of your natural body build. Perhaps you come from a family of slender folks, and it is easy for you to remain thin, even without much exercise. Maybe it has never occurred to you that your long, irregular cycles are related to being slender. If you are eating a vegetarian or vegan diet, either of these could possibly be at the root of your cycle or fertility problems. Or perhaps you are the type of person who cannot seem to eat well when stressed, and you are under fairly constant, though not necessarily intense, stress. Smoking cigarettes is yet another contributor to underweight, though there are many other serious reasons to quit.

If you are prone to diarrhea when eating certain foods, intestinal disorders or food allergies could be a factor. An intolerance to gluten, a protein found in wheat, rye, and barley, is called celiac disease, and could be responsible for low body weight and low body fat. (Celiac disease is discussed in Chapter 10.) If recurring bouts of diarrhea are part of your low body weight or low body fat, it's important to discuss it with a doctor.

> **Your exercise regimen could be the cause of short luteal phases,
> long cycles, anovulatory cycles, or no cycles at all.**

Vigorous exercise can decrease your body fat and increase your muscle mass while you maintain a completely normal weight for your height. You may enjoy the challenge of getting in shape to run a marathon, or maybe you are a dedicated dancer, gymnast, swimmer, or basketball player. Or perhaps you had regular cycles but were overweight, and you began dieting. As you have progressed toward your goal, to your surprise your periods have gotten irregular or stopped altogether!

Even though anorexia nervosa, bulimia, and **female athlete triad** (menstrual irregularities, disordered eating, and bone loss in female athletes) have gotten much media attention, you don't need to have any of these psychological disorders in order to have low body fat. Any situation that causes you to take in or to absorb fewer calories than you need will sooner or later result in low body fat, and it will result in long cycles or no cycles at all. Psychological factors do not need to be involved.

OTHER CONSEQUENCES OF LOW BODY FAT. No matter what the reason, if caloric intake is inadequate, a woman who loses her cycles is at risk for loss of bone mass, stress fractures, and eventual osteoporosis. Constant restriction of calories by female athletes in order to attain athletic goals also contributes to fatigue, stress, and depression.[45] Correcting your cycle irregularities through improved nutrition and weight gain will contribute to a better quality of life, both in the short term and in the long term.

ARE YOU UNDERWEIGHT? The popular **Body Mass Index** (BMI), which uses only height and weight to determine normal body weight for all ages and both sexes, has a number of limitations. It does not take into account bone structure; that is, whether you are big-boned, medium-boned, or small-boned. The BMI does not take into account the source of the weight—fat versus muscle. Muscle is heavier than fat, so if you are a trained athlete, your BMI may be normal but you may be "underfat." It does not take into account the natural changes that occur with age, as muscle is lost and body fat is gained.

 Your natural family planning chart gives you better information than your BMI as to whether or not you have adequate body fat for optimum fertility.

If you have normal temperature levels, normal mucus patterns, ovulations that occur somewhere around Days 14 to 18, and normal luteal phase lengths, you probably have adequate body fat, even though you may be quite slender and active. A small-boned woman may have a rather low BMI, but her chart will reveal whether or not her cycles are normal. If, on the other hand, your ovulations are usually delayed, perhaps to Day 20 or more, you may be somewhat "underfat" despite a BMI in the normal range. When this occurs with a normal luteal phase length (twelve to sixteen days), just gaining three to five pounds will very likely cause ovulation to occur sooner.

If your charts are showing a short luteal phase, especially after delayed ovulation, the cause could also be from vigorous exercise, too.[46] Cutting back on exercise and improving your nutrition in order to reduce the stress on your body will almost certainly improve your cycle. Of course, no cycles at all when you are underweight or "underfat" is also good evidence that you need to make changes in your exercise level and your overall food intake to bring your body fat up to normal.

DIETING AND LOSS OF CYCLES

Even women of supposedly "ideal" weight may experience loss of menses or delayed ovulation because they, too, are underweight! I have counseled several women with total amenorrhea for months after sensible weight loss. These women were emphatically not over-dieting. Yet regaining just a few pounds restored the cycle. For example, a young woman who had previously conceived easily consulted me after her physician could offer no explanation for her prolonged **amenorrhea** (loss of periods) of eight months' duration. She had recently lost forty pounds through a sensible diet plan, and she was maintaining her "ideal" weight. I advised her to regain just a few of the lost pounds. In less than three months, after she had regained seven pounds, she conceived the child for whom she had been hoping.

STRATEGIES FOR WEIGHT GAIN

Fortunately, cycle irregularities and infertility caused by low body fat are reversible. One of the most important factors in correcting such cycle problems is simply recognizing the lack of body fat as the cause.

If you love to exercise, you don't need to quit. Instead, cut back on the amount of exercise, or substitute a milder form of exercise so that some of your normal body fat can return. Perhaps you could rest one extra day per week, or shorten the duration of your workouts. Your chart will show your progress, as your cycles will become more normal.

Women who are athletic and have been restricting their food intake to meet athletic goals often are deficient in all the major nutrients, especially dietary fats, including the essential fatty acids, and dietary protein.[47] Review Chapter 1 of this book and make a true effort to eat enough good food to regain your body balance. Be sure to include adequate fat in your diet; for example, whole-fat dairy foods, nuts, and meat that is not overly lean. Those foods will also provide protein, which is needed for both muscle and bone. Starchy vegetables such as white potatoes and sweet potatoes, and grains of every type are also helpful to gaining weight. Try to eat more frequently, perhaps adding healthy snacks in addition to regular meals.

At the same time, make sure that you are getting plenty of good vitamins, minerals, and essential fatty acids through supplements, as recommended in Chapter 3. Athletic women who are underweight are prone to deficiencies of the B vitamins, including vitamin B12 and folate.[48] Bone-building nutrients, including calcium, magnesium, and vitamin D, are particularly important.[49]

Do you tend not to eat if you are stressed? One way of decreasing stress is to get more sleep or at least more rest. See Chapter 4, "Increasing your Energy & Decreasing Your Stress," for more information on managing stress. Finally, if you have an eating disorder such as anorexia, bulimia, or female athlete triad, let those who love you and care for you assist you in finding a compassionate, nutritionally-oriented medical doctor or psychologist.

MEDICAL INTERVENTION FOR INFERTILITY RELATED TO LOW BODY WEIGHT

If you are a thin or athletic woman who is experiencing infertility related to very long cycles, short luteal phases, anovulatory cycles, or amenorrhea, I urge you not to undergo medically-induced ovulation (Clomid or similar medications) until you have gained sufficient body fat through more food and less exercise. You are much more likely to conceive on your own when your body weight and body fat content is normal. Even more important, normal weight gain during pregnancy is vital to a healthy outcome for both mother and baby. Starting at a naturally fertile body weight will help you throughout the pregnancy, especially if you are a woman who finds it difficult to gain weight.

SUMMARY—CHAPTER 8

1 Cycle irregularity and infertility are related as a continuum, and therefore the self care for irregular cycles and infertility is the same.

2 Several common causes of cycle irregularity and infertility may be seen on the chart. Short luteal phase, thyroid problems, and underweight or low body fat all affect the charted signs. It's possible for more than one of these to occur at the same time.

3 Short luteal phase may be improved by the same strategies that are helpful to PMS. Consider the use of Optivite PMT, ProCycle PMS, or Fertility Blend.

4 Low thyroid function (hypothyroidism) can sometimes be improved through better nutrition and supplements. It is common after childbirth, and it sometimes resolves on its own. If improvement occurs, the levels of temperatures will rise, and better mucus and bleeding patterns will occur. In some cases, medical intervention is necessary, and thyroid hormone replacement can restore normal cycles and fertility.

5 While iodine is essential to thyroid function, excess iodine has been implicated in autoimmune thyroiditis. Restaurant food is often highly seasoned with iodized salt, a source of excess iodine to be considered.

6 Hyperthyroidism is much less common than low thyroid function. It is seen on the chart through higher-than-normal basal temperatures. Hyperthyroidism is not likely to respond to nutrition, and medical care is necessary.

7 Underweight or low body fat can delay ovulation, cause short luteal phase, or result in the complete absence of cycles. Often just gaining a few pounds with good diet is enough to improve the cycle. Reducing excessive exercise may be necessary.

9

[He] fills your days with good things, so your youth is renewed like the eagle's.

— Psalms 103:5

POLYCYSTIC OVARY SYNDROME (PCOS) & OVERWEIGHT WITHOUT PCOS

We are currently in the midst of an explosion of interest in and research regarding polycystic ovary syndrome (PCOS). Diet, exercise, vitamins, minerals, and probiotics are now being studied in relationship to this all-too-common hormonal disorder. Equally important, the relationship between PCOS and low thyroid function (hypothyroidism) is a promising area of research. Such research offers real hope and direction for cycle irregularity and infertility related to PCOS.

PCOS, which often but not always occurs with overweight, is the first topic of this chapter. However, you can be overweight or obese without PCOS. Being overweight, even without any tendency to PCOS, can also disrupt the cycle in some but by no means all women, as the second part of this chapter explains.

PCOS

CHART MANIFESTATIONS OF PCOS

Long to very long cycles, often with less-fertile mucus patches interspersed with more-fertile mucus;

short luteal phases (when ovulation does occur)

painful periods

complete lack of cycles

miscarriage

infertility

TABLE 9
POSSIBLE SYMPTOMS OF PCOS AND RELATED HEALTH RISKS

If the basal temperatures are very low (preovulatory temperatures averaging 97.3°F or less), see also "Low Thyroid Function" in Chapter 8. Low thyroid function has been implicated in PCOS.

SYMPTOMS OF PCOS (REPRODUCTIVE)	SYMPTOMS OF PCOS (OTHER)	RELATED RISK FACTORS
Long cycles	Acne	Depression
Anovulatory cycles	Obesity	Non-insulin-dependent diabetes
Amenorrhea	Hirsutism (excess body hair)	Cardiovascular disease
Enlarged ovaries	Carbohydrate intolerance	Elevated blood cholesterol
Infertility		Autoimmune thyroid disease

UNDERSTANDING PCOS

DEFINING PCOS. The simplest way to define **polycystic ovary syndrome**, also known as polycystic ovarian disease (PCOD) is to call it a reproductive dysfunction in which a woman ovulates infrequently or not at all because her ovarian follicles become arrested in their growth and secrete "male" hormones. Many small follicles accumulate on her ovaries—hence the name—causing the ovaries to enlarge. Besides the menstrual cycle disruption due to the arrested follicle development, abdominal obesity and **hirsutism** (a masculine pattern of body hair) are often part of the symptoms.

PCOS tends to begin early in a woman's reproductive years and to continue chronically.

However, PCOS is a complex problem, not an "all or nothing" condition. It may be mild, or it may be severe. A woman can have PCOS and ovulate more or less regularly. She can have PCOS and not be overweight or have hirsutism. She can also have PCOS with or without infertility. It may begin later in her reproductive years rather than earlier. The variation in the severity of the disorder partly explains the variation in the symptoms. Equally as important, a woman can have irregular cycles without PCOS; she can be overweight without PCOS; and she can have hirsutism without PCOS. She can even have cysts on her ovaries due to factors other than this syndrome! For example, PCOS is not at all the same as the single large **follicular cysts** that women of child-bearing age occasionally experience. It's no wonder that PCOS is often unrecognized. Yet women who use natural family planning find it much easier to recognize PCOS.

Despite controversy regarding what actually constitutes the syndrome, a medical consensus statement on the diagnosis of PCOS was created by researchers with expertise in the disease. The diagnosis of PCOS now depends on a woman having at least two of the following three conditions:

(1) Chronic anovulation (cycles without ovulation, infrequent ovulation, or no cycles)

(2) Evidence of elevated "male" hormones, whether through clinical signs such as hirsutism or through blood tests

(3) Multiple small cysts on the ovaries, as confirmed by ultrasound.[1]

Please note that overweight, though very common in PCOS, is not a necessary part of the diagnosis.

UNDERLYING CAUSES OF PCOS

PCOS is a complex hormonal disorder most often characterized by elevated levels of the hormones insulin, LH, and androgens ("male" hormones), all of which contribute to the dysfunction of the ovaries.

LH is necessary to mature the follicle, but abnormal secretion of this hormone, along with and possibly stimulated by elevated insulin, causes the follicles to stop growing prematurely. At the stage of arrested growth, the follicles secrete androgens. These "male" hormones disrupt the cycle further, and cause some women to develop a masculine pattern of hair growth.

INSULIN RESISTANCE. The abnormality in which many of the body's cells decrease in their ability to respond to insulin is called **insulin resistance**, and it is a major factor in PCOS.[2] The receptors for insulin on the cells fail to transmit the vital message that insulin normally signals, which is to allow the cells to admit glucose. To compensate, the pancreas secretes high levels of insulin so that the cells do get their glucose. Some cells still have trouble getting enough glucose, but there is another complicating factor—the high levels of insulin cause other problems, because not all cells become insulin resistant.

Here's an analogy to explain insulin resistance: Imagine that you have to shout to give directions to a crowd of people who are hard of hearing. While that may help those people to respond, your shouting may cause misunderstandings among others around you with normal hearing. Is there an emergency? Should they work harder? Your voice is like the insulin giving directions to the cells. Skeletal muscle cells are known to become insulin resistant, so they may benefit from the high insulin "shouting." But some cells in the ovary do not become insulin resistant, and they respond abnormally to the high insulin levels.[3] This analogy also explains the tendency to weight gain, because fat cells which do not become insulin resistant respond to the high insulin levels by "working harder"—taking in glucose excessively and storing it as fat. And when that happens, the brain cells (which do not need insulin's signal) get deprived of their share of glucose, leading to low blood glucose symptoms of fatigue, brain fog, depression, and craving for food.

HYPOTHYRODISM. New research is "connecting the dots" between PCOS and low thyroid function. Both PCOS and hypothyroidism are common hormonal disorders of women. Low levels of thyroid hormone can indirectly lead to elevated testosterone in women, interfering with the cycle and causing masculinizing symptoms.[4] Both PCOS and hypothyroidism can be related to weight gain, insulin resistance, and immune dysfunction.[5] In a recent case-controlled study of eighty women with PCOS, 22% also had clinically-diagnosed **autoimmune thyroiditis** (versus only 1.25% of controls who did not have PCOS).[6] According to researchers interested in the relationship between PCOS and hypothyroidism, "Polycystic-appearing ovaries are a clinical feature of hypothyroidism, though hypothyroidism should be excluded before diagnosing PCOS disorders."[7]

RISK FACTORS ASSOCIATED WITH PCOS. High insulin levels, insulin resistance, and glucose intolerance are risk factors for a number of other conditions, including abdominal obesity, **non-insulin-dependent diabetes** (type 2 or "adult-onset" diabetes), and high cholesterol levels which predispose to heart disease. These risk factors affect women with PCOS, and they are caused by the insulin resistance and high insulin levels rather than by the irregular or absent cycles. Many researchers now consider PCOS to be one more manifestation of a constellation of conditions such as those just mentioned, all caused by insulin resistance.[8] These conditions are collectively called **metabolic syndrome**.

SELF-HELP STRATEGIES FOR PCOS

There is good news, though, when it comes to PCOS. It responds to lifestyle changes aimed at improving "insulin sensitivity," which is the opposite of insulin resistance. Insulin sensitivity is the normal condition, meaning that the body's cells sense and respond to insulin as they should.

When insulin sensitivity improves, the cells get the glucose they need, and the damaging high levels of insulin naturally drop. It's a "win-win" situation for the entire body.

To understand insulin sensitivity, consider the previous analogy of the hard-of-hearing people. If those people could somehow hear better, they will respond to your directions much better. In turn, you will naturally lower your voice. And the others around you with normal hearing will no longer be confused and overstimulated by your shouting. When insulin sensitivity improves, insulin levels naturally drop, and PCOS improves. The guidelines that follow are helpful to PCOS mainly because they help improve your insulin sensitivity.

1) CONSIDER THE POSSIBILITY OF HYPOTHYROIDISM. Whether or not low thyroid function contributes to PCOS or occurs along with PCOS, the possibility of hypothyroidism should be investigated. Your basal body temperatures are an excellent clue as to your thyroid function, as explained in Chapter 8, under the subtopic "Low Thyroid Function." I have counseled women with symptoms and cycle irregularities typical of PCOS; in many cases the basal temperatures have been quite normal, but in others the temperature patterns were significantly below 97.3°F, even in the range of 96.5°F. Very low temperatures point to low thyroid function.

2) LOSE WEIGHT IF YOU ARE OVERWEIGHT. A key self care step for women with PCOS is to lose weight.[9] Of course losing weight is a struggle for just about everyone who needs to do so, but losing only a modest amount of body weight can significantly improve your cycle regularity and your fertility. For example, a study in Great Britain showed that dropping only 5 percent of body weight resulted in improved cycle regularity in nine of eleven obese women with PCOS, as well as five pregnancies in seven previously infertile women with PCOS. Women who lost less than 5 percent of their body weight showed no such improvement.[10]

Weight loss in obese women improves insulin sensitivity, and insulin levels in fact dropped in the women in this study who lost weight and regained cycle regularity and fertility.[11] Incidentally, a 5 percent weight loss in a 200-pound individual is only a 10-pound loss. Moreover, dropping just a moderate amount of weight also improves other aspects of PCOS: it lowers androgen levels, cholesterol levels, and the number of ovarian cysts.[12]

While losing a modest amount of weight is recommended by virtually all researchers involved with PCOS, there is no consensus as to what kind of weight-loss diet is best. Some researchers have concluded that a high-fiber, moderate protein, healthy-fats diet is the best,[13] while others recommend a diet that is relatively high in protein (at least 40% of calories from protein), because of the effect of protein on suppressing the appetite.[14] An extensive recent review of many research studies has led the reviewers to report "improvements in the majority of reproductive, metabolic, and psychological features of PCOS after weight loss with all dietary compositions evaluated in this review. This indicates weight loss is crucial for improving the presentation of PCOS, regardless of the means of achieving weight loss."[15]

The authors of *The Fertility Diet*, which is based on research from the ongoing Nurses' Health Study, recommend that you use a sensible diet plan that works best for you, whether it is low in fat or low in carbohydrates. The diet plan that helps you to be satisfied with fewer calories is the best one for you.[16] These doctors emphasize avoiding *trans* fats, which increase the risk of ovulatory infertility,[17] including PCOS.[18] They also encourage you to avoid liquid calories (soft drinks and juices), which have the same negative effect.[19] They devote an entire chapter of their book to reviewing popular diet books and plans, and offer their own common-sense, nutritionally-sound weight-loss advice. (See "Further Reading.")

3) AVOID FOODS THAT RAPIDLY ELEVATE BLOOD GLUCOSE LEVELS. High blood glucose levels are the trigger for the secretion of insulin. Some foods and eating patterns stimulate the release of insulin more than others. The **Glycemic Index** is a ranking of foods, based on how rapidly they increase blood sugar levels and therefore insulin. In general, simple sugars and refined starches are highest on the list and should be avoided. Breakfast cereals, bread, rice, white potatoes, and corn are examples. Apples, pears, ice cream, and milk are fairly low in their ability to trigger a release of insulin.[20]

Surprising? In general, refined starches and sugars by themselves will quickly do what you don't want—raise the blood glucose levels. On the other hand, fats, proteins, and fiber slow the digestive processes down, which results in a slower release of glucose into the blood, stimulating less insulin. That explains why ice cream, a food containing quite a bit of sugar, is lower on the Glycemic Index than plain whole wheat bread or brown rice. The protein and fat in ice cream slow the release of the glucose into the blood. Interestingly, the Nurses' Health Study researchers found that one or two servings daily of full-fat dairy, such as ice cream, reduced the risk of ovulatory infertility, including PCOS. They attribute this effect to the natural cow estrogens in the fatty portion of milk products, since cows are often pregnant when milking, and pregnancy is a time of high estrogen production. They observed no such effect with skim milk products.[21]

Should you avoid eating healthy but high-glycemic foods? Not necessarily. Instead, cut down on junk foods such as soft drinks, packaged pastries, fast foods, and candy. Combine healthy whole grains, fruits, and vegetables with foods containing protein and natural fat (for example, cheese, eggs, meat, fish, or nuts). As an example, a baked white potato has a high glycemic index, but eaten with butter or as part of a meal containing meat, its ability to elevate blood sugar is greatly reduced. Review the "Twelve Rules for Better Nutrition" in Part 1 for further information on healthy eating. For more information on the Glycemic Index, go to www.glycemicindex.com.

4) STRICTLY AVOID NUTRASWEET AND OTHER ARTIFICIAL SWEETENERS. Many people were amazed and skeptical when research published in the prestigious medical journal *Circulation* showed that drinking only one soft drink daily, whether sugared or diet, significantly increased the rates of obesity, insulin resistance, and cardiovascular problems related to high insulin levels (metabolic syndrome).[22] Diet drinks alone were evaluated in another large study; again, daily drinking of diet sodas was associated with metabolic syndrome, leading the researchers to conclude that "Diet soda consumption, either independently or in conjunction with other lifestyle behaviors, may lead to weight gain, impaired glucose control, and eventual diabetes."[23] How can diet drinks, which contain virtually no calories, promote weight gain and insulin resistance?

Answers to that question were proposed as long ago as 1990. That year, the distinguished medical consultant H.J. Roberts, M.D., in reviewing the literature and his own clinical experience related to aspartame (NutraSweet), reported that aspartame as well as other artificial sweeteners caused weight gain in some people. He offered several explanations for this paradoxical finding. For example, the very taste of sweetness reflexly triggers insulin release. However, insulin, released in the absence of real, calorie-containing food, abnormally lowers blood glucose levels, which in turn stimulates hunger.[24] Dr. Roberts also referred to research showing that the amino acid phenylalanine, which forms 50 percent of the aspartame molecule, raises the levels of insulin and promotes insulin resistance.[25]

Cutting-edge research recently published in *Nature* shows that artificial sweeteners can unfavorably alter the type of bacteria living in the intestines, and that such "bad" bacteria can produce glucose intolerance in humans.[26] These researchers assert that the use of artificial sweeteners must be reassessed, based on their association with abnormal intestinal bacteria and metabolic disturbances.

---

5) TAKE COMPREHENSIVE VITAMIN, MINERAL, AND ESSENTIAL FATTY ACID SUPPLEMENTS. Because so many nutrients are involved in PCOS and related health issues, a high-quality, comprehensive multivitamin/multimineral along with essential fatty acids and a good probiotic is a basic starting point. ProCycle PMS covers many key nutrients for PCOS: vitamin A, the B group, vitamin C, and optimum amounts of selenium and chromium. (See "Resources" and "Appendix A".) However, you will need to supplement other nutrients along with it.

The B vitamins are central to PCOS self care. The large Nurses' Study provided evidence that multivitamins containing B vitamins, especially folate (in the form of folic acid), reduce the occurrence of ovulatory infertility, including PCOS.[27]

Vitamins B6, B12, and folic acid reduce levels of the amino acid **homocysteine**, which in excess is harmful to cells. Elevated levels of homocysteine are a risk factor for cardiovascular disease and insulin resistance, and homocysteine levels are elevated in women with PCOS.[28] Administration of B-group vitamins reduced homocysteine levels in women receiving **metformin**, a drug that increases insulin sensitivity and is used for treating PCOS.[29]

In another study, supplementing B vitamins reduced homocysteine levels and improved pregnancy rates more than metformin in women with PCOS.[30]

MYO-INOSITOL FOR PCOS

Very large amounts of the B vitamin myo-inositol (also called inositol) have been shown to improve many aspects of PCOS in several studies. In one double-blind trial, insulin sensitivity improved, while insulin levels, testosterone levels, blood pressure, and plasma triglycerides all dropped. These effects occurred after use of 4,000 mg (4 g/day) of myo-inositol was taken daily by women with PCOS for three to four months.[31] In another study, a slightly different form of inositol, D-chiro-inositol (1g/day), was compared to myo-inositol over a six-month period. The smaller amount of D-chiro-inositol had the same positive results as the myo-inositol, except that the D-chiro-inositol lowered testosterone levels more.[32] Myo-inositol has been shown to increase progesterone and decrease prolactin.[33] Four grams per day of myo-inositol also greatly reduced the incidence of gestational diabetes in pregnant women with PCOS.[34] Certainly you should have the approval of your health care professional before using this amount of this vitamin, and it is well to remember that vitamins and minerals work together, not alone.

Vitamin D3 may be especially beneficial to women with PCOS, because low levels of this vitamin correlate with high body weight and with insulin resistance.[35] Low levels of vitamin D may be related to depression in women with PCOS.[36] Getting summer sunshine is wonderful way to get more vitamin D. Light-skinned individuals, though, have to take extra care not to burn, and dark-skinned individuals actually need more sun exposure to make vitamin D3. However, because people wear clothes, work indoors, or live in a northern climate, supplementing vitamin D is necessary for almost everyone. Around 2,000 IU/day is a good range to aim for.

Magnesium (1,000 mg/day), chromium, and vanadium are minerals that are helpful to increase insulin sensitivity. Using the previous analogy, they can be considered natural "hearing aids" which enable the cells to respond normally to insulin. A recent double-blind study on the effects of 200 mcg of chromium daily on insulin levels in women with PCOS resulted in a very significant decrease in insulin levels, and a very significant increase in insulin sensitivity.[37] Dr. Julian Whitaker recommends 30 mg/day of vanadium for help with insulin resistance related to overweight.[38]

The hard-to-get omega-3 fatty acids improve the cells' sensitivity to insulin.[39] EPA (720g/day and DHA (480 g/day), given in capsule form under double-blind conditions for eight weeks, improved blood glucose levels, insulin levels, blood lipids, and levels of an important hormone called **adiponectin**.[40] A similar double-blind study, using slightly less EPA and DHA for eight weeks, also resulted in increased levels of adiponectin.[41] Adiponectin improves insulin sensitivity and has anti-inflammatory effects, and it is often lower than normal in women with PCOS. Adding fish oil (about 5 g/day) may be beneficial to PCOS for more than one reason since fish oil is a rich source of EPA and DHA.

The richest source of the omega-3 essential fatty acid, alpha-linolenic acid, is flax oil. Flax oil, which is a food, can be taken by the spoonful; 1–2 teaspoons per day (5–10 grams; or 5-10 1-gram capsules) is sufficient. You may prefer capsules due to the taste of flax oil; though not particularly unpleasant, most Americans are unaccustomed to it. Cod liver oil (1–2 teaspoons daily), which contains omega-3 fatty acids, vitamin A, and vitamin D may also help with infertility related to PCOS.[42] The antioxidant vitamin E (200-400 IU) is an essential vitamin to take if you supplement the essential fatty acids, as it prevents oxygen damage to these valuable yet fragile molecules.

6) TAKE A GOOD PROBIOTIC SUPPLEMENT. Amazing new research is revealing how profoundly the intestinal bacteria affect overall health, whether for better or for worse. **Gut dysbiosis** refers to an excess of harmful intestinal bacteria or a lack of "friendly" bacteria. Among other negative effects, gut dysbiosis can lead to obesity,[43] and it may be a significant underlying factor in PCOS.[44] When the gut bacteria get out of balance, yeast organisms in the gut can increase abnormally. **Yeast overgrowth** refers to health problems that occur when normally harmless yeast cells get out of control. They can cause infection, allergic reaction, or inflammation due to the toxins they produce. Carolyn Dean, M.D., authored a chapter in *The Yeast Connection and Women's Health* titled, "Understanding the Weight Connection." (See "Further reading.") She makes the case that yeast overgrowth contributes to overweight, especially belly fat that is hard to lose.[45] Taking a good probiotic supplement is a powerful way to improve your **microbiota** (the microscopic organisms in your intestines), increasing the friendly bacteria, which in turn crowd out both bad bacteria and yeast. See "Yeast Overgrowth/Gut Dysbiosis" in Chapter 10 for more information.

7) SERIOUSLY UNDERTAKE A REGULAR EXERCISE PROGRAM. Regular aerobic exercise helps most people to lose weight, but even if exercise does not enable you to lose weight, here is some great news—your insulin sensitivity nevertheless will very likely increase significantly.[46] So don't give up if the weight will not come off as fast or as well as you would like; exercise makes a positive difference even if it does not show on the scales! Brisk walking for half an hour four or five times a week is an example of moderate exercise with beneficial effects on insulin sensitivity. Try combining such brisk walking with taking stairs instead of elevators, parking far away from shop entrances, and other such small but cumulative changes to increase your activity.

 Higher-intensity exercise, including weight-lifting, may make a greater difference to your weight as well as to your insulin sensitivity and overall health, but a gradual start with a routine that fits into your lifestyle is the best way to begin.

Regular exercise has another benefit—it also lowers levels of the harmful homocysteine in women with PCOS. When homocysteine levels decrease, the risk of cardiovascular problems also decreases.[47]

AN ENCOURAGING ANECDOTE. The Couple to Couple League received the following letter a few months after I published an article in their *Family Foundations* magazine regarding nutrition for PCOS. Not every woman will have the quick and dramatic change that this writer did, but many who try the strategies for PCOS suggested above will be pleased with their improved cycles and fertility.

> After more than a year and a half of infertility after discontinuing the pill, I was finally diagnosed with polycystic ovary syndrome in March of this year. My doctor told me that natural conception would be "highly unlikely." My husband and I were very disappointed, since we had no interest in using fertility drugs and were uncertain about adoption. Then I read Marilyn Shannon's article in *Family Foundations* on the role of sugar in relation to ovarian function. I decided to take her advice of taking flax oil capsules and eliminating sugar from my diet. I purchased the book *Get the Sugar Out!* [See "Further Reading."], and was amazed at how much sugar was in my current diet. The book pointed out not only the pitfalls of foods with high amounts of sugars, but also discussed how to eliminate foods that the body quickly converts to sugar, such as foods made with white flour and starches. Upon reading the book, I was amazed to find out how high in sugar my otherwise healthy, low-fat diet truly was.
>
> Within days of beginning my new diet regimen, I ovulated for the first time in years. I was surprised not only that the suggestions were helpful, but also how quickly and dramatically the changes were. I experienced my first thermal shift ever only a matter of days after eliminating sugar from my diet.
>
> My dietary changes not only resulted in ovulation, but also conception as well. My husband and I are both shocked and elated. The baby is due in March and we could not be happier.
>
> Thanks again to CCL for the wonderful nutritional advice for women suffering from PCOS. I am still in disbelief as to how such small changes in my diet made such a dramatic change in my fertility![48]

OVERWEIGHT WITHOUT PCOS

Many women who are significantly overweight have normal cycles and high fertility. In fact, in many cases having several children has contributed to the problem with overweight! On the other hand, overweight, even without the androgens ("male" hormones) and long cycles of PCOS, can be at the root of other cycle problems or infertility.

PCOS OR NOT?

Women who are overweight without PCOS tend to have a "pear-shaped" figure; that is, much of their excess body fat is carried mainly in their hips and thighs. In contrast, overweight women with PCOS usually carry much of their excess body fat around their waist, the so-called "apple" shape. Estrogens are responsible for the pear shape, while androgens promote the apple shape.

PCOS often causes long or very long cycles, and often a masculine pattern of body hair (hirsutism). If you are dealing with a weight problem, body shape, cycle regularity, and whether or not you have a tendency toward hirsutism are all clues as to whether or not PCOS is part of the picture. If you are in doubt, a gynecologist can determine if you have PCOS.

CHART MANIFESTATIONS OF OVERWEIGHT WITHOUT PCOS

Being overweight without having PCOS can cause

short luteal phase

poor mucus patterns

poor temperature rise

amenorrhea or

infertility with or without regular cycles

You might also wish to consider "Luteal Phase Deficiency" in Chapter 8. If your basal temperatures are very low (preovulatory temperatures averaging about 97.3°F or lower), please refer to "Low Thyroid Function" in Chapter 8.

BODY FAT AND HORMONES. Body fat is essential to female fertility. Fat is a metabolically active tissue which produces its own hormones. Body fat converts circulating androgens, which are naturally produced by the adrenal glands, into estrogen. In many women, though, too much body fat contributes to elevated levels of estrogen. Elevated estrogen levels interfere with the function of the corpus luteum, decreasing progesterone. Excess estrogen can also interfere with thyroid function by blocking the receptors within the body cells that respond to thyroid hormone.[49] The slowdown of metabolism that occurs when thyroid function decreases encourages storage of more body fat, which in turn increases estrogen levels more. The problems caused by elevated levels of estrogen, called **estrogen dominance**, have been well documented: weight gain, PMS symptoms, uterine fibroid tumors, fibrocystic breasts, and a higher risk of breast cancer.[50] As you can probably guess, losing weight is an important strategy to limit estrogen dominance.

WEIGHT-LOSS DIETS FOR OBESITY. A consensus as to which type of diet plan is best to lose weight is finally developing, after years of debate. That consensus is this: the type of diet that is most helpful to *you* is the best diet for *you*. Almost every informed person agrees that no matter whether you emphasize more animal protein or more vegetables and fiber, whole natural foods are far preferable to sugary foods, refined starches, or foods containing the damaging *trans* fats.

Even though you may have overweight without PCOS, the strategies numbered in the previous topic, "PCOS," are applicable to you as well. Even myo-inostiol has been shown to restore cycles and increase progesterone in some women who are overweight without PCOS.[51]

NUTRITIONAL SUPPLEMENTS. Because estrogen dominance is related to overweight without PCOS, look for nutritional supplements that are aimed at increasing progesterone levels and decreasing estrogen levels. The supplements listed for PMS in Chapter 6 may be most helpful to you. These include Optivite PMT, ProCycle PMS, or Fertility Blend. |I especially prefer ProCycle PMS, as it contains 200 mcg of chromium. Chromium helps with the problem of insulin resistance, which also affects overweight women without PCOS. For a list of ingredients of all of these, see Appendix A. Add flax oil (about 5–10 g/day) and/or fish oil (5 g[1 teaspoon]daily).

SOME NOTES ABOUT INFERTILITY. If you are overweight and are having difficulty becoming pregnant, be careful to lose weight slowly with wholesome nutrition and regular exercise. Attempt to overcome hypoglycemia and sugar cravings with regularly timed meals of whole plant and animal foods (see Chapter 1) and appropriate supplements (see Table 7, Chapter 3). As is true of overweight women with PCOS, you should not despair of losing all the weight necessary to attain your "ideal" weight, but should just set a modest goal, such as ten pounds. Finally, you and your husband should not overlook less obvious factors that may also contribute to your infertility. Please see Appendix B, "Focus on Infertility," for other self care suggestions to improve your chances of conceiving.

SUMMARY—CHAPTER 9

1 Polycystic ovary syndrome (PCOS) is one manifestation of a constellation of hormonal and metabolic dysfunctions which are related to insulin resistance, the body's inability to respond properly to the hormone insulin.

2 PCOS may be related to or may occur along with hypothyroidism.

3 PCOS affects the reproductive hormones, so it is diagnosed through any two of the following: (1) irregular or absent cycles, (2) evidence of excess "male" hormones, and/or (3) enlarged or polycystic ovaries.

4 PCOS may be improved by weight loss, dietary modifications, vitamin, mineral, essential fatty acid, and probiotic supplements, along with a regular program of exercise. Avoiding artificial sweeteners is a recommended strategy.

5 While overweight is often associated with PCOS, overweight without PCOS can also disrupt the cycle. In cases in which the excess weight is carried more in the hips and thighs, as opposed to the belly, it may contribute to excess estrogen.

6 Weight loss on a healthy diet may be very helpful, but women with overweight without PCOS should look for signs of low thyroid function and short luteal phase on their charts, and address these issues directly as well.

OTHER FACTORS THAT MAY AFFECT CYCLE REGULARITY OR FERTILITY

10

> But the Lord said to Abraham: "Why did Sarah laugh and say, 'Will I really bear a child, old as I am?' Is anything too marvelous for the Lord to do?"
>
> — Genesis 18:13-14

The two previous chapters dealt with hormonal or other problems that are well known to affect cycle regularity or fertility. Luteal phase deficiency, thyroid dysfunction, underweight, PCOS, and overweight can all do so. When they do, it's usually in a predictable way. For example, a slender, athletic woman can expect to see a delay in ovulation if she loses excess body fat. A woman with a tendency to hirsutism and overweight can suspect that PCOS is contributing to her long cycles and irregular mucus patterns. Very low body temperatures with irregular mucus patterns lead you to consider whether low thyroid function might be involved. Poor temperature rise with only a few days of elevated temperatures indicate luteal phase deficiency.

However, there are a number of less obvious factors that may affect your cycles or your fertility, and they are worth investigating if you are having problems with either. This is especially true if your chart or body weight doesn't help you judge what might be the problem. But even if your chart suggests underweight, low thyroid, or so forth, some of the factors described below might also be involved.

YEAST OVERGROWTH/GUT DYSBIOSIS

"You're not going through life alone!" That's the way microbiologists like to introduce their students to the microorganisms, mostly bacteria, that live within the human digestive tract, respiratory tract, skin, and vagina. The study of the human microbiota, as these organisms are collectively called, took a huge step forward in 2007, when the National Institute of Health instituted the Human Microbiome Project, an initiative whose goal has been to genetically identify the thousands of types of microbes which inhabit the human body. The spin-off of this research is boosting our understanding of health and disease in unexpected ways, even, for example, correlating the type of bacteria in a woman's intestines with her risk of breast cancer, with obesity, and with the health of her pregnancies.[1] The microbiota is involved in the development of the immune system and in inflammation. While an individual's genetics, age, and sex are unchangeable factors which affect the health of the microbiome, diet and medications are controllable factors that even more profoundly affect the microbiota.

In short: healthy nutrition and lifestyle choices can improve the microbiota, and can positively affect your fertility, your pregnancies, your body weight, and even your risk of cancer.

Awareness of gut dysbiosis, or the wrong type of organisms in the intestines, expanded greatly when the late William Crook, M.D., authored *The Yeast Connection* in 1983. He wrote that several health problems of women may be related to yeast organisms in the digestive tract which cause infection, allergic reactions, or toxic reactions.

Reproductive problems related to yeast overgrowth that Dr. Crook named included PMS, vaginal infections, and vulvodynia (genital pain in women), low thyroid function, endometriosis, low sexual desire, pain with intercourse, overweight, and female infertility, as well as chronic prostatitis in men. He named use of the birth control pill as a risk factor for yeast problems in women.

Throughout several editions of the book, spanning nearly twenty years, Dr. Crook continued to make his case, yet he was always careful to state that yeast overgrowth, or **candidiasis**, as it is more formally called, was not necessarily the actual cause of any of these reproductive problems, but that yeast might very well be an important contributing factor.[2]

The research published since the Human Microbiome Project began makes it plain that yeast organisms aren't the only source of gut problems. The wrong types of bacteria, or not enough of the right types, can also create digestive system problems that in turn affect the entire body.

But even if yeast is not actually at the root of the problems mentioned above, the diet that Dr. Crook and other "yeast-aware" health professionals recommend will certainly help you to improve your health. It will help you replace bad gut bacteria with friendly bacteria. It will increase the value of the food you eat, because it eliminates most sugar and emphasizes whole, natural foods. It will help you to discover hidden allergies that might be involved in your health issues. And the recommended nutritional supplements will help you to overcome deficiencies that may or may not be related to yeast overgrowth.

SYMPTOMS. Yeast overgrowth or gut dysbiosis may be involved with reproductive problems in both sexes. But the symptoms of yeast overgrowth go well beyond problems of reproduction, and they may also occur in children. They include the symptoms summarized in Table 10.[3]

TABLE 10
Symptoms of Yeast Overgrowth

REPRODUCTIVE SYMPTOMS	OTHER SYMPTOMS
Vaginal infections	Extreme fatigue or lethargy (the feeling of being drained)
Premenstrual Syndrome (PMS)	Depression
Vulvodynia (genital pain in women)	Inability to concentrate
Low thyroid function	Headaches
Endometriosis	Skin problems (such as hives, athlete's foot)
Low sexual desire	Gastrointestinal problems (especially constipation, abdominal pain, diarrhea, gas or bloating)
Pain with intercourse	Muscular and nervous system symptoms (including aching or swelling in your muscles and joints, numbness, burning or tingling)
Overweight	Respiratory symptoms
Female infertility	Hyperactivity and recurrent ear problems [in children][2]
Chronic prostatitis in men	

In women, repeated vaginal yeast infections are a major sign of this disorder, but it is possible to have yeast overgrowth without such infections.

Its symptoms also overlap with those of PMS, though yeast overgrowth is not as closely related to the cycle as is PMS. The strong link to reproductive dysfunction in women makes this disorder worth investigating if you feel inexplicably unwell over a prolonged period, or if you are having trouble overcoming the reproductive problems which have been associated with yeast overgrowth.

If you have enough of the symptoms listed above to believe that yeast might be involved with your health problems, the next step is to get a copy of *The Yeast Connection and Women's Health* by Dr. Crook and Dr. Carolyn Dean, M.D., who has continued Dr. Crook's work. Or, you can go to Dr. Dean's website, www.yeastconnection.com. Score yourself using the yeast questionnaire, which covers these symptoms in detail. If your score puts you in the "probable" or "almost certain" class, you will very likely be helped by an anti-yeast diet and supplements.

HOW YEAST CAUSES PROBLEMS. Yeast overgrowth occurs when the common and usually harmless fungus, *Candida albicans*, reproduces excessively within the body. It may invade body tissues, as it does in vaginal yeast infections and in oral thrush, but it may also make trouble by causing allergic reactions. Toxins that the yeast produce may contribute to inflammation. Yeast overgrowth contributes to **leaky gut syndrome**, a descriptive name that refers to intestinal walls inflamed because of yeast or other factors. Whole undigested food molecules can be absorbed through the leaky gut into the blood, triggering allergic reactions. Because of this relationship, controlling yeast overgrowth may benefit individuals with allergies.

LIFESTYLE CAUSES. What causes the normally harmless *Candida albicans* to get out of hand in the gut? The chief predisposing factors involved in yeast overgrowth are listed in Table 11, in the approximate order of importance:

TABLE 11
Possible Causes of Yeast Overgrowth[4]

Use of antibiotics, which kill the normal, healthy bacteria that live in the intestines, where they naturally discourage yeast. Long-term use of tetracycline for adolescent acne in particular can set the stage for yeast overgrowth.

A diet which is high in sugary and starchy foods, including sweet fruits. Sugar feeds yeast organisms.

Use of oral contraceptives (birth control pills), or other hormonal birth control. The synthetic estrogen and progestogens in birth control pills cause changes in the vaginal wall which allow yeast to multiply more rapidly, causing vaginal yeast infections.

Use of cortisone and related drugs (prednisone, for example). Because these drugs by design suppress the immune response for therapeutic purposes, the immune system may be less able to keep yeast under control.

Hormonal fluctuations in women, including those of the menstrual cycles or those of pregnancy.

LIFESTYLE STRATEGIES FOR YEAST OVERGROWTH. Getting off antibiotics if at all possible, getting off the birth control pill, and getting off other steroid medications such as cortisone or prednisone will get you started on the right track. If you are on antibiotics for acne, please see "Acne" in Chapter 16, "Questions & Answers, Part 2." Could you substitute nonsteroid anti-inflammatory drugs (NSAIDs) for steroid anti-inflammatory medications? For safe and highly effective natural birth control, please contact the Couple to Couple League for Natural Family Planning, the publishers of this book, to learn how to use the Sympto-Thermal Method (www.ccli.org).

NUTRITION FOR YEAST OVERGROWTH. Improved nutrition is the next major line of defense against yeast overgrowth. Anti-yeast nutrition works on the principles of cutting off the yeast's food supply (sugar and refined starches), reducing the intake of yeast-containing foods, re-establishing healthy bacteria in the intestines to naturally crowd out the yeast, and providing the body with excellent nutrition to decrease inflammation and to bolster the immune system.

There's a good analogy to help understand yeast overgrowth: Friendly bacteria are like grass; they naturally grow in the intestines like grass on a healthy lawn. Of course, like grass, they need some maintenance. Yeast organisms and bad bacteria are like weeds, unnecessary but harmless in small numbers. If, though, the grass is burned out or otherwise damaged or destroyed, what grows back first? The weeds, of course, and without the healthy grass to crowd them out, they take over. That's yeast overgrowth, or gut dysbiosis caused by bad bacteria. Taking in friendly bacteria in supplement form or eating high-quality yogurt is like planting grass seed. This is especially important after taking antibiotics, which "burn out" the good bacteria as well as the bad. Eating sugary foods and taking steroid drugs such as oral contraceptives and cortisone is like feeding the weeds! Eating foods which support gut health and taking vitamins, minerals, and essential fatty acids is like fertilizing the lawn; good nutrition promotes the friendly bacteria so that they crowd out the bad bacteria and yeast organisms, keeping them at a harmless level. Seed, weed, and feed![5]

DIET. Most important is sharply reducing sugary, processed foods, white flour, and sweets such as honey and maple syrup. Avoid artificial sweeteners, since they promote the wrong type of bacteria in some people.[6] Emphasize foods that feed healthy bacteria. Such foods, called **prebiotics** are fiber-rich plant foods, especially those rich in soluble fiber: sweet potatoes, garlic, flax seed, onions, asparagus, and Jerusalem artichoke. The fiber of other vegetables and beans feeds a healthy microbiome as well. Unless your yeast problem is severe, whole grains and not-too-sweet fruits can be used in moderation.

ALLERGENS. At the same time, look for food allergies that might be increasing inflammation; many people with yeast problems have both known and unrecognized food allergies. The most common food allergies are to dairy products, wheat, corn, eggs, and fish. Broad elimination diets are helpful if you are not sure if you are allergic to various foods. For example, you can strictly avoid all dairy products and all grains for a month or more and note the results. Do you feel better? If so, you begin to add back various foods until you find the trigger foods that may be causing allergic reactions. The books recommended at the end of this section have more specific information on how to eliminate foods and equally as important, how and when to reintroduce them. By the way, many individuals with yeast problems are also sensitive to airborne allergens, such as mold in damp rooms. Because of this, treating the yeast may help with chronic sinus inflammation.

FRIENDLY BACTERIA SUPPLEMENTS. Probiotics is the term for friendly bacteria that are taken as supplements to "reseed" your intestines. Friendly bacteria not only crowd out the yeast, but they also crowd out unfriendly, disease-causing bacteria involved in gut dysbiosis. **Bifidobacterium** and **Lactobacillus** are examples of friendly bacteria available in supplement form. Look for a brand containing a mix of live bacteria, with numbers of live organisms listed as several billion per tablet or capsule. Tablets or capsules coated so that the bacteria survive the stomach acid are preferable.

WHAT IF YOU MUST TAKE AN ANTIBIOTIC?

Supplementing probiotics if you must take an antibiotic is one of the most effective ways of preventing yeast overgrowth related to antibiotic use. Take the probiotic supplements daily during the time that you are taking the antibiotic, if possible three hours or more before or after you take the antibiotic. Take the probiotic faithfully for at least several days after using the antibiotic.

Probiotics promote health in a number of ways. They reduce inflammation in the gut. They help prevent vaginal yeast infections and even bladder infections.[7] They enable the liver to rid the body of toxins more effectively. This includes helping the liver to get rid of excess estrogen, a most beneficial function.[8] Lowering levels of estrogen may be the chief reason that treating yeast overgrowth improves female reproductive function.

VITAMINS, MINERALS, AND ESSENTIAL FATTY ACIDS. Magnesium, vitamin B6, zinc, and essential fatty acids such as those found in cod liver oil and flax oil may prevent candidiasis or promote healing of it. Vitamin A is also useful. Multivitamins and minerals in amounts quite similar to those in Table 7 (Chapter 3) are also recommended by Dr. Crook and Dr. Carolyn Dean.[9]

HERBAL REMEDIES. A number of herbal remedies are helpful, including grapefruit seed extract (500 mg three times daily),[10] which is safe for pregnant and nursing mothers, babies, and children. Oregano extract (200 mg/day)[11] is another excellent choice to reduce yeast problems. Other herbal remedies are available at health food shops.

Diet and supplements alone may control moderate cases of yeast, but severe overgrowth may require management with anti-candida drugs prescribed by a "yeast-aware" medical doctor. To use the previous analogy, such drugs are like herbicides which specifically target the weeds while sparing the grass.

For completely documented but concise information on this subject, refer to "Chronic Candidiasis" in *The Encyclopedia of Natural Medicine*, revised 3rd ed., by Michael Murray, N.D., and Joseph Pizzorno, N.D. Dr. William Crook and Dr. Carolyn Dean's *The Yeast Connection and Women's Health* has a more informal tone, but deals more extensively with women's reproductive health than any other source. If yeast is a concern to you, it will help you with every aspect of recovery, from the initial restricted elimination diet to weight loss to maintenance of your health. Dr. Jacob Teitelbaum's *Beat Sugar Addiction Now!* treats sugar cravings as a manifestation of yeast overgrowth, and has concise, practical advice on how to overcome it by overcoming yeast overgrowth. I especially like his step-by-step, day-by-day, multiple foods elimination diet (See "Further Reading" and www.yeastconnection.com.)

DISCONTINUING BIRTH CONTROL PILLS OR OTHER HORMONAL BIRTH CONTROL

Congratulations on your decision to discontinue birth control pills or other hormonal contraceptives! You have taken a giant step toward better health. As hormone specialist Diana Schwarzbein, M.D., has written, you cannot achieve optimum hormonal balance while you are on the pill, because hormones interact with each other.[12] Some of the problems that you may have experienced while on the pill include mood swings, weight gain, breast tenderness, and scant menses or absent periods.

On the other hand, when you discontinue birth control pills, your body may have to go through a period of readjustment to its own natural hormones. Coming off the pill or other artificial hormones used for contraception may be followed by delayed ovulation, a pattern of constant less-fertile mucus, and heavy menses. As an NFP instructor, I have seen many charts from women who have recently discontinued hormonal birth control. My experience has been that about half of them have very regular cycles immediately after coming off the pill, whereas the other half have one, two, or three irregular cycles of adjustment, especially cycles with poor mucus patterns.

DIET AND SUPPLEMENTS FOR BETTER CYCLES POST-PILL

 Many women who are coming off the pill view it as an opportunity to improve their health generally.

Whether or not your cycles are immediately regular, why not read through Part 1 of this book and consider general dietary improvements? Eating more fresh whole foods, reducing your intake of sugary treats, and avoiding artificial sweeteners are good places to start. Use the 80-20 rule (Rule 12 in Chapter 1) so that you don't get discouraged. Aim for improvement, not perfection!

When it comes to vitamins, minerals, and essential fatty acids, research evidence shows that oral contraceptive users have a significant decrease in vitamin B12[13] and folate,[14] vitamin B6[15], vitamin E, and beta-carotene levels in their blood.[16] They have a significant decrease in the essential fatty acids and in the healthy EPA.[17] They have an increase in vitamins A and D, which drop once the pill is discontinued.[18] Use of the pill is also associated with higher levels of the "bad" LDL cholesterol levels and lower levels of the "good" HDL cholesterol.[19]

Dr. Ellen Grant, a British medical doctor who formerly conducted research on the birth control pill but who now considers them unsafe, recommends zinc, magnesium, essential fatty acids, vitamin E, and B vitamins for those recovering from pill use.[20] Any of the multivitamin/multimineral brands suggested in Chapter 3 contain the zinc, magnesium, B vitamins and vitamin E recommended by Dr. Grant. Professional Pre-Natal Formula, ProCycle PMS, or Optivite all come close to "covering all the bases," but if you choose to use Optivite, you may wish to include extra folate or folic acid, at least 400–800 mcg in addition to the 200 mcg in the full dose. (See "Appendix A" and "Resources.") Cod liver oil contains the fatty acid EPA as well as vitamins A and D, which both drop after the pill is discontinued. Fish oil also has positive effects on blood cholesterol composition.

IMPROVING OTHER PILL-RELATED PROBLEMS

The pill worsens PMS in some women. It has been associated with yeast overgrowth. Chapter 6 covers strategies to overcome PMS, and "Yeast Overgrowth/Gut Dysbiosis" is discussed in this chapter. If you were on the pill to lighten heavy bleeding or to reduce menstrual cramping, you will find very effective natural answers to these problems in Chapter 7. If you were on the pill to "regulate" your cycle, try referring to the section on low thyroid function, underweight, overweight, or other relevant sections of Chapters 8 and 9 to get to the root cause of your cycle irregularities. If you have been using the pill in an attempt to overcome acne, you may be interested to read Chapter 9, which covers polycystic ovary syndrome (PCOS). The high levels of "male" hormones typical of PCOS are a major trigger for acne. See also Chapter 16, "Questions & Answers: Part 2" for nutrition to help overcome acne.

SENSITIVITY TO NIGHT LIGHTING

When I was a first-year graduate student, I worked in a lab dedicated to understanding the pineal gland and its major hormone, **melatonin**. The graduate students investigated the link between day length, light-dark cycles, and reproductive readiness in birds, frogs, snakes, and lizards. In these animals, the pineal gland serves as the biological coordinator between the day length and the ability of the animal to reproduce at the most favorable time of year. Most vertebrates, including humans, produce the hormone melatonin from the pineal gland in response to changes in light and darkness.

In many animals as well as in humans, when light hits the eyes, it sends a neural message to the pineal gland, located within the brain, which decreases the production of melatonin. Oppositely, when it is dark, melatonin rises rapidly.

In many mammals, birds, and reptiles, naturally high levels of melatonin inhibit the reproductive hormones. That explains why birds cannot reproduce in the fall and winter when the days are short and the nights are long; their melatonin levels are high, inhibiting reproduction. It explains why, as the day length increases and the nights grow shorter, birds regain their reproductive capability and are able to mate and produce young in the spring. The longer day length reduces the production of melatonin.

WOMEN AND MELATONIN. What about human beings? Since humans are capable of reproducing all year around, it's clear that day length is not the chief factor in human fertility. Yet ongoing research is investigating whether melatonin levels affect cycle regularity and fertility in women.[21]

 When human beings are in a very dark environment, melatonin levels rise rapidly.

When light, even dim light, hits the eyes, it reduces melatonin output. Bright light does so better than dim light, so that light reduces melatonin output in a "dose-dependent" fashion—more light, less melatonin. The increase in melatonin in the dark seems to be one reason why it's easier to sleep in the dark than in the light, since melatonin promotes sleep.[22]

Is melatonin pro- or anti-fertility in women? Accumulating research suggests that the right amount promotes fertility, whereas either too much or too little can inhibit the fertility cycle. For example, in women who are physically stressed by intense exercise or anorexia nervosa (the disordered eating pattern that results in underweight), cycle irregularities such as delayed ovulation, short luteal phases, anovulatory cycles, and complete absence of cycles occur. In such women, melatonin levels are abnormally high and prolonged during the night. In Finnish women who live relatively close to the North Pole, where winter nights are extremely long, winter melatonin levels are high and LH (the hormone of ovulation) levels are low.[23]

Conversely, though, since artificial lighting is an integral part of modern life, many women may have too *little* melatonin for optimal reproductive health. A number of studies have shown that women who work night shifts are more prone to breast cancer compared to women who work day shifts. Night shift work tends to reduce melatonin levels, since people work with the lights on. Melatonin is a powerful antioxidant in itself, but there is another link. When melatonin is too low, estrogen rises.[24] Interestingly, nighttime melatonin levels naturally fall during premenopause and remain at their lowest levels in women after menopause.[25] This may explain the decrease in sleep quality that many women experience after menopause.

NIGHT LIGHTING AND NFP. Since 1976, Joy DeFelice, R.N., director of the Natural Family Planning Program at Sacred Heart Medical Center, Spokane, Washington, has studied the effect of eliminating nighttime illumination on the menstrual cycle and on fertility in women who use NFP. She has found that eliminating light from the sleeping area can improve cycle irregularity and infertility. Women who have carefully reduced night lighting in their bedrooms have experienced improvement in their cycle lengths, their bleeding patterns, their mucus patterns, and their temperature patterns, including longer, more normal luteal phases. Such changes generally occur within three menstrual cycles of reduced night lighting. Pregnancy among couples previously experiencing infertility has been achieved following elimination of night lighting, and early miscarriage rates have been reduced by eliminating night lighting while sleeping.[26]

Do you wonder how small amounts of light at night can adversely affect a woman's fertility? Light rays are quite capable of penetrating the eyelids, and in dim light, the retina is exquisitely sensitive even to very low levels of illumination. A special neural route from the eyes sends information about lighting to the pineal gland, reducing melatonin. Getting rid of the light increases melatonin, and sufficient melatonin increases progesterone levels,[27] which may be a major factor in the results Mrs. DeFelice reports.

PRACTICAL CONSIDERATIONS. For most women, the sources of night illumination in the bedroom are easily identified and controlled.

> Smart phones, tablets, laptops and computer screens end up in the bedroom all too often, so make it a point to get them out, at least an hour before bedtime.

Hall lights, digital clocks, street lights, headlights, moonlight, and so forth need to be dealt with. An irregular bedtime does not seem to be a factor in this phenomenon, provided the woman receives sufficient hours of darkness, and getting up in dim light for short periods to care for a child or to use the bathroom does not disrupt the protocol.[28]

In rare cases, women who do not show improved menstrual cycles after three cycles of night darkness may respond to a temporary regimen of reduced night lighting during all nights except for three nights of low to moderate illumination. These three nights begin two days after more-fertile mucus begins. However, for those who have recently discontinued birth control pills, have experienced a miscarriage, are ending the natural infertility of breastfeeding, or are bottle-feeding a new baby, Mrs. DeFelice does not recommend the regimen of three nights with lighting, but only the constant night darkness. In these situations, the cycles should be allowed to "settle down" on their own for six months before trying the temporary addition of night lighting.[29]

NUTRITION AND MELATONIN. Caffeine reduces melatonin, and caffeine plus night lighting profoundly reduces melatonin.[30] Since melatonin is a natural sleep aid, this may account for what you have probably observed—caffeine late in the afternoon or evening disrupts your sleep. The effect of caffeine on melatonin may also help to explain the effect of caffeine consumption on pregnancy achievement and miscarriage, discussed in the topic that follows.

Supplements of niacin (100 mg), vitamin B6 (75 mg), magnesium (500 mg), and calcium (1,000 mg) are recommended by Julian Whitaker, M.D., author of *Health and Healing* (see "Further Reading") in order to boost the natural production of melatonin.[31]

It is possible to purchase supplements of melatonin at most pharmacies. At least one study suggests that supplements of melatonin of 1 to 3 mg may be beneficial to infertile women.[32] However, in young women in their fertile years (under age 40), the best way to increase melatonin is to do as Mrs. DeFelice's studies have indicated—get rid of night lighting. Besides melatonin, the pineal secretes other factors which might also be a valuable part of the observed effect of reduced night light. For women in perimenopause and afterward who are interested in better sleep only, the same advice holds. However, if three months of careful elimination of night lighting have not improved your sleep, you may wish to try melatonin supplements, as suggested in the question and answer on this subject in Chapter 4. If you do wish to use melatonin supplements, especially if you are trying to achieve a pregnancy or are breastfeeding, seek the counsel of your healthcare practitioner.

OTHER FACTORS THAT AFFECT MELATONIN. Melatonin levels can be affected by some drugs, including nonsteroidal anti-inflammatory agents, steroids, some anti-depressants, beta blockers, calcium channel blockers, and tobacco. Alcohol early in the evening may decrease melatonin, but right before bed may increase it.[33] Exposure to natural daytime sunshine, which decreases melatonin production, may actually cause melatonin to "rebound" at night, a positive effect.

Mrs. DeFelice has published a booklet, "The Effects of Light on the Menstrual Cycle: Also Infertility, Clinical Observations," that explains why and how to eliminate night lighting in order have more regular cycles and improved fertility (see "Further Reading"). Will it work for you? People vary considerably; for example, many women have regular cycles and normal fertility despite the presence of night lighting.

> **You will not know whether or not your menstrual cycles will improve in response to reduced night lighting unless you give it a try.**

If nothing else, though, carefully making your bedroom very dark will probably improve your sleep. Enough rest has many benefits!

Keep in mind that sleep, facilitated as it is by darkness and melatonin, is a basic physical need that cannot be replaced with better nutrition. Likewise, higher melatonin levels and improved sleep cannot make up for poor nutrition. Diet, exercise, and stress should be considered as well as night lighting when cycle irregularities or infertility occur. I have been disappointed to see NFP clients work hard to eliminate night lighting from their bedroom without removing junk food from their kitchen!

CAFFEINE CONSUMPTION

Whether or not caffeine consumption affects fertility has been a controversial topic for quite some time. As long ago as 1988, a systematic study concluded that women who used more than the equivalent of one cup of coffee per day took significantly longer to conceive than did those who used less, and high caffeine users experienced longer delays in conceiving than did lower level users.[34] This finding was quickly confirmed by other researchers who studied large numbers of women.[35] However, other studies have found no such relationship.[36]

The issue of caffeine consumption and fertility is again timely due to a large, well-designed more recent study that found that more than 200 mg of caffeine daily, the amount in two average cups of coffee, increased the risk of miscarriage.[37] This new information is relevant to any woman who is hoping to become pregnant.

COULD THIS BE YOU? I once counseled a woman who was experiencing secondary infertility of about eighteen months. I suggested that she cut out sugar and caffeine, eat nutritiously, and try to drop a few pounds, as she was somewhat overweight. She conceived two months later and reported that the only change she had made was to reduce her coffee consumption from six or seven mugs per day to one or one and a half cups daily. She also reported that in the year previous to conception, her cycles had become longer and longer, causing her, a non-NFP user, the inconvenience of repeated pregnancy testing.

If you are astounded that anyone could consume so much coffee, you are probably not a caffeine "addict;" if you didn't bat an eye, perhaps you should cut down on your caffeine! This is true even if you are not presently experiencing any direct adverse effects.

Heavy caffeine users may be attempting to overcome fatigue related to hypoglycemia. Emphasis on the B vitamins, especially folate (or folic acid; about 2,000 mcg/day of either), is helpful. Your meals and snacks should contain a mix of protein, complex carbohydrates, and natural fats. Limiting sweet treats as much as possible is another great help to overcoming low blood glucose.

TEA DRINKING

There is one surprising finding when caffeine consumption has been studied for its effect on fertility: Consumption of tea has been associated with an *increase* in fertility. Tea generally contains considerably less caffeine than coffee or sodas. In addition, it contains "polyphenols" which are healthy to the chromosomes. It's also possible that tea drinkers have a generally healthier lifestyle than others, according to the researchers who observed this relationship.[38] And some types of tea, such as green tea, are particularly rich in antioxidants, which contribute to fertility.

If you are experiencing cycle irregularity or any type of infertility, I recommend that you reduce caffeine-containing foods, drugs, and beverages to the equivalent of two cups of coffee per day. More information on caffeine is contained in Rule 7 and Table 6, in Chapter 1. Caffeine consumption also lowers melatonin levels, especially when illumination levels are high. You may wish to refer to the previous section, "Sensitivity to Night Lighting."

CELIAC DISEASE/GLUTEN INTOLERANCE

Once thought to be a rare disease that began in childhood, celiac disease is now estimated to affect at least one in 100 people worldwide, and many adults with it go undiagnosed.

Celiac disease is now recognized as a cause of cycle irregularity, infertility, recurrent miscarriage, low birth weight babies, and preterm birth.[39]

This genetically-determined disease is caused by a specific intolerance to gluten, a protein found in wheat, rye, and barley, and in oats which are processed on equipment that has been used for these grains. In individuals with celiac disease, even tiny amounts of gluten cause a reaction in the small intestinal wall that results in inflammation mediated by antibodies. Inflammation in this vital organ damages it, leading to the inability to absorb nutrients from food properly, thus causing nutritional deficiencies that impact the entire body.

SYMPTOMS. Untreated celiac disease can cause digestive upsets, including nausea, abdominal pain, diarrhea, and constipation. It often leads to weight loss. Anemia is an important problem that can occur with it,[40] perhaps because so many vitamins and minerals are needed to make red blood cells. It may cause the feeling of being "tired all over," as well as irritability or mood swings. On the other hand, in some people it may produce few symptoms, but it can affect fertility.[41]

Even once it is treated, celiac disease may underlie cycle irregularity and unexplained infertility, which may be related to the multiple nutritional deficiencies that occur as a result of damage to the small intestine. The awareness of celiac disease as a possible cause of infertility has greatly increased, but if you have any doubt as to whether or not you may have this disease, you should request medical tests to diagnose it.

DIET FOR CELIAC DISEASE. There is effective treatment for celiac disease. It is the absolute and lifelong avoidance of wheat, rye, and barley, any foods containing them, as well as avoidance of oats, which apparently are often contaminated by wheat dust when processed. When gluten is strictly avoided, over time the inflammation of the intestinal wall subsides.

If tests show that you have celiac disease, you will need a dietitian's assistance to help you become aware of which foods you can eat and which you cannot, as many processed and restaurant foods contain gluten. It will be an adjustment, but your newfound health and vitality will motivate you to continue to avoid gluten as is necessary to control the disease. There are many, many whole natural foods that you can eat: meat, poultry, fish, milk, eggs, fruits, vegetables, beans, nuts, and even grains such as corn and rice. And you have no doubt observed, it's become easy to obtain gluten-free alternative foods such as gluten-free cake mixes, even in ordinary grocery stores.

As your health improves on a gluten-free diet, gaining weight if you have been underweight will improve your cycle regularity. However, weight gain alone may not be sufficient to restore optimal health, ideal cycles, and fertility. Overcoming vitamin and mineral deficiencies related to damage to the intestinal wall is a key step in improving cycle regularity and fertility in women with celiac disease.

VITAMINS, MINERALS, AND OTHER SUPPLEMENTS. Harvard School of Public Health researchers Drs. Chavarro and Willett, in *The Fertility Diet*, hypothesize that even when gluten is strictly avoided, past damage to the intestinal wall results in ongoing deficiencies of folate, iron, vitamin D, vitamin K, and other micronutrients that are involved with fertility. They offer evidence that the infertility that may occur with celiac disease is somehow related to low levels of the B vitamins folate and vitamin B12. They summarize published anecdotes of women with untreated celiac disease and infertility who became pregnant soon after taking large doses of folic acid daily.[42]

Vitamin, mineral, and essential fatty acid supplements are especially valuable if you are trying to overcome cycle irregularity and infertility. It is quite easy to find supplements labeled "gluten free." However, it is important to start to take supplements slowly, so that they help to heal, not to irritate, your small intestinal wall. The assistance of a nutritionally-oriented physician is a must as you begin supplements.

Ideally, you would take all supplements as listed in Chapter 3. Whether or not you are actually able to do so depends on the health of your intestines and on your doctor's recommendations. If you are dealing with infertility, folate (folic acid) in the amount of 2,000-4,000 mcg per day may be especially helpful, and is safe and beneficial during pregnancy. Vitamin B12 (1,000 –2,000 mcg/day) and zinc (15–30 mg/day) also assist folate in its beneficial effects on fertility, and are helpful in achieving pregnancy.

RELATED CONSIDERATIONS. As you consider your chart, look for specific signs of cycle irregularity that are discussed elsewhere in this book. For example, the anemia which is so common in women with celiac disease may contribute to heavy bleeding, which in turn contributes to painful periods. Chapter 7, "Shorter, Lighter and Pain-free Periods," has information on nutrition for overcoming anemia.

> **Often related to celiac disease is underweight due to poor absorption of food molecules; underweight from any cause will result in long cycles or no cycles at all.**

Or, if your basal temperatures are low (average preovulatory temperatures of 97.3°F or below), see "Low Thyroid Function" in Chapter 8. If you continue to have cycle irregularities, make sure your physician looks for other problems that may occur unrelated to the celiac disease. In summary, if your cycles and fertility do not respond to diet and supplements aimed at eliminating gluten, do not overlook other factors that may be involved.

A LITTLE CAUTION

Some people are sensitive to gluten, and feel much better when they avoid wheat products and the other sources of gluten. However, allergies to wheat and celiac disease are not the same thing. The recent public awareness of gluten intolerance has made many people choose to avoid gluten. A side effect of the market demand is that it's now quite easy to get gluten-free foods that are high in sugar and low in vitamins and minerals. If you choose to go gluten free, perhaps to see if it helps you feel healthier, make sure that you are improving your overall nutrition with a variety of whole natural foods as well as targeted supplements.

If you would like practical information on implementing a gluten-free diet, go to the Celiac Disease Foundation at www.celiac.org and the National Celiac Association at www.nationalceliac.org. Still, the many available websites are no substitute for personal care from a doctor and dietitian, at least as you get started on the road to recovery.

PERIODONTAL DISEASE

New research links gum disease (periodontal disease) to cycle irregularity,[43] infertility,[44] and pregnancy problems such as pre-clampsia and low birth weight.[45] The cause versus the effect is not clear: Does gum disease cause inflammation or infection that affects the reproductive organs of the woman, or is gum disease a marker for inflammation that causes reproductive problems? The answers are not in yet, but the association between the gum disease and reproductive problems will most likely be strengthened with further research.

How does this affect you? First, periodontal disease is usually preventable with regular professional teeth cleaning and regular check-ups. Should you suspect gum disease, the good news is that periodontal disease is very treatable and curable with good dental care. In addition, you can now purchase tablets of "friendly" oral bacteria to combat the "bad' bacteria that may colonize your mouth, contributing to dental cavities, bad breath, and gum disease. And nutrition may make a difference, as the anecdote below illustrates.

I counseled a woman in her early thirties who had experienced infertility and several miscarriages after two children were born to her. When I suggested a chewable multivitamin, she remarked that she had difficulty chewing, because she had lost several molars. Loss of teeth is a late symptom of periodontal disease, and in some cases a lack of vitamin C is related to loss of teeth. This is so because collagen, the threadlike protein that binds teeth to the bone, requires vitamin C for its synthesis. I recommended emphasis on vitamin C, which is necessary for the synthesis of progesterone as well. This woman went on to have four more children, which she credited to her improved overall nutrition.

AGE-RELATED INFERTILITY/INFERTILITY OF UNKNOWN CAUSE

Based on my experience in counseling NFP and nutrition, I now recommend a specific nutritional strategy for women who are over 40 and are having difficulty conceiving or maintaining a pregnancy. Such over-40 problems occur because of the age-related decline in the quality of the ova (eggs).

**I also recommend this same strategy for women of any age
with stubborn infertility of unknown cause.**

However, if you are also dealing with overweight, underweight, endometriosis, short luteal phase, or any of the many other possibilities discussed previously, be sure to address those issues at the same time—your problem may not be completely age-related.

Please refer back to the Introduction to Part 2, which explains that, amazingly, the unfertilized ovum must complete its cell division, called meiosis I, during the two days prior to ovulation. As the ova age, their ability to do this properly declines, contributing to infertility, early miscarriage without proper development of the newly conceived child, and even Down syndrome. In addition, the reproductive hormones FSH and LH decline in the early years of premenopause, so that their hormonal "push" of the ovum to complete meiosis I may be insufficient.

The vitamins, minerals, and essential fatty acids listed below are intended to accomplish two ends: first, to provide the body with the nutrients needed to produce adequate progesterone. If progesterone levels during the second half of the cycle are normal, it is likely that FSH and LH in the first half of the cycle are also normal. Studies cited in Chapters 6 and 8 show that vitamin B6 and vitamin C can raise progesterone levels. Other B vitamins and the mineral magnesium support the activities of vitamin B6.

The second goal is to provide the ovum itself with nutrients known to be involved in meiosis and cell division. These nutrients include folate (folic acid), vitamin B12, zinc, and the essential fatty acids, particularly the omega-3 alpha linolenic acid. Vitamin E is an antioxidant that reduces the oxidation of the essential fatty acids. Coenzyme Q10 in the form of ubiquinol is an antioxidant, but it also enables cells to use energy effectively. The ovum is a metabolically active cell with high energy requirements.

DIET. Improve your overall diet, as outlined in Chapter 1, with special attention to avoiding *trans* fats, aspartame (NutraSweet) and other artificial sweeteners, caffeine, and sugary treats. If you are overweight, whether extremely overweight or just moderately so, try to lose some weight—perhaps 10 pounds. If you are underweight, you will need to gain weight.

SUPPLEMENTS. Consider vitamins, minerals, essential fatty acids as in Chapter 3, including these higher amounts of the following daily (see next page):

Vitamin B6	300 mg[46]
Folate (folic acid)	4,000 mcg[47]
Vitamin B12	1,000 mcg[48]
Vitamin C	1,000-3,000 mg
Vitamin E	400-800 IU
Zinc	15-50 mg
Flax oil and/or fish oil	5-10 g (1-2 teaspoons)
Coenzyme Q10 in the form of ubiquinol	5 g (1 teaspoon)
Probiotic capsule	200 mg/day[49]

You can start with any of the vitamin brands recommended in Chapter 3. Then add these additional nutrients so that the daily overall total is at the level listed here. Vitamin B12 is easily available in small, flavored tablets that can dissolve under your tongue. Folic acid or methyl folate, the preferred natural form of this B vitamin, is available in 400, 800 or 1,000 mcg tablets. You will need to take several to achieve the higher dose.

NIGHT LIGHTING. If you can reduce the night lighting in your bedroom, as described in "Sensitivity to Night Lighting" above, you may be able to increase your melatonin levels, which in turn, may help to normalize your progesterone levels.

IMPORTANT NOTE: If you get pregnant using these guidelines, do not discontinue them during the pregnancy! It is not wise to "pull the rug out" from yourself nutritionally once you achieve pregnancy. All of these are safe for use during pregnancy, but of course you should work together with a doctor who is knowledgeable about the benefits of good nutrition.

A TRUE SURPRISE PREGNANCY. Here is an article that I wrote for The Couple to Couple League's *Family Foundations* magazine.

> As members of CCL, we tend to think of surprise pregnancies as breaking the rules, ignoring the rules, or rarely, a method failure—any of which could result in an unintended pregnancy. There is another "true surprise" pregnancy, though—the one that follows infertility. Ron and I have experienced our very first surprise pregnancy this way. At age 47, I am now five months pregnant! Our youngest biological child was born when I was 41. My cycles returned during breastfeeding about the time I turned 43, but even though I have ovulated more or less regularly, it certainly appeared

that my fertile years were over. Of course I took my own advice, but to no avail. When I was 45 we applied for adoption, and and within a year we adopted a baby son from overseas. My interest in achieving pregnancy dropped once he was in my arms, and I stopped charting. I could honestly say that after the adoption, my recurring periods had no more meaning to me than they did when I was single. We did nothing to avoid a pregnancy, but were completely convinced that it would not happen. In fact, we were confidently discussing the possibility of initiating a second adoption in another year or two.

Meanwhile, my cycles became quite irregular when I was 46—my first sign of approaching menopause. They straightened out again for several cycles until the following summer when another long cycle began. Since I wasn't charting, I didn't know for sure what was happening, but I thought to myself, a bit tongue-in-cheek, "Here comes menopause again!" I started charting, but even before I had 21 high temperatures charted, I was convinced that the rapid physical changes were indicative of a healthy pregnancy. By God's grace all is well so far, my health is excellent, and we are anticipating the birth in early May. Ron and I are beside ourselves with surprise and happiness.

Did nutrition make any difference? One can never say for sure. I take vitamins daily similar to what I recommend for infertility, mostly because it makes such a difference in my energy level to do so. In May or June, however, I started taking 1,000 mcg of vitamin B_{12} daily, again for the energy. In August, when I conceived, I was taking all my vitamins especially carefully, including flax oil, folic acid [2,000–3,000 mcg], and the whole laundry list. I have done some reading and in fact have been able to verify that B_{12} is important for fertility. Who knows? When my doctor, who was truly astounded, asked me what I thought might have made the difference, I answered sincerely, "The Lord."[50]

This article preceded the birth of a healthy baby daughter, two months before I turned 48. I never requested an ultrasound during the pregnancy, yet I felt confident that the baby would be healthy. If you are interested in the research that helped give me that confidence, please refer to Chapter 12, "Repeated Miscarriage & Birth Defects."

SUMMARY—CHAPTER 10

1 A number of seemingly unrelated health problems or situations may interfere with cycle regularity, or they may contribute to infertility without obvious changes in the cycle at all. They include:

1) yeast overgrowth, in which the usually harmless intestinal fungus, *Candida albicans*, causes infection, allergic reactions, or reactions to toxins;

2) discontinuing birth control pills or other hormonal birth control;

3) sensitivity to night lighting, which apparently can affect fertility by decreasing the hormone melatonin;

4) excess caffeine consumption;

5) celiac disease, in which an abnormal reaction to the protein gluten in certain grains damages the small intestine, resulting in multiple nutritional abnormalities;

6) periodontal (gum) disease; and

7) age-related infertility, the natural life progression that results in hormonal changes and poor ovum quality.

2 Each of these may respond to specific nutritional or other strategies aimed at overcoming them.

PREGNANCY & POSTPARTUM NUTRITION

11

Ideally, pregnancy is a time of great joy, anticipation, and wonder. It is a miracle — a child, the fruit of your love, developing within you! There is sweet anticipation on sharing the secret with others, donning your maternity clothes for the first time, and feeling the first fluttery kicks. You are already a mother, and your protective instincts are already powerfully engaged. What you eat, what medicines you take, and what type of exercise you engage in are all done with your growing baby constantly on your mind and in your heart.

No one needs to convince you what good nutrition means to your unborn baby. But more than at any other time in your life, what you eat, how much you eat, and what supplements you take will also make an immense difference in how much you enjoy your pregnancy. However, even if excellent nutrition does not give you the energy you would like, or does not prevent morning sickness, stretch marks, or some of the other annoyances of pregnancy, it will enable your baby to develop the healthiest nervous system and immune system that he or she can. Good nutrition is the best insurance that your baby will be born at full term and at a healthy weight. Good nutrition will help you feel your best during the postpartum period so that you can delight fully in that all-too-fleeting time when your newborn is so tiny and helpless.

PREGNANCY

HOW LONG SHOULD YOU PREPARE BEFORE PREGNANCY? There is no absolute answer to the question of how long you should work to improve your nutrition before trying to become pregnant. It depends on your health at the time. Many women's health advocates recommend about three months of preparation, including taking prenatal vitamins. If you have cycle problems such as short luteal phase or polycystic ovary syndrome, implementing the self-help strategies in the earlier chapters of this book for two or three months gives you time to reap the benefits of improved nutrition. If you are coming off birth control pills or other hormonal birth control, it's prudent to let your own hormones readjust for three months as you improve your nutrition and start taking good supplements. If you have been sick with an illness that has caused you to lose weight, such as pneumonia, two or three months gives you time to recover your health and regain your weight. If you are significantly overweight, you may wish to try to get into a better body balance before becoming pregnant.

On the other hand, if you are in good health and are already eating nutritious foods, starting your prenatal vitamins and other supplements at the beginning of the cycle before the one in which you hope to conceive is certainly adequate. I also believe that waiting just one cycle is adequate for women who have unfortunately experienced an early miscarriage, as long as it has not been complicated by heavy blood loss or surgical intervention.

But what if you decide, on short notice, that you would like to conceive this month? Or what if you discover you are pregnant, quite by surprise? Right then is the best time for you to fully implement a diet and supplements aimed confidently at the healthiest pregnancy possible.

NUTRITIONAL PREPARATION FOR PREGNANCY. As you prepare for pregnancy, cut down on sugary treats and soda pop (especially avoid diet drinks[1]), and limit caffeine to the equivalent of two average cups of coffee daily.[2] Replace poor food choices with healthy food, as outlined in Part 1 of this book.

> In a new Australian study, researchers showed that women who ate a diet characterized by fish, meat, fruit, and whole grains for the twelve months before pregnancy had a significantly lower risk of a premature birth compared to women who had eaten a high fat, high sugar, fast-food diet with refined grains.[3]

Avoid *trans* fats, and make sure you have sources of the essential fatty acids, as explained in Rule 3, Chapter 1. Pay special attention to nutritional choices aimed at stabilizing your blood glucose levels, as described in Rule 6, Chapter 1. A natural-foods diet will make you confident that you will give your baby the best start possible. Beginning your pregnancy with good blood sugar control as a result of good diet will also go a long way toward decreasing morning sickness.

No doubt you are aware that the B vitamin folic acid has been shown to reduce the incidence of several types of serious birth defects called neural tube defects. A large body of research on the effectiveness of folic acid in preventing such problems has indicated that supplementing this vitamin for several weeks before conception and until the end of breastfeeding is most beneficial.[4] That is why the beginning of the cycle or two *before* the one in which you hope to conceive is the best time for you to start your vitamins, unless you have already been taking at least 400 mcg of folic acid (and preferably more, especially if you are an older mother or are dealing with infertility).

FOLIC ACID OR FOLATE?

New research has shown that a substantial number of people have genetic variations which makes it less efficient for them to convert folic acid, the common but synthetic B vitamin, into folate, the natural form. Folate, in the form methyl folate, bypasses the problem. The question becomes, "How much methyl folate should I use, since the original studies of this B vitamin's effectiveness against birth defects, miscarriage, preterm birth, and infertility were all done using the synthetic folic acid?" At this time there is very little research on supplements of methyl folate and its role in preventing birth defects. While we can assume that folate works at least as well, right now there is no researched reason to take a smaller dose of folate compared to the amount of folic acid that has been studied and recommended. It is my opinion that using methyl folate is a better option than using folic acid, even though there is a large body of excellent research on the benefits and safety of folic acid. If you choose to take methyl folate, I believe that you should use the same amount as has been studied using folic acid. Please see Chapter 12 for details on this topic.

But do not supplement just folic acid or folate. Take a comprehensive multivitamin/multimineral and essential fatty acids supplement, as recommended below. As one British researcher wrote in a review article on supplements for pregnant women: "Since the Medical Research Council study in 1991 on folic acid and the prevention of neural tube defects, it has become evident that there are nutrients in supplement form that can have a significant impact on the outcome of pregnancy. Folic acid is only one of the B vitamins, but what about all the nutrients that are contained in food?"[5]

MORNING SICKNESS

The nausea and vomiting of morning sickness can take enjoyment out of even the most eagerly-awaited pregnancy. More importantly, though, it can be severe enough to cause you to lose weight early in pregnancy. Fortunately, it usually subsides by the second trimester, when you really need to increase your intake of good food to meet the growing needs of your baby and yourself.

Nausea and vomiting of early pregnancy are often related to low blood glucose, which in some women stimulates the vomiting center in the brain.

A diet rich in protein foods, vegetables, fruits, and grains, without sugary junk food, will naturally tend to stabilize blood sugar. Ideally, such a diet would be started well before you get pregnant. However, even if you have morning sickness already, you may find that you actually do feel better after you eat small meals of protein, carbohydrate, and natural fat. This is often true despite the fact that your appetite may be poor and you just do not feel like eating.

Adrenal exhaustion, described in Chapter 4, may also be a factor in morning sickness, because healthy adrenal glands support normal blood glucose levels and normal blood pressure. I have noticed that many women with morning sickness have low blood pressure, which may explain why some women say that frequently eating salty foods early in pregnancy helps them. Rereading Chapter 4 and implementing its nutritional recommendations to the extent that you are able may help you. All of the recommendations within that chapter are safe for pregnant women.

SUPPLEMENTS FOR MORNING SICKNESS. Studies show that vitamin B6 is effective in reducing morning sickness.[6] Taking 50–300 mg daily is helpful in pregnancy, but make sure to get your doctor's approval first, especially if you take more than 200 mg daily.[7] Magnesium works together with vitamin B6, and 500-1000 mg per day in the easily available chelated forms is valuable. (See Chapter 3 for information on chelated minerals). Complete vitamin/mineral supplements are useful to keep blood glucose levels steady, but often they contribute to nausea by irritating the stomach. If this is true for you, take only the supplements that you can with a meal at the time of day you feel best. Folic acid or folate and vitamin B6 are the most important supplements in early pregnancy. Folic acid reduces the risk of prevents birth defects, but it also supports fasting blood glucose levels and therefore may help with morning sickness.

My dear friend Ann had her ninth baby at age 43. She and I took our kids swimming at a beautiful wooded lake on a sunny summer day when her new baby boy was just two weeks old. Ann looked and felt wonderful, and the baby was a really content little guy. She mentioned that during this pregnancy, she took a prescription vitamin pill for morning sickness that reduced her morning sickness from a "7 or 8" on a scale of 1 to 10 during her previous pregnancies, to a "2 or 3" this time. This product, called PremesisRx, contains 75 mg of vitamin B6, 1,000 mcg of folic acid, and 200 mg of calcium carbonate as a buffer against stomach upset. (She also took additional folic acid.)

Ginger, in the amount of 1 g daily, helps some women to overcome morning sickness and is safe to use during pregnancy.[8] Capsules of ground ginger root are available at health food shops and can be taken with meals or made into a tea.

 Digestive enzymes, available at health food shops, reduce nausea in some women by promoting digestion of food by the stomach and intestines. Do give these a try—you may be surprised at the difference they make!

If you know you are sensitive to certain foods, for example, gluten-containing foods, by all means avoid them! That small amount that you can tolerate when you are not pregnant may cause you real digestive distress when you are pregnant.

MYTHS ABOUT MORNING SICKNESS. Morning sickness is not in the least psychological in origin—you already know that if you have had it!—but sometimes others who have never experienced it may imply that it is. If you have had it, you probably agree that the name itself is a myth, because it can happen at any time of the day or even all day long.

The traditional name, morning sickness, is based on the fact that most people's blood sugar levels are lowest when they wake up in the morning, and low blood glucose stimulates nausea in some people.

Morning sickness is certainly not a "healthy sign," as some doctors tell women. Yes, it does indicate that the hormonal changes of pregnancy are well underway, but many women, myself included, have had several healthy pregnancies without even an hour of this distressing, demoralizing condition. Nor is it inevitable, even if you have had it during past pregnancies—consider my friend Ann's improvement. And if you are prone to it, the nutritional strategies discussed here can make it far less severe.

My booklet, *Managing Morning Sickness*, has more information on this topic. (See "Further Reading.) However, if you cannot keep your food down and gain weight with self care as you begin the second trimester, your doctor's treatment is essential for your health and for that of your baby.

DIET DURING PREGNANCY

There is simply no substitute for nutritious food during pregnancy to ensure both your health and your baby's. As an expectant mother, your need for protein increases progressively, especially as you enter the second half of your pregnancy. Your need for calories increases as well, so that your body can use the protein for the baby's rapid growth and for your own increased blood volume, uterine size, and so forth. Not enough overall calories causes protein to be "burned" as fuel, rather than used as an essential building material for mother and child. On the other hand, enough calories but not enough protein foods cannot do the job either. You absolutely need both— adequate protein, and enough overall calories from carbohydrates and natural fats.

PREECLAMPSIA (TOXEMIA OF PREGNANCY). You may have wondered why prenatal care includes blood pressure monitoring and urine checks more and more frequently as you approach your due date. These are done in order to detect early signs of a potentially serious problem, **pre-eclampsia**, or metabolic toxemia of late pregnancy. **Toxemia**, as it is still often called, can be recognized clinically by high blood pressure and protein in the urine. Severe edema (fluid retention) often occurs with it.

If early signs of toxemia occur, the expectant mother is usually advised to rest in order to help keep her blood pressure down, and to limit salt in order to reduce the edema. If the situation worsens, the doctor frequently induces labor or performs an emergency caesarian section to prevent the dangerous stage that follows, called **eclampsia**. If it is left untreated, eclampsia can progress from seizures to coma, and even to death of the mother and unborn child.

Perhaps you know a woman who has had her labor induced early due to her elevated blood pressure and other abnormalities, even though it meant that the baby was born several weeks prematurely. The induction of labor was not undertaken lightly. The attending physicians had to weigh the risk of eclampsia against the long-term problems that often occur when a baby is born too early. That's how serious toxemia of pregnancy is. Inducing labor can prevent a disaster.

> **As with so many other things in life, prevention is infinitely preferable to dealing with the problem once it has occurred.**

Avoiding toxemia is by far the best strategy, yet toxemia along with premature induction of labor to avoid the effects of this disease is distressingly common.

THE BREWER DIET TO PREVENT TOXEMIA. The late Tom Brewer, M.D., spent a long career advocating the use of a healthy daily diet aimed at preventing toxemia in pregnant women. The diet he developed is high in protein and rich in plant foods, and he implemented it successfully with thousands of women in various parts of the United States. As part of his dietary plan, he specifically advised pregnant women against restriction of weight gain.[9]

The Brewer diet is simple to learn and is made up of ordinary foods. It recommends the following daily: One quart of milk, two eggs, one or two servings of meat or fish; two servings each of dark green vegetables and a vitamin C source; five servings of grains or starches, three servings of fats and oils, and one source of vitamin A.[10] These recommendations, with minor modifications, serve as the basis of Table 12, "Suggested Daily Food Goals for Pregnant and Nursing Women" (see pages 204-205).

Dr. Brewer additionally recommended that pregnant women salt their food to taste, drink plenty of water, and eat at least one snack daily. His website, The Blue Ribbon Baby Pages (www.blueribbonbaby.org), contains further information on this topic and includes a checklist that you can use to make certain you have eaten all the recommended foods daily. It also contains food substitutions for a lacto-vegetarian or vegan diet.

> As you begin your pregnancy, the hearty intake of food recommended by the Brewer diet is neither necessary nor possible, but as you get into the second and especially the third trimester, your appetite picks up and eating healthy food becomes almost a craving!

ALLERGIES TO MILK OR EGGS. If you are allergic to milk, it is important to realize that it is a major source of protein and you need to compensate for avoiding it. You can substitute two 3-ounce servings of lean meat or fish for one quart (four glasses) of milk. It is best to supplement calcium, along with magnesium and vitamin D, if you do not use dairy products.

Eggs have a number of wonderful nutrients in them, so much so that my midwife used to refer to them as "big vitamin pills." However, one 3-ounce serving of meat can replace the protein of two eggs.

OVERWEIGHT WOMEN. I am always troubled when I hear a woman recount a story that goes like this: "I was overweight when I got pregnant. My doctor told me to gain no more than 30 pounds. I really tried to keep my weight down. But by seven months, I already had gained the full 30. The doctor told me in no uncertain terms that I had

TABLE 12
SUGGESTED DAILY FOOD GOALS FOR PREGNANT AND NURSING WOMEN

WHOLE GRAINS

5 servings daily

(1 serving = 1 slice bread or ½ cup cooked cereal)

Whole grain bread	Whole grain breakfast cereal	Whole grain pancakes	Tortillas
Oatmeal		Whole grain pasta	Bagels
Rice	Quinoa		

DAIRY/EGGS

6 servings daily

(1 serving = 8 oz. milk, 2 oz. cheese, 1 egg)

Whole milk	Cheese	Kefir
Yogurt	Ice cream	Eggs

COMPLETE PROTEIN

1-2 servings daily

(1 serving = 4 oz. meat)

Poultry	Pork	Dairy + Grain
Fish (preferably twice weekly)	Lamb	Dairy + Legume
Beef	Grain + Legume (Peas, beans, peanut butter, nuts, lentils)	

YELLOW FRUITS AND VEGETABLES

1 serving daily

(1 serving = ½ cup cooked or 1 cup raw)

Carrots	Sweet potatoes	Mangos	Peaches
Squash	Pumpkin	Apricots	Cantaloupe

TABLE 12 (CONT.)
SUGGESTED DAILY FOOD GOALS FOR PREGNANT AND NURSING WOMEN

LEAFY GREEN VEGETABLES

3 servings daily

(1 serving = ½ cup cooked or 1 cup raw)

Lettuce (leaf, Romaine, Bibb, iceberg)	Endive	Kale
	Beet greens	Cole crops (cabbage, broccoli, Brussels sprouts, cauliflower, kohlrabi)
Spinach	Alfalfa sprouts	
	Asparagus	
Escarole	Chard	

VITAMIN C SOURCE

2 servings daily

(1 serving = 1 medium fruit or ½ cup berries)

Citrus fruits (oranges, grapefruits, tangerines)	Tomatoes	Peppers
	Melons	Potatoes
	Berries	

UNSATURATED OILS

3 serving daily

(1 serving = 1 tablespoons)

Monounsaturated	**Polyunsaturated**	**Both**
Olive oil	Soy oil *	Canola oil *
		Sesame oil
Peanut oil	Walnut oil *	
Unprocessed peanut butter	Safflower oil	
	Sunflower oil	* Source of the essential
Avocado oil	Corn oil	omega-3 alpha-linolenic acid.

This table may be photocopied, covered with adhesive backed clear plastic and taped to your refrigerator. Check off the boxes daily with a dry erase marker.

gained my quota. So I really cut down, just as much as I could. I started swelling, and my blood pressure went sky high. They did an emergency C-section at seven and a half months. My baby was in neonatal intensive care, and I had to pump milk and bring it to the hospital. It was really a stress all the way through."

Dr. Brewer made a distinction between gaining weight on junk food and carbohydrates versus weight gain based on his protein-rich diet. He pointed out that women who are obese or overweight when they get pregnant still need to eat healthy food daily and that pregnancy is not the time to diet. On the other hand, women who begin their pregnancies while overweight or obese may find that with his diet plan, they in fact do not gain much weight, or may even lose a little, which in such a case is not a problem.[11]

Unfortunately, studies of how weight gain, or lack of weight gain, affects pregnancy in women who are obese still fail to include consideration of what type of diet these women were eating.[12] How much of the diet is carbohydrate or fat versus protein? During pregnancy, it makes an immense difference.

UNDERWEIGHT WOMEN. If you are overly thin, part of your preparation before pregnancy should be an earnest attempt to bring your weight up. Once you become pregnant, working towards the Brewer ideal should be your goal. While some health experts state that 25–35 pounds of weight gain is adequate, an additional 10 or 15 pounds (35–50 pounds total) may be completely normal and healthy for a thin or slender woman.

MAINTAINING YOUR FIGURE. If you are troubled by the idea of "losing your figure" or by the time it takes to lose weight after childbirth, remind yourself that you are feeding your baby's developing brain every day. You are forming your baby's immune system with what you eat. A woman's body is designed to store several pounds of fat during pregnancy. This is necessary for the health of both mother and baby, and the fat reserves are gradually nursed away over a period of a few weeks or months.

> **Failure to gain enough weight on good food is the leading cause of low birth weight and prematurity, both of which may have lifelong physical and mental consequences for the baby.**

IF YOU HAVE ALREADY GAINED "TOO MUCH." What about the woman in the previous anecdote? What should you do if you have already gained "too much" weight, yet still have two or three months to go? The answer is straightforward: whether you were of normal weight, overweight, or obese when you got pregnant, you need to continue nourishing your baby and eat especially the protein and other nutrients that both you and your baby must have. There is no substitute for daily, nutritious food and the need for overall calories and protein is highest during the last trimester.

RESEARCH ON NUTRITION FOR PRE-ECLAMPSIA. Unfortunately, the role of actual food type—protein versus fat or carbohydrates—is ignored in major research studies concerned with preventing pre-eclampsia. A number of different vitamins, minerals, and fatty acid supplements have been studied for their effect on toxemia, but except for the B vitamins, most have ended with disappointing results.[13]

One study assessed the effect of a high-fiber diet on the risk of developing toxemia. While fruits, vegetables, low-fat and high-fat dairy products were evaluated, overall protein intake was not. Nevertheless, the authors did observe that foods rich in fiber, such as cereal, whole-grain bread, low-fat dairy, and fruits and vegetables were generally associated with a reduced risk of toxemia.[14]

Other studies indirectly confirm Dr. Brewer's work. One study found that women with a low intake of milk had a higher risk of developing toxemia (pre-eclampsia), and those with the lowest milk intake were most likely to suffer from the dangerous eclampsia. The researchers observed that two and one-half glasses of milk daily was average for women who had pre-eclampsia, and noted "an evident protective effect" against pre-eclampsia of five glasses of milk daily; that much milk consumption lowered the risk of toxemia almost *five times*. Yet the discussion centered on the role of calcium, and the authors stated, "The mechanisms by which calcium may prevent pre-eclampsia are still unknown."[15] They then noted that other large studies in which calcium was supplemented did not reduce the risk of toxemia.[16] Two and one-half glasses of milk daily average about 20 grams of protein; five glasses, about 40 grams. How is it that the role of protein in preventing toxemia can be overlooked even when it is staring you in the face!

In another study, the pattern of eating fish, meat, chicken, fruit, and whole grains was associated with a reduced risk of preterm birth, while eating a high sugar, high fat, refined grain, and fast-food diet was associated with an increased incidence of premature birth.[17]

"The Blue Ribbon Baby Pages" (www.blueribbonbaby.org) have all of the information you need to know about what and how much to eat when you are pregnant, even if you have had problems with previous pregnancies. It will help you whether or not you are milk intolerant or eat a vegetarian diet. You may also wish to read Dr. Brewer's classic book, *What Every Pregnant Woman Should Know: The Truth about Diet and Drugs in Pregnancy.* (See "Further Reading.")

PERIODONTAL DISEASE AND PRE-ECLAMPSIA. New research has linked gum disease (periodontal disease) to an increased risk of pre-eclampsia.[18] If you have not had regular dental care, with regular professional teeth cleaning, be sure to see your dentist, preferably before you become pregnant. With treatment by a dentist, periodontal disease can be cured. Beyond saving your teeth, it may help prevent toxemia. Certainly when your teeth are healthy and pain-free, it is easier to chew and eat the healthy foods you need during pregnancy, but the bacterial infection and inflammation themselves contribute to the problems caused by periodontal disease.

VITAMIN AND MINERAL SUPPLEMENTS DURING PREGNANCY

 Both over-the-counter prenatal vitamins as well as prescription prenatal vitamins vary widely in their potencies, so you need to read labels whether or not your prenatal supplement is under prescription.

In fact, prescription prenatal vitamins are often surprisingly low in potency. I recommend supplements in amounts similar to those listed in Table 7, Chapter 3. Professional Pre-Natal Formula comes the closest of any supplement I know to meeting all the needs for pregnant women. It is labeled for six tablets per day, allowing you to adjust your intake downward if you wish, or if you cannot tolerate a full dose.

ProCycle PMS is also safe and healthy for pregnancy, though it contains no iron. You may need to supplement iron separately if tests show that you need more. Optivite PMT is also safe for pregnancy, and may even reduce nausea and vomiting.[19] It contains only 200 mcg of folic acid per full dose, so additional folate or folic acid must be added. (See "Appendix A" and "Resources.")

If you have taken other vitamins, minerals, or a product such as Fertility Blend to achieve pregnancy, do not stop taking them now! You need the nutritional support for your hormones more than ever. With your doctor's approval, you can continue Fertility Blend.[20] You could combine it with a two-thirds or three-fourths dose of Professional Pre-Natal Formula, Optivite, or ProCycle.

One of the principles of this book is that vitamins, minerals, and essential fatty acids work together to maintain health. Nowhere is this principle more evident than during pregnancy, as more and more new studies illustrate. Here are some important examples of this.

THE BIG B'S: FOLIC ACID, VITAMIN B12, AND VITAMIN B6. Supplements of folic acid (the synthetic form of folate) decrease the risk of neural tube birth defects, including spina bifida and anencephaly. (See Chapter 12 for more on this topic.) But folate plays other important roles in pregnancy. It is involved in cell division and has a vital role in the implantation, development, and health of the placenta, which develops from a single cell into an organ weighing over a pound.

Low levels of folate have been found in women who have had preterm births, pre-eclampsia (toxemia),[21] and abruption of the placenta, the dangerous situation in which the placenta separates from the uterus, threatening mother and fetus.[22]

Supplements of multivitamins containing folic acid in the second trimester lower the risk of pre-eclampsia,[23] and large amounts of folic acid supplements (3-9 mg/day) reduced the incidence of premature birth in women who had an early onset of pre-eclampsia.[24]

However, folate works together with two other B vitamins—vitamin B12 and vitamin B6—to support important biochemical processes necessary to protein metabolism. These three B vitamins decrease the overproduction of a potentially harmful amino acid, homocysteine. Homocysteine is under intense study to understand its role in several different diseases, including heart disease. With reference to pregnancy, there is a growing acceptance of the possibility that homocysteine is the actual chemical that causes neural tube defects.[25] Homocysteine is elevated in women who have pre-eclampsia.[26] In addition, it has been implicated in early miscarriages, intrauterine growth retardation (failure of the fetus to grow normally), and low birth weight babies.[27] These topics are explored more fully in Chapter 12.

What does this research mean to you? Multivitamin supplements which contain folic acid, vitamin B12, and vitamin B6 are preferable to folic acid or methyl folate supplements alone. Taking such supplements before pregnancy helps if you cannot tolerate vitamins during the first trimester, and taking complete supplements throughout your pregnancy, along with good diet, should give you confidence in your own health and that of your baby.

FOLIC ACID AND IRON. Supplementing folic acid together with iron is more effective than iron alone in enabling pregnant women to overcome iron-deficiency anemia.[28] Folic acid and iron may also help to reduce an annoying problem, **restless legs syndrome**, which some women develop during pregnancy.[29] See Table 7, Chapter 3, for recommended amounts.

FOLIC ACID AND VITAMIN B12 FOR ENERGY. Some women feel much better when they take larger amounts of folic acid than the usual 400 mcg. Some international organizations and researchers recommend ten times that amount (4,000 mcg) or more (5,000 mcg) beginning before pregnancy for women who have had a child with a neural tube defect[30] or for all women's prenatal vitamins.[31] I recommend that you try up to 4,000 mcg daily of folic acid or folate if you are an older mother, or if you struggle with fatigue during your pregnancy. In addition, Dean Raffelock, D.C., and Robert Rountree, M.D., authors of *A Natural Guide to Pregnancy and Postpartum Health*, recommend for "severe fatigue during or after your pregnancy, try taking up to 5,000 mcg of vitamin B12. This is a safe way to energize your body, and it will not harm your baby."[32] You will very likely find that small tablets of 1,000 mcg of vitamin B12, dissolved under your tongue, contain enough vitamin B12 to enable you to overcome pregnancy fatigue. If you can obtain it, prefer the natural form of B12, methylcobalamin.

VITAMIN B6 AND MAGNESIUM FOR EDEMA. Texas physician John Ellis, M.D., spent years studying the relationship between vitamin B6 deficiency and various disorders, including pregnancy edema, toxemia, and eclampsia. The following excerpts from his book, *Vitamin B6: The Doctor's Report*, summarize the results of his clinical experience:

> Numerous signs and symptoms appear during pregnancy that are responsive to B6. These include painful neuropathies in the fingers and hands, swelling (edema) in the hands and feet, leg cramps, hand and arms "that go to sleep," and, most of all, B6 is a factor in the prevention and treatment of toxemia of pregnancy and the convulsions of eclampsia...Edema of pregnancy, long discussed in both medical and lay circles, has become so common that many doctors have come to accept it as being normal during pregnancy, and patients have grown resigned to suffering through it. It is not normal at all. It is not normal at any time. The patient feels bad. There is nothing healthy about being swollen with fluids. Based on my investigations with 225 pregnant women on B6 therapy, in most cases vitamin B6 will completely relieve and prevent edema of pregnancy as it has been known to the scientific community. This is a large statement, but it has been proved over and over. Because of the skepticism that some readers may entertain, it would be wise to repeat that in these 225 cases no diuretics were given to any patient, and there was no restriction on either salt or fluids.[33]

Dr. Ellis presented a series of conclusions based on his research, including emphasis that salt restriction is not necessary when vitamin B6 is adequate, and that the babies born to mothers who have taken large doses of B6 do not show increased need for this vitamin. He also noted the role of magnesium, which works synergistically with vitamin B6:

> ...All pregnant women should have at least 50 milligrams of B6 [daily] as a supplement throughout their pregnancies, and many of them will require considerably more than that. All pregnant women should also receive at least 500 milligrams of magnesium daily, and with the appearance of the signs of toxemia the magnesium should be increased to 1,000 milligrams daily.[34]

While I consider this older research valuable enough to recommend here, please note that there is no substitute for adequate protein to prevent toxemia of pregnancy. However, vitamin B6, like folate and vitamin B12, does improve the use of protein in the body through its effect on reducing homocysteine. During my own pregnancies, I found that Dr. Ellis's findings were true for me—for example, I can confirm that the numbness of the hands that some women complain of is much improved by vitamin B6.

**In addition, vitamin B6, along with other B vitamins,
is helpful to preventing "brain fog."**

PUTTING IT ALL TOGETHER: The following anecdote, contributed by a young medical student, illustrates the beneficial effects of adequate supplements during pregnancy:

My wife and I were expecting our third child. Both of our older children had been born at home, and our plans were to deliver this child at home as well. However, a potentially serious problem presented an obstacle to a safe delivery at home. Despite care in maintaining good nutrition, in each of the other two pregnancies my wife had retained water and experienced nausea far beyond the normal length of "morning sickness." In addition, she had other related problems, such as tingling and numbness in her fingers and hands, joint aches and pains, elevated blood pressure, and a general feeling of not being well. These symptoms had occurred earlier in the second pregnancy than the first, and now, in the third, were occurring earlier still; she was only in the fourth month of pregnancy and had already gained 35 pounds. We both felt strongly that she had been only slightly better than a marginal candidate for home delivery with the last baby, and that if she wasn't in substantially better health with this pregnancy (largely because 6-1/2 years had passed, and she was now 30 years old with a family history of diabetes), it would not be safe to have this baby at home. However, we were even less enthusiastic about a hospital birth.

As we were in the middle of this quandary, I had the opportunity to discuss the subject with the author, with whom I taught a class weekly. She shared with me information on the importance of good multi-vitamin supplements, and recommended a balanced nonprescription prenatal multivitamin. [The full dose of this supplement contained 75 mg/mcg of most B vitamins, 100 mg of B6, 450 mg of magnesium, and other vitamins and minerals in amounts similar to those in Table 7, Chapter 3. Professional Pre-Natal Formula is very similar.]

As soon as my wife began taking these vitamins (and I mean within one day), she began shedding excess water, and experienced a visible improvement of the edema in her hands and feet. She lost nearly six pounds in the first week, and continued to improve until we could see the veins on the tops of her feet. Her blood pressure remained normal, there was no numbness, and she only occasionally felt nauseous. The improvement was so pronounced that we no longer felt reservations about continuing with plans for a home birth.

The effectiveness of this improvement in nutrition was demonstrated very pointedly some weeks later, when we ran out of the vitamin supplement, and found that the health food store where we had purchased them was also out of stock. In the week that my wife was out of this supplement, she quickly became fatigued, nauseous, and edematous [swollen with fluid]. As soon as we had obtained a new supply and she had begun to take them regularly again, the problems disappeared.

My wife enjoyed excellent health throughout the remainder of the pregnancy, and delivered a healthy baby boy at home.[35]

OTHER STRATEGIES TO REDUCE EDEMA

Good multivitamin/multiminerals, combined with an excellent diet, really help to reduce water retention and swelling. But here are some more tips to prevent edema: eat more protein and reduce extra carbohydrates if you are retaining fluid. Drink plenty of water, which in itself is a natural diuretic. Do not sit for too long, and elevate your feet when you rest. Keep cool! Try going wading in deep, cool water. The cool water causes vasoconstriction of the blood vessels in the skin, a change that generally stimulates the kidneys to produce more urine. The actual pressure of the water on the body also signals the kidneys to excrete extra fluid. If you cannot go wading, try soaking your feet in tall buckets of cool water.

FISH OIL AND FLAX OIL SUPPLEMENTS

FISH AS BRAIN FOOD. A recent research article noted that the advice for pregnant women to limit their seafood consumption due to the possibility of toxins, especially mercury, may be counterproductive. Why? The less seafood pregnant women consume, the higher the risk that their children will have developmental problems, including those involving fine motor skills, communication, and social skills. The researchers concluded that based on their large study, "risks from the loss of nutrients were greater than the risks of harm from exposure to trace contaminants in 340 g [12 oz., or three 4-oz. servings] seafood eaten weekly."[36] That is, mothers who ate more than the government-recommended amounts of seafood had children with better developmental outcomes from six months of age until eight years of age, which was the age limit of the study.

Why should seafood matter when there are many other sources of protein? In this case, it's not the protein. It is the DHA found in fish that is critical to the brain development of the fetus in the womb. If DHA is insufficient, neuron-to-neuron connections in the developing brain are not made properly.

Seafood is a good source of many nutrients, but instead of worrying about mercury and avoiding fish, as so many women do,[37] use the Internet to access recommendations as to the least contaminated species of fish. (See the question and answer on this topic in Chapter 5.) However, supplementing with certified contaminant-free, good-tasting cod liver oil is another option that is supported by new research. Supplements of fish oil enhance the development of the brain of the baby before birth; in fact, the need for DHA is highest during the last trimester of pregnancy, when the baby's brain is growing the fastest. Such supplements may even reduce the risk of premature birth, especially in women who have had premature babies previously.[38]

FISH OIL AND FLAX OIL SUPPLEMENTS. Drs. Raffelock and Rountree, in *A Natural Guide to Pregnancy and Postpartum Health*, recommend an amount of purified fish body oil that supplies 150–300 mg of DHA and 180–300 mg EPA daily.[39] They do not recommend fish liver oil because of the vitamin A content, but I disagree with them on this point. The amount of fish liver oil with these amounts of DHA and EPA is in the range of only one-half teaspoon daily (3 1-g capsules), and the vitamin A in fish liver oil of this amount is only 350–600 IU, very far below the limit of safety for a pregnant woman, which is 8,000–10,000 IU of true vitamin A.[40]

These doctors also recommend a tablespoon of ground flax seed daily.[41] This is equivalent to about 1 teaspoon or five 1 g capsules of flax oil, which is a source of the essential omega-3 fatty acid, alpha-linolenic acid. They recommend the same for postpartum women, especially those who are breastfeeding. In any case, be sure to take about 400 IU of vitamin E as an antioxidant to protect these valuable oils.

THE POSTPARTUM TIME

Life changes profoundly when the new baby arrives! The entire family dynamic is reshuffled. If it is the first child, the husband and wife become parents. A single child becomes a big brother or sister. The current baby becomes an older sibling. Schedules change; sleep patterns are disrupted; visitors come and go. The mother is entirely focused on her new baby, ideally with help from caring relatives and friends. It is easy for everyone to forget that profound hormonal changes are occurring in the new mom. There is simply no other situation in healthy human physiology that comes remotely close to the speed and magnitude of the hormonal readjustments that happen to a new mother.

Mom's first meal after labor and birth is the best meal many women have ever had! I still savor the memories of the biggest and tastiest pizza I ever ate, which our best neighbors brought to our home after a very long labor and birth of our third child, Stephen. These neighbors had kept our two older children at their home during the labor and birth, but they arrived soon afterwards with the kids (and the pizza). Here is the story they told us: When Ron finally called them with the news, they told John, who was six, and Rosemary, who was four, that Mom and Dad had had a baby boy, and so now they had a new baby brother. "But I wanted a girl brother!" Rosemary wailed.

EMOTIONAL NURTURING. When it comes to "postpartum nutrition," the emotional nurturing of the mother comes first. Birth is an intense physical stress; the adjustment to the new baby is an intense emotional stress; and the excitement of it all is an intense overall stress, albeit a positive one.

> **Having trusted helpers around who know how to reduce stress will provide the mother with joyful memories for the rest of her life.**

Conversely, thoughtless remarks that she might construe as a criticism during this hormonally and emotionally unsettled time will easily upset her. The new mother needs complete support, as much rest as she can get, and the positive assurance that everything around her is being taken care of. One of the nicest things that you can do for a new mother is to drop off a meal, spending a few minutes to congratulate the family and admire the baby.

BREASTFEEDING NUTRITION

The physical stress of late pregnancy far exceeds the physical stress of breastfeeding. Before the baby is born, you are not only eating for him (or her), but you are also breathing oxygen for him and excreting his wastes. You are carrying him around in an internal bathtub "24/7," as they say. As a breastfeeding mother of a young baby, you are now only eating for him, and carrying him some of the time. But that's a job, too! Ideally, as you get started, you should have the assistance of at least one experienced, compassionate, encouraging woman who has nursed her own babies successfully.

 Water is the first nutrient that you need as a breastfeeding mother, and you need to make sure you are drinking enough, whether or not your sense of thirst is a reliable guide.

FLUIDS. Just as you can judge your baby's fluid intake by his or her wet diapers, you can get a sense of the adequacy of your own input by your output. When you are fully breastfeeding, you are producing about a quart or more of milk daily. Nevertheless, you should be producing as much urine as before you were pregnant. That means you need to drink considerably more than when you were pregnant. Many women experience a distinct sensation of thirst when the baby first latches on—it relates to the hormonal response of milk "letdown." Keep a large water bottle handy so that you can drink plenty of water before that sensation fades.

DIET. You will likely find that your appetite drops after the birth compared to when you were pregnant. It's usual to lose some weight immediately, and then to gradually lose the "baby weight." A modified version of the Brewer diet will serve you well as you breastfeed. High-quality protein and natural fat in the diet are the most important of the major nutrients for milk production. If you are tolerant of milk, you will probably agree that "milk makes milk." On the other hand, if you do not drink milk or use dairy products, substituting two servings of meat or fish for a quart of milk enables you to keep up your protein.

About 50 percent of the calories that breast milk provides come from fats. The fat composition of breast milk reflects the mother's diet. Eating *trans* fats is to be avoided, as they end up in the breast milk. Using olive oil or other expeller-pressed oils helps to provide the fatty acids that the baby requires.

Plenty of nursing mothers find that certain foods they eat make their babies fussy, but that doesn't mean that a food that seemed to bother your older child will necessarily bother the newest one. Lists of foods that bother some babies often include caffeine-containing drinks and foods, spicy foods, and gas-producing vegetables. As your baby gets older, foods that you may have had to avoid earlier may be fine for you to eat.

SUPPLEMENTS. Fish oil (or flax oil or both) will continue to nourish your baby's growing brain now that he or she is born. Your breast milk will contain the valuable DHA that enables proper development of your baby's brain tissue, as long as DHA is available through your diet. Use about the same amounts of fish and flax oil as recommended in the preceding section on pregnancy. You need at least as much of the essential fatty acids when you are breastfeeding as when you are pregnant.

Good vitamins, minerals, and essential fatty acids will nourish both you and your baby. Supplements, such as those in Table 7, Chapter 3, or as recommended in the preceding section on supplements for pregnancy, will help you meet your own increased nutritional needs as well as those of your baby.

POSTPARTUM THYROIDITIS

At some point after giving birth, often before the baby is six months old, a small percentage of women experience thyroid problems.

About one to four months after the birth, some new mothers (approximately 4 percent) develop an overactive thyroid gland. They may feel heart palpitations and fatigue, both of which develop rather rapidly. They may develop a small, painless goiter (an enlarged thyroid gland). About two-thirds of such women will return to normal on their own, or they may actually go on to develop *low* thyroid function.[42]

Approximately 2–5 percent of women develop low thyroid function (hypothyroidism) about four to eight months postpartum, but sometimes even earlier. Often it corrects itself on its own by the time the baby is a year old, but replacement of thyroid hormone may be necessary, at least temporarily. Of the women who develop either overactive thyroid or hypothyroidism after giving birth, about one-third develop permanent hypothyroidism, which must be treated medically.[43]

THE NFP CHART

I have observed very low temperatures, often in the range of 96.8°F and below, on the charts of some women with young babies, reflecting the low thyroid function that may occur postpartum. I have also seen the temperatures rise over a period of two weeks to a month after such women have supplemented vitamins, minerals, and essential fatty acids as recommended in Chapter 7 under the topic "Low Thyroid Function." If you see very low temperatures on your chart, whether or not you are breastfeeding and whether or not you have had your periods return, give the supplements recommended in Chapter 7 a try for a month or two. However, you should be in touch with a medical doctor as well.

Mary Shomon, author of *The Thyroid Hormone Breakthrough*, explains postpartum thyroid problems thoroughly in an excellent chapter dedicated to this topic. (See "Further Reading.") For example, she explains how women with previous thyroid problems may have to be tested regularly after they have a baby because their needs for thyroid medication may change. She explains how either hyper- or hypothyroidism can reduce milk production in a nursing mother, and offers strategies to increase milk output.

HAIR LOSS. Mary Shomon also makes the distinction between the hair loss that is common after a woman has a baby versus hair loss that is a symptom of low thyroid function. In addition to comprehensive multivitamin/multimineral supplements, she recommends 500 mg of evening primrose oil daily to overcome hair loss.[44] However, if you are nursing your baby, instead of evening primrose oil, I recommend flax oil (five to ten 1 g capsules or 1–2 teaspoons daily), along with vitamin E (400 IU). Eating a couple of eggs daily will also provide a source of sulfur, which is beneficial to hair growth.

OVERCOMING POSTPARTUM BLUES

ADRENAL FUNCTION. If you are dealing with the "three-day baby blues," or other minor anxiety or depression related to birth, please read Chapter 4, "Increasing Your Energy & Decreasing Your Stress." During pregnancy, the placenta produces large amounts of hormones which stimulate your adrenal glands to produce their hormones. In the right amounts, adrenal hormones help you to feel good if you are otherwise healthy. However, once the placenta is lost after birth, your adrenal glands lose that stimulation and need to readjust to this change. If the adrenal hormone cortisol is too low, it can contribute to depression. The B vitamins, vitamin C, and the minerals zinc, selenium, manganese, and magnesium are all involved in supporting the adrenal glands, as are the omega-3 fatty acids from flax oil and fish oil. Nutrition aimed at improving the ability of the adrenal glands to produce their hormones is discussed in Chapter 4.

SLEEP. Don't overlook the role of sleep if you are dealing with baby blues. Sleep directly helps the adrenal glands to recover. Your spouse, a trusted relative, or a friend can help you rest by caring for other children, and perhaps for the baby, so that you can get the sleep you need. Enough sleep is a key issue in preventing or overcoming postpartum mood problems. However, if you are breastfeeding, do not use melatonin supplements as a sleep aid.[45]

THYROID FUNCTION. It's possible that your thyroid gland is the source of the postpartum fatigue, depression, anxiety, or "brain fog" that may develop while your baby is young. Postpartum thyroiditis, described above, could be the underlying cause, especially if you see very low temperatures on your NFP chart. If you have had previous thyroid problems, you will need to have your thyroid function re-evaluated. *The Thyroid Hormone Breakthrough* addresses the link between hypothyroidism and postpartum depression.

NATURAL PROGESTERONE. Supplements of natural progesterone are helpful to many women who experience postpartum mood problems. The late Dr. John R. Lee recommended small amounts of over-the-counter progesterone cream for nursing mothers with the baby blues, in the range of 10 to 15 mg daily.[46] Drs. Raffelock and Rountree recommend the same, but in addition they caution against artificial progestins, and especially against the artificial hormones in birth control medications.[47] In any case, discuss natural progesterone supplements with your doctor, and be aware that supplements of oral "micronized" natural progesterone are available by prescription.

A PRACTICAL HANDBOOK. Dr. Raffelock and Dr. Rountree's book, *A Natural Guide to Pregnancy and Postpartum Recovery*, is a unique resource if you have struggled with postpartum depression or anxiety and are looking for effective self care options. (See "Further Reading.") Very readable, it has many practical recommendations for preventing or overcoming postpartum mood problems. It explains in laymen's terms several topics of nutrition that you may have heard about but have not had explained.

In particular, the information on leaky gut syndrome and on the role of the liver in detoxifying wastes and ingested toxins is excellent. While its focus is on nutrition, it also covers the topic of using natural hormones to recover health.

SUMMARY—CHAPTER 11

1 Diet and supplements aimed at stabilizing the blood sugar are the best strategies to prevent or lessen morning sickness. Vitamins B6 and folic acid (folate) are both helpful to blood sugar control.

2 During pregnancy, there is no substitute for a protein-rich diet that also supplies enough calories. Eating such a diet reduces the risk of pre-eclampsia, as well as other complications of pregnancy such as prematurity.

3 Comprehensive vitamin, mineral and fatty acid supplements are the next priority. Folic acid (folate) is well known to prevent certain birth defects, but it also helps prevent other problems, such as preterm birth, pre-eclampsia, and abruption of the placenta. In various health functions it works together with iron, vitamin B12, and vitamin B6. Vitamin B6, along with magnesium and other B vitamins, is helpful for preventing swelling (edema) that occurs so commonly in pregnant women. The nutrients found in fish and fish oil are vital to the healthy development of the unborn baby's brain.

4 Once the baby is born, "emotional nurturing" of the mother is as important as her physical nutrition.

5 Extra fluids are essential to the breastfeeding mother, and her supplements should be similar to that of a pregnant woman. Plenty of protein in the diet is necessary to promote the production of breast milk, but the amount of overall calories needed is generally less while breastfeeding than while pregnant.

6 Postpartum thyroiditis occurs in some women after childbirth, and is usually temporary. Postpartum blues may respond to nutrition aimed at restoring adrenal gland function. Postpartum health also depends on enough sleep.

REPEATED MISCARRIAGE & BIRTH DEFECTS

12

You formed my inmost being; you knit me in my mother's womb. I praise you, because I am wonderfully made; wonderful are your works! My very self you know. My bones are not hidden from you, when I was being made in secret, fashioned in the depths of the earth.
— Psalms 139:13-15

If you have had personal experience with either of these topics, I am sorry for the sadness it has brought you. May you find courage and especially hope in the face of your disappointment and heartache. Let me emphasize that the purpose of this chapter is not to stir up "what if's" or "if only's," those self-doubts that parents so often experience after the loss of an unborn child or the birth of a child with a life-threatening birth defect. Even experts seldom know with certainty the underlying cause of a particular miscarriage or a particular birth defect, and even the most optimistic agree that not all prenatal loss or developmental errors will ever be prevented.

But knowledge is power, and knowing the risk factors and ways to reduce them enables you to "change the things you can, and accept the things you cannot change." My goal is to point out known risk factors and to offer nutritional or other lifestyle strategies so that you can look forward to another pregnancy with confidence and joy.

MISCARRIAGE

Miscarriage refers to the loss of a child after conception but before twenty weeks of gestation. (Such a loss after that time is termed stillbirth.) "Early miscarriage" refers to a loss that occurs in the first trimester of pregnancy, about the first twelve weeks. For a number of reasons, the first trimester is the most common time of pregnancy loss. About 12 to 15 percent of confirmed pregnancies end in miscarriage.[1] Very early miscarriage, occurring before a woman is aware that she is pregnant, is another possibility, but it is difficult to estimate accurately how frequently it occurs.

Having two consecutive miscarriages occurs in about 3 percent of women,[2] and having three consecutive miscarriages occurs in about 1 percent of women.[3] Experiencing three consecutive miscarriages is recognized as a clinical problem and is called recurrent miscarriage, but two miscarriages in a row may be considered recurrent as well. The statistics on the frequency of recurrent miscarriage are reassuring in one sense—even though the heartbreak of miscarriage is all too common, it is the exception to have even two in a row.

 Women who have experienced a miscarriage can usually have good hope that their next pregnancy will result in a full term baby.

CAN THE RISK OF MISCARRIAGE BE REDUCED? The answer is yes; research literature confirms this. Nutrition has an important role to play in reducing the incidence of miscarriage. Other lifestyle factors such as smoking affect the chance of having a miscarriage. Some risk factors, such as older age of the mother, cannot be changed. Nevertheless, there are definite self care steps you can take, even if you are in a situation of higher risk. Both the nutrition for overall health in Part 1 of this book and the information aimed at overcoming specific reproductive problems covered in Part 2 apply importantly to reducing the risk of miscarriage. The discussion of pregnancy nutrition in Chapter 11 is especially applicable to preventing pregnancy loss.

CAUSES OF MISCARRIAGE

There are a number of known causes of miscarriage, though in many cases what triggered a particular miscarriage is never discovered.

OVUM QUALITY

More and more, you will hear the term **ovum quality** or **egg quality** when fertility or miscarriage is discussed. This is a vital topic, because many miscarriages actually result from events that occur before the unfertilized ovum is ovulated. How so? Amazingly, the unfertilized ovum must complete a critical cell division, called meiosis I, during the 24 hours before ovulation. Meiosis I is the cell division that converts the ovum from a **diploid** cell containing 46 chromosomes to a **haploid** cell containing 23 chromosomes. Meiosis I serves the vital role of preparing the ovum for fertilization with a sperm, which is also a haploid cell containing 23 chromosomes. The newly conceived child, then, has 46 chromosomes, 23 from each parent. Forty-six is the normal chromosome number.

If meiosis I occurs properly, then ovum quality is good, and the ovum can be fertilized and the newly-conceived child is likely to develop normally. However, if this cell division does not occur as it should, the unfertilized ovum will contain too many or too few chromosomes. In most cases, fertilization cannot take place because the chromosomal abnormality is too great. Sometimes, though, conception does occur, but the genetically abnormal child, tiny as it is, cannot develop properly and within a few days or weeks, it passes away. In such a case an early miscarriage will ensue, usually without evidence of a fully formed embryo.

Proper completion of meiosis I in the few hours before ovulation depends on the hormonal "push" and timing of FSH and LH, as well as on nutrients that are known to promote efficient cell division. The "Introduction to Part 2" discusses this topic in more detail, and "Age-Related Infertility/Infertility of Unknown Cause" in Chapter 10 lists the nutrients that are most helpful to promote proper cell division during meiosis.

IMPLANTATION. About a week after conception, the tiny embryo must implant into the lining of the uterus, the endometrium, in order to tap into the mother's nutrient provisions. Successful implantation depends on a thick, healthy endometrium, which in addition to adequate nutrition, depends on hormones, especially progesterone. If the endometrium is not well developed, or if the embryo cannot attach properly, an early miscarriage may occur within a few days or weeks.

HORMONAL SUPPORT. Progesterone levels are affected by other hormones, including thyroxine (thyroid hormone), estrogen, and cortisol. Hormonal imbalances contribute to miscarriage. Some of these may respond, at least in part, to improved nutrition or body weight; in other cases medical intervention is needed.

OLDER AGE OF THE MOTHER. As you are probably aware, the risk of miscarriage rises as a woman ages. The quality of her ova tends to decline with age, and her reproductive hormones change.

OTHER FACTORS. Physical problems with the uterus, such as fibroid tumors, can interfere with proper implantation and formation of the placenta, leading to miscarriage. Problems with blood clotting are yet another factor. Infections such as sexually transmitted disease or damage from them can be contributing factors. Rarely, there are genetic factors involving both parents that affect the embryo. If a woman has been infertile, she is unfortunately at a higher risk for miscarriage if she becomes pregnant. Yet infertility treatment itself raises the incidence of miscarriage,[4] making self help for overcoming infertility an important first step.

GENERAL GUIDELINES TO PREVENT MISCARRIAGE

If you have particular reasons to be concerned about pregnancy loss, the ideal time to attempt to prevent it is during the two to three months before and after conception.

If possible, use the three preconception months to improve your diet and begin multi-viamin/multimineral supplements, as outlined in Part 1 and Chapter 11 of this book.

DIET. How important is a healthy diet? In a large population study of British women, pregnant women who ate fresh fruits and vegetables daily had a rate of miscarriage only half as high as women who did not do so. Eating dairy products frequently also related to a reduced risk of miscarriage. The authors did not consider these foods as specific "anti-miscarriage foods," but rather interpreted eating such nutritious foods often as evidence of an overall well-balanced diet.[5] Consumption of *trans* fats has been shown to be related to a small but significant increase in miscarriage.[6] Cut your intake of *trans* fats by reading labels and avoiding packaged foods containing processed fats, such as pastries and candy bars.

VITAMIN AND MINERAL SUPPLEMENTS. Taking vitamins, especially multivitamins containing folic acid or iron, reduced the miscarriage rate by half compared to women who did not do so.[7] In another study, vitamin B12 deficiency was found to relate to fetal loss, and supplementing it in deficient women restored fertility and reduced the number of miscarriages, even among women who had suffered many recurrent miscarriages. In a published medical anecdote, one woman with undiagnosed vitamin B12 deficiency had had seven miscarriages without a single term birth. After taking vitamin B12, she quickly became pregnant and went on to have a total of three full term births in a row.[8]

Virtually every vitamin and mineral is involved in some aspect of pregnancy, literally from "A to Zinc." Comprehensive supplementation, as suggested in Chapters 3 and 11, is far preferable to taking just one or two vitamins or minerals as you prepare for pregnancy.

BODY WEIGHT, MEDICATIONS, AND LIFESTYLE FACTORS. If you are underweight or overweight or if you are coming off the pill, use the appropriate parts of this book to help yourself attain a better body weight or a better hormonal balance. Before you become pregnant is also the best time to eliminate unhealthy habits such as smoking or excess alcohol consumption.

Cut your caffeine intake to the equivalent of two cups of coffee per day, as more than 200 mg of caffeine daily has been associated with an increased risk of miscarriage. More caffeine increases this risk.[9] Be careful that any medications you take are acceptable for use during early pregnancy. If necessary, make arrangements to minimize exposure to workplace toxins. Exposure to heavy metals, organic solvents, pesticides, and many other chemicals may increase the risk of miscarriage.[10]

If you have a history of miscarriage, you may wish to try eliminating night lighting, as explained in Chapter 10 under the topic of "Sensitivity to Night Lighting." Exposure to light affects the hormone melatonin, which in turn may affect progesterone levels.

STRESS AND MISCARRIAGE. The role of stress in miscarriage is not well established, but one study has shown that women who had very early miscarriages did have higher levels of the adrenal stress hormone cortisol.[11] With or without such research, pregnancy is itself a stress, though a healthy and natural one. Reducing other stressores if you are able is prudent.

There is no doubt that many women in their childbearing years are under a great deal of stress. How do you decrease it? First, eat the best diet you can, and take your vitamins and minerals. Get enough sleep, or at least lie down and rest in a darkened room if you have trouble sleeping. If you get very little exercise, try to find a way to incorporate some moderate exercise into your routine. Conversely, if you are exercising excessively, cut down on it. It is a stress to your body, even if you enjoy it. Instead, exercise moderately, and find a slower, more relaxing physical activity that you can enjoy to take the place of overly demanding workouts.

Most important of all, if you are planning to become pregnant and are under great stress, do your best to eat as much good food as you know you need, even if your appetite is very low. When under stress, many women just don't feel like eating, and the stress of low blood glucose creates a vicious cycle that adds more stress. You can stop that cycle by eating small, healthy meals, even if you just don't feel like it. Use your bathroom scale to check your progress.

Finally, see Chapter 4, "Increasing Your Energy & Decreasing Your Stress" for nutrition to support adrenal health. Supporting your adrenal health decreases your body's response to stress even when you can't remove the actual stressors in your life. And try not to stress out over your daily stress! Work to reduce physical stresses, such as poor nutrition, inadequate sleep, and inadequate (or excessive) exercise, and you will find that the daily stresses of life feel much more manageable. Your cortisol levels will also drop.

SPECIFIC RISK FACTORS FOR MISCARRIAGE

If your charts show problems such as very short luteal phase, low thyroid function, or other irregularities discussed in the previous chapters of this book, you may wish to wait up to three months to conceive as you work to improve them.

LUTEAL PHASE DEFICIENCY. Abnormal levels of FSH or LH before ovulation may ultimately result in the formation of a corpus luteum which releases insufficient progesterone for an insufficient number of days. This is called luteal phase deficiency, and it appears on the NFP chart as fewer than the normal number of postovulatory elevated temperatures. In addition, the abnormal FSH and LH may cause ovulation of an immature egg, as described above. In such a situation pregnancy may be difficult to achieve, but even if it does occur, the newly conceived life may not be capable of normal development, or the corpus luteum may not produce enough of the progesterone necessary to sustain the pregnancy. Repeated early miscarriage is a known consequence of luteal phase deficiency.[12]

In Chapter 8, the topic "Luteal Phase Deficiency" explains the relationship between luteal function, the charted signs of fertility, and certain nutrients. This information is pertinent to you if you have observed short luteal phase cycles—cycles with less than ten to twelve days of elevated temperatures. It may also help you if you have experienced an unexplained early miscarriage, especially if fetal development did not occur.

> **In the case of an early miscarriage, you may have been told that you had a "blighted ovum," or an "empty sac" pregnancy, or that the miscarriage was the result of a "random genetic error." But a precious child was conceived and was lost, despite these clinical terms.**

The information above on ovum quality pertains to this situation. Please refer to "Age-Related Infertility/Infertility of Unknown Cause" in Chapter 10 for a comprehensive list of all the nutrients that are most helpful to improve short luteal phase as well as ovum quality.

LOW THYROID FUNCTION. The thyroid gland, which sits at the base of the neck, produces hormones that stimulate the function of most of the body's cells.

> **When the thyroid hormones are too low, they can cause a number of female reproductive problems.**

Infertility and miscarriage are among these problems. Thyroid hormones produced by the mother affect the embryo and fetus from a very early stage of development, including implantation and formation of the placenta. Early miscarriage, stillbirth, prematurity, and developmental problems with the baby's nervous system are other consequences of low thyroid function in a pregnant mother.[13]

Nutrition can improve thyroid function, as explained in Chapter 8, under the topic "Low Thyroid Function." If your charts shows signs of low thyroid function, especially basal temperatures in the range of 97.3°F or below in the preovulatory phase, implement nutrition aimed at improving thyroid function, but also look for medical assistance. Even if you need to take thyroid hormone replacement, improved nutrition can enable your own thyroid gland to function better.

If you already take thyroid medication because of low thyroid function, before you become pregnant you should make sure that your prescription is up to date for your current needs.

Thyroid hormone replacement greatly reduces the incidence of miscarriage in women who need it, but not if the level of replacement is too low.[14]

You will also need your thyroid levels monitored as your pregnancy progresses. *The Thyroid Hormone Breakthrough* devotes an excellent chapter called "Pregnancy Challenges" to women with thyroid dysfunction. (See "Further Reading.")

POLYCYSTIC OVARY SYNDROME. Polycystic ovary syndrome (PCOS), discussed in Chapter 9, may cause an increased risk of miscarriage. Apparently it is the **insulin resistance** that is the culprit, and improving insulin resistance may provide effective treatment.[15] However, women who have elevated levels of androgen ("male" hormones) are at an increased risk for miscarriage, even if they do not have full-blown PCOS.[16] In either case, please refer to Chapter 9 for an explanation of insulin resistance as well as the nutritional strategies to overcome it. Overcoming insulin resistance also helps to decrease the production of androgens.

Moderate weight loss, regular exercise, a low-sugar diet, and vitamin and mineral supplements are the self care means of dealing with the problems of insulin resistance and high androgen levels that underlie PCOS.

OBESITY. Obesity increases the risk of miscarriage and stillbirth.[17] It is very easy for researchers who report such data simply to suggest that obese women who are contemplating pregnancy lose weight, but if it were so simple, such women already would have done so! Yes, try your best to manage your weight problem, but above all eat the healthy foods you need and take high quality supplements before and during your pregnancy. Once you become pregnant, do not begin dieting in an attempt to lose weight. On the other hand, eating healthy foods, especially adequate protein and natural fat, may make it so that if you are obese, you can have a healthy pregnancy without much weight gain.

UNDERWEIGHT. Low body weight or low body fat can result in infertility and complete absence of cycles, but they can also cause or be related to short luteal phase and low thyroid function, especially if a woman is excessively athletic. If an underweight woman or a woman with low body fat becomes pregnant, she has a higher risk of miscarriage compared to women of normal weight.

A large study of women in the United Kingdom who had early miscarriage showed that having a body mass index (BMI)

of less than 18.5 increased the risk of miscarriage.[18] This is equivalent to a weight around 110 pounds in a woman whose height is 5 ft., 5 in.

THE LIMITS OF THE BODY MASS INDEX (BMI)

BMI is an inexact estimate of appropriate body fat, and your chart gives you better information about possibly being underweight. For example, if you are small-boned but have regular cycles, you probably have adequate body fat for your frame, even though your BMI seems rather low. Or, you may be slender, and your ovulations may be a few days later than average, but if your luteal phase is at least twelve days in length and your temperature levels are normal (preovulatory temperatures averaging around 97.3° to 98.2°F), it's my opinion that your body weight is adequate for healthy hormones and a healthy pregnancy. On the other hand, if you perform vigorous muscle-building exercise and have replaced body fat with muscle, you could lack sufficient body fat despite having a normal BMI. Often delayed ovulation, a short luteal phase or low basal temperatures will reveal this stress to your body. As discussed in Chapter 8 under the topic "Underweight or Inadequate Body Fat," bringing your body fat up, often by just a few pounds, will restore normal charts. What is the right weight for you? The weight at which your charted cycles are normal!

CELIAC DISEASE. Celiac disease is a disorder in which the body's immune system reacts to gluten, a protein found in wheat, rye, and barley. It causes inflammation of the small intestine, and consequently decreases the absorption of nutrients. Apparently, because of the nutrient deficiencies, including iron-deficiency anemia, untreated celiac disease is responsible for a high risk of repeated miscarriage.

 Treatment of celiac disease with a strict gluten-free diet has been shown to reduce the incidence of miscarriage to as low as that of the general population.[19]

The prevalence of celiac disease is higher than was once thought, and the disease may be "silent" in terms of obvious gastrointestinal problems. If you have had recurrent miscarriages without explanation, you should have your doctor arrange for a test for this disorder. See Chapter 10 for more information about celiac disease and the supplements that are helpful in overcoming nutritional deficiencies that may occur because of it.

CLOTTING DISORDERS. In some women, abnormal antiphospholipid antibodies increase blood clotting abnormally. This disorder, called **antiphospholipid syndrome**, decreases blood flow to the placenta during pregnancy, and the result may be recurrent miscarriage in such women. Low-dose aspirin during pregnancy is often recommended to decrease the clotting and therefore the risk of miscarriage. Omega-3 fatty acid derivatives from fish oil (4 or 5 g of mixed EPA and DHA daily) have been used in two studies to achieve the same effect, and the omega-3 treatment was as effective as aspirin in enabling women with antiphospholipid antibodies to carry their pregnancies to term.[20]

> **While the anti-inflammatory properties of fish oil are becoming better known, you should discuss this alternative with your doctor if you have reason to believe that you may have a clotting disorder.**

Fish oil, though, is an excellent supplement for most women before and during pregnancy.

UTERINE PROBLEMS. Anatomical problems within the uterus can interfere with implantation of the embryo or growth of the fetus. One such problem is **fibroid tumors**,[21] which are benign growths within the muscle layer of the uterus. Endometrial growths called polyps are another possibility. Occasionally a woman is born with a uterus that is abnormally separated into two halves. If necessary, surgery to correct the uterine anatomy can help prevent future problems in a woman who has had miscarriages due to this abnormality.[22] However, it is wise also to consider your overall health and your chart so that other problems such as the ones just discussed are not overlooked.

AGE-RELATED MISCARRIAGE. Increasing age of the mother, especially past age 35, is a well-established risk factor for miscarriage. Nevertheless, estimates on the risk of miscarriage as related to age vary. One researcher estimated the risk of miscarriage at age 37 to be 20 percent, at age 44 to be 30 percent, and at age 48 to be 40 percent of all pregnancies.[23] A large British study found that women had no age-related risk before age 35, but between age 35 and 39, their risk was 75 percent higher compared to the low-risk years of 25 to 29. Once over age 40, these women's risk of miscarriage progressed to five times greater than at age 25 to 29.[24]

Much of the problem that occurs as a woman ages has to do with the quality of her remaining ova, and delays in becoming pregnant often occur as well. Please see Chapter 10's topic, "Age-Related Infertility/Infertility of Unknown Cause," for specific nutritional and other lifestyle recommendations for achieving pregnancy when age is a factor. These are exactly the guidelines that I recommend to reduce the risk of age-related miscarriage, because they are intended to provide the ova with the nutrients they need and to support healthy progesterone levels as well.

HOLDING HOPE DESPITE POSSIBLE LOSS

In counseling women in their 40s who would like to have more children despite having had a recent miscarriage, I encourage more than just nutrition. There is a kind of internal courage, an emotional resolve, that is required. That is, if you are hoping to have more children, you need to hold the hope for another child firmly against the pain and fear of another loss.

I counseled a woman who consulted me after having two miscarriages in a row in her early forties. She had given birth to five children without difficulty when she was younger, and she told me that she could not bear the grief of another miscarriage. What could I say? If she avoided a pregnancy, she would never experience such a loss again. But she would never have the chance for the joy of giving birth to another child again, either. Yes, we discussed nutrition, and she closely followed the guidelines that I recommend for older mothers (see Chapter 10). After she gave birth to her sixth child, she contacted me to share the wonderful news. She said that what made the greatest difference to her was the counsel that she would need courage to try again. She went on to have a second "over-40" baby as well.

PREVIOUS MISCARRIAGES. A history of miscarriages in itself is considered a risk factor for miscarriage, though many women who have experienced it, even with their first pregnancy, go on to give birth to several full-term babies without any other losses. Keep in mind that studies that report such data involve women who have not specifically implemented nutritional or lifestyle strategies aimed at reducing their particular risks for miscarriage, as discussed here.

INFERTILITY. It is apparent that there is a relationship between infertility and miscarriage; it is known that women who take longer to conceive are more prone to miscarriage. What does that mean to you? First, if you are having a problem with infertility, do all the self-help steps listed in Appendix B, "Focus on Infertility." You will be healthier for it, and better health will reduce your chance of miscarrying, as you can see from the research above.

Equally as important, if you seek medical care for your infertility, keep up the good nutrition! You will respond best to medical care if you are as healthy as you can be. Finally, if you become pregnant while using the nutritional or other self-help suggestions in this book, do not discontinue them. All recommendations in this book are safe and healthy for pregnancy, unless a nutritionally-aware doctor has counseled you otherwise. To discontinue good nutrition or whatever else has seemed to help—weight gain, weight loss, reduction of night lighting—could interfere with your hormones during the vulnerable first trimester.

BIRTH DEFECTS

Are you ready to be encouraged? The amazing research that follows should help you put aside the unfounded fears that so many women have about giving birth to a baby with a major birth defect. In short, when it comes to reducing the risk of *many* different birth defects, the B vitamin folate, supplemented in the synthetic form of folic acid, has a leading role, but as you will see, not the only role.

NEURAL TUBE DEFECTS

It has been firmly established in the last thirty years that supplements of folic acid greatly reduce the incidence of birth defects that are collectively referred to as "neural tube defects," even in mothers who have had a previous child with such a developmental error.

Neural tube defects are a major cause of death among newborns, second only to congenital heart defects.[25]

There are several types of neural tube defects, including **spina bifida**. When spina bifida occurs, the child may require several surgeries in order to prevent fluid accumulation around the brain (hydrocephalus) and to promote the ability to walk. **Anencephaly**, or failure of the brain to develop normally, is an even more severe neural tube defect than spina bifida. Sadly, anencephaly usually results in stillbirth or death soon after birth.

> While the following discussion focuses on supplements, daily diet and body weight are factors in preventing birth defects.

A "prudent" diet, including fruits and vegetables, yogurt, whole-wheat bread, and fish, along with folic acid supplements, has been shown to reduce the incidence of neural tube defects and also congenital heart defects more than folic acid supplements alone.[26] Also, obesity of the mother at the time of achieving pregnancy seems to weaken the effect of folic acid supplementation in preventing neural tube defects.[27]

FOLIC ACID, MULTIVITAMINS, AND OTHER BIRTH DEFECTS

FOLIC ACID AND OTHER MAJOR BIRTH DEFECTS

Folic acid and multivitamin supplements around the time of conception not only reduce the incidence of neural tube defects, but they also significantly reduce the risk of congenital heart defects, which are the leading cause of death of newborns. In addition, folic acid and multivitamins taken before and during pregnancy have substantially reduced the occurrence of oral facial clefts (such as cleft lip or cleft palate), urinary tract defects, limb formation defects, omphalocoele (a defect of the intestines and umbilical cord), and even childhood brain cancers and leukemia.[28]

FOLIC ACID, VITAMIN B12, AND VITAMIN B6. Ongoing research is shedding light on the nutrients in multivitamins that might be involved in the reduction of birth defects in the babies of women who take folic acid along with a multivitamin. It is known that **folate** (the natural form of this nutrient) works together with two other B vitamins—vitamin B12 and vitamin B6—to reduce the production of the amino acid homocysteine. It is beyond the scope of this book to explain the biochemical details, but in low concentrations homocysteine is normal to the cells. If folate, especially, or the other two B vitamins are deficient, homocysteine builds up and creates havoc within cells. For example, it causes problems within the linings of the blood vessels, making it a risk factor for cardiovascular disease. This also explains why it is harmful to the placenta, which is a vascular organ.

> When it comes to pregnancy, homocysteine may be the actual culprit involved with the birth defects listed above, as well as with problems such as abruption of the placenta.[29]

In addition to vitamin B12 and vitamin B6, the mineral zinc works along with folate. Vitamin C is necessary for the absorption of folate. It's probable that several nutrients found in multivitamins together make a difference in preventing birth defects.

FOLIC ACID OR FOLATE?

As pointed out in previous chapters, new research confirms what researchers of the 1980's postulated: Some people have genetic variations which make it less efficient for them to use convert folic acid, the common but synthetic B vitamin, into folate, the natural form. Folate, in the form **methyl folate**, seems to bypass the problem. Methyl folate is now easily available at health food shops. The question becomes, "How much methyl folate should I use, since the original studies of this B vitamin's effectiveness against birth defects, miscarriage, preterm birth, and infertility were all done using the synthetic form, folic acid?" At this time there is very little research on supplements of methyl folate and its role in preventing birth defects.

While we can assume that folate works at least as well as folic acid, right now there is no researched reason to take a smaller dose of folate compared to the amount of folic acid that has been studied and recommended. It's my opinion that using methyl folate is a better option than using folic acid, even though there is a large body of excellent research on the benefits and safety of folic acid. If you choose to take methyl folate, my suggestion is that you use a minimum of 2 mg [2,000 mcg] and a maximum of 4 mg [4,000 mcg]. You may wish to work up gradually to 4 mg, as the side effects of large amounts can include temporary anxiety that subsides soon after the dose is reduced. In the text that follows, you will see that I recommend methyl folate, even though in referring to scientific studies, I must use the term "folic acid," since that was the supplement that was actually studied.

FOLATE AND OTHER SUPPLEMENTS: WHEN SHOULD YOU START TAKING THEM? Since the neural tube forms by 22–28 days after conception (one to two weeks after a woman misses her period), it is clear that folate should be started *before* conception in order for it to prevent neural tube defects. How long before conception? Some researchers have suggested three weeks, others eight weeks, and still others three months before conception. A two-to-three-month preparation time may be ideal, but many pregnancies are unplanned—or planned on very short notice!

 The best insurance is for every woman who might become pregnant to supplement folate and a multivitamin/multimineral as part of her daily good health habits.

However, beginning supplementation just as soon as you realize that you might be pregnant is the next best strategy. So if you discover you are pregnant by surprise, don't delay. Start the folate immediately.

FOLATE AND OTHER SUPPLEMENTS: WHEN CAN YOU DISCONTINUE THEM? Many researchers suggest that folic acid be supplemented until twelve weeks of pregnancy, but because this vitamin decreases the risk of intrauterine growth retardation, pre-eclampsia, abruption of the placenta and fetal death, "it seems highly advisable to administer folic acid during the second and third trimester of pregnancy in order to prevent hyperhomocysteinuria [elevated homocysteine levels] which in many cases could be partially or totally responsible for the vascular damage [to the placenta]."[30]

As noted, multivitamins have been shown to reduce the occurrence of childhood cancers, but in at least one large study of childhood brain cancers, the effect occurred only if the vitamins were taken in both the first and second trimester of pregnancy, and a greater effect (an astounding 50 percent reduction) occurred if the multivitamins were taken during the third trimester as well.[31]

FOLATE: HOW MUCH? Since 1992, the U.S. Public Health Service has recommended that all women who may become pregnant take 0.4 mg [400 mcg] of folic acid daily. In addition, the U.S. Centers for Disease Control in 1991 recommended that women who have had a previous child with a neural tube defect or who are otherwise at high risk should take 4 mg [4,000 mcg] of folic acid when they are trying to become pregnant, and for the first twelve weeks of pregnancy.[32]

CANADIAN FOLIC ACID RECOMMENDATIONS FOR WOMEN WITH RISK FACTORS FOR BIRTH DEFECTS

The Society of Obstetricians and Gynaecologists of Canada (SOGC) Clinical Practice Guideline (2015) has updated, comprehensive recommendations based on critical review of nearly two hundred studies of folic acid and birth defects. SOGC first recommends a folate-rich diet for all women. Such a diet includes broccoli, spinach, Brussels sprouts, peas, corn, lentils, and oranges.

For all women at high risk for folate-related birth defects, they recommend 4 mg [4,000 mcg] of folic acid daily beginning three months before conception and continuing until twelve weeks of pregnancy; thereafter 0.4 mg [400 mcg] to 1.0 mg [1,000 mcg] until after birth and completion of breastfeeding. A male partner who himself has had a neural tube birth defect or who has fathered a previous child with a neural tube defect puts a woman in this high risk group.

For women with moderate risk, SOCG recommends 1,000 mcg folic acid beginning three months before conception, and 400-1,000 mcg folic acid from twelve weeks of pregnancy until breastfeeding is complete. Moderate risk factors include family history of folate-sensitive birth defects—heart defects, limb reduction, cleft palate, urinary tract errors, and hydrocephaly. Diabetes, both type I and type II, puts a woman into the moderate risk group. Crohn's disease, celiac disease (gluten enteropathy), gastric by-pass surgery and other causes of malabsorption from the digestive system are also moderate risk factors. The drug metformin is one of several medications that put a woman into the moderate risk group.

For women with low risk; that is, no family history of folate-sensitive birth defects, SOGC recommend 400 mcg folic acid beginning two to three months before conception until the end of pregnancy and completion of breastfeeding.

They note that folic acid does not mask vitamin B12 deficiency, but recommend that B12 should be taken as part of their recommended multivitamin regime during this time of life. Their guidelines further note that folic acid has not been shown to either promote or prevent breast cancer, and may possibly lower the risk of ovarian cancer in women who take it. They cite inconclusive evidence that folic acid supplementation around the time of conception results in a reduced risk of autism.[33]

The previous SOCG Clinical Practice Guideline (2007) recommended a multivitamin of unspecified potency,[34] noting only that true vitamin A (retinol) should not exceed 10,000 IU per daily dose, as it has been associated with birth defects.[35]

A review article by Canadian researchers of The Hospital for Sick Children in Toronto, Canada echoes these recommendations.

They point out that even though controlled studies show that 800–1,100 mcg daily of folic acid is adequate to protect women from having a child with a folate-related birth defect, in practice women do not unfailingly take their vitamins.

For example, even women who describe themselves as motivated to take vitamins averaged less than 60 percent compliance in taking their vitamins in a controlled study. These authors believe that larger amounts of folic acid, together with "impaired compliance" (hit-or-miss taking of vitamins), will enable many more women to avoid having a child with a birth defect. Finally, in addressing the safety of large amounts of folic acid, they state that "case-control and some prospective studies have repeatedly shown a 20–30 percent decline in cancer associated with folic acid."[36]

Finally, Chrisopher J. Schorah, the lead investigator of the seminal MRC Vitamin Study (1983-1991),[37] which was cut short because of its overwhelming evidence that folic acid reduced the incidence of neural tube defects, recently wrote, "The MRC Vitamin Study showed that about 80 percent of neural tube defects could be prevented by taking 4 mg [4,000 mcg] immediately before pregnancy. Subsequent work showed that this achieved a greater degree of protection than with 0.4 mg (400 mcg) indicating that all women planning a pregnancy should take a 4 mg pill daily (or the more readily available 5 mg), not 0.4 mg [400 mcg] as currently recommended. This would mean recommending the same dose for women in general as for women who have already had a neural tube defect pregnancy, for whom 4 mg [4,000 mcg] is already the standard dose."[38]

Why would this outstanding researcher suggest that all women contemplating pregnancy take the higher dose of folic acid? For most women, having a child with a neural tube error is the first sign they have of their high risk status. Given the safety of folic acid and the severity of the problems it prevents, I concur with Schorah's opinion, at least when it comes to preparing for late-30's or over-40 pregnancies—4.0 mg [4,000 mcg] folic acid or folate.

FOLIC ACID AND TWINNING. A large Hungarian study that was done to add evidence that folic acid reduces the risk of having a child with a neural tube defect was re-evaluated in 1994, and the original researchers reported a 40 percent increase in the incidence of twinning among women who had taken folic acid around the time of conception.[39] However, scrutiny of these results by other investigators revealed that women in the study who conceived while using fertility drugs accounted for 40 percent of the multiple births.[40]

Several other studies followed to address this issue. A very large Chinese study showed no effect on twinning when women took 400 mcg of folic acid daily around the time of conception,[41] but a Swedish study showed a doubling of the rate of fraternal twinning among women who used folic acid, mostly in the same amount.[42] Another large Hungarian study evaluated women who had taken on average large doses of folic acid (6,000 mcg daily) along with multivitamins, and only a very small increase in the incidence of twinning was seen.[43]

FOLIC ACID AND MISCARRIAGE. Studies have shown that low folate status in women increases the risk of miscarriage, which apparently relates to elevated levels of homocysteine.[44] It came as a surprise in 1997 that the same Hungarian researchers who re-evaluated their studies on the effect of folic acid on twinning also reported a 16 percent increased occurrence of miscarriage. These researchers speculated that folic acid might actually decrease the occurrence of neural tube defects by the improbable route of causing unborn children with such developmental errors to be "selectively" miscarried.[45]

This disturbing hypothesis stirred up the interest of other researchers, some of whom suggested that if such data were accurate, another hypothesis is that folic acid and multivitamins may enable what would have been a very early, undetected miscarriage to continue long enough to be recognized as such.[46] In light of the research on the beneficial effect of folic acid and multivitamins on the health of the placenta, that hypothesis seems much more likely, and in fact the original Hungarian researchers did offer this possibility to explain the increase in miscarriages that they observed. They also noted a pro-fertility effect of folic acid; there were more pregnancies and more births to the women who supplemented folic acid compared to those who did not.[47] When more pregnancies occur, the opportunity for miscarriage also increases.

A 2005 review of several studies which investigated the relationship between miscarriage and folic acid, as well as the studies on twinning, ends with the following: "It is reassuring that data do not support the reports that folic acid supplements increase the occurrence of miscarriage or multiple births because women of childbearing age in many countries are advised to take folic acid supplements daily to prevent NTDs [neural tube defects]. Women of reproductive age and their health care providers can support the periconceptional folic acid supplementation without concern that this practice will increase the occurrence of multiple births or miscarriage."[48] As noted previously, a large study of early miscarriage in British women showed that taking multivitamins before pregnancy reduced the incidence of miscarriage by half.[49]

A large, recent, carefully-controlled study comparing women taking small amounts of folic acid (0.4 mg [400 mcg] versus taking large amounts of folic acid (4.0 mg [4,000 mcg]) in order to reduce the incidence of oral cleft birth defects reported that there was a small but nonsignificant decrease in the occurrence of miscarriage in the women who took the larger amount of folic acid.[50]

DOWN SYNDROME

Down syndrome is a genetic disorder that occurs at the time the child is conceived. Instead of having 23 pairs of chromosomes, 23 from each parent, the child has three number 21 chromosomes; thus, **trisomy 21**, the genetic name for Down syndrome. Children with this disorder have developmental disabilities, including cognitive impairment, and they may have physical health problems such as poor immune function, low muscle tone, hypothyroidism, and sometimes heart defects.

Compared to many genetic diseases, though, Down syndrome may be considered a mild disorder.

 With the care of a loving family and the support of health professionals and educators, many children born with Down syndrome can expect to have good health, go to school, and grow to happy adulthood.

The Human Genome Project has led to increased understanding of the various manifestations of the syndrome, and in turn, treatment for individuals with Down syndrome has improved.

NUTRITION FOR INDIVIDUALS WITH DOWN SYNDROME. Before considering prevention of Down syndrome, I would like you to be aware that there is nutritional therapy available to treat children and adults with this genetic disorder. A nutritional supplement called Nutrivene-D has been designed for newborns, children, and adults with Down syndrome.

Nutrivene-D is intended to compensate for specific metabolic defects that occur because of the trisomy 21 error, which affects all cells. A major problem is excessive oxidative stress on the body's cells, including the brain cells. High oxidative stress occurs because the extra chromosome 21 causes cells to overproduce oxidized cellular wastes faster than they can get rid of them. To compensate, Nutrivene-D contains large quantities of antioxidants: vitamins A, C, E, beta-carotene, selenium, coenzyme Q10, and alpha-lipoic acid. Another challenge occurs because children with Down syndrome do not produce enough of the structural protein collagen to promote proper muscle tone and joint stability. Certain amino acids have been included in Nutrivene-D to enable connective tissue cells to produce more collagen. Folic acid and B vitamins are also part of the formula, again compensating for particular metabolic deficiencies.[51]

> While I have not had personal experience with a child with Down syndrome, I wholeheartedly encourage parents of children with Down syndrome to consider the targeted nutritional therapy discussed above as an adjunct to the medical, educational, and social assistance you no doubt already have in place. To gain a fuller understanding of the biochemical challenges that people with Down syndrome face, as well as the possibilities for solving some of these through nutrition, see the website of pediatrician and geneticist Lawrence Leichtman, M.D., of Virginia Beach, Virginia, who treats children with Down syndrome using targeted nutritional therapy as well as other approaches. If you are interested in more information as well as updated research, see www.lleichtman.org/tni.shtml and www.nutrivene.com.[52] (Both are listed in "Resources.")

CAN THE RISK OF DOWN SYNDROME BE REDUCED? The greatest risk factor for conceiving a child with Down syndrome is older age of the mother. Even so, having a baby with Down syndrome is much more common in younger mothers since they have many more babies overall. Research has not answered this question definitely, but there are several very hopeful studies that, in fact, point to the same nutrients that decrease the risk of neural tube defects—folate and others which work together with it.[53]

The genetic error that results in Down syndrome occurs in the hours shortly before ovulation, when the unfertilized ovum completes meiosis I, as explained in the Introduction to Part 2 and at the beginning of this chapter. During meiosis I, the ovum normally divides so that instead of 23 pairs of chromosomes, it contains only 23 single chromosomes.[54] In what is called a nondisjunction error, the two 21 chromosomes stick together. When the ovum is fertilized, then, trisomy 21 occurs. About 95 percent of Down syndrome conceptions occur because of improper cell division in the unfertilized ovum as opposed to the sperm.[55] Among its other functions, folate is necessary for the events of meiosis to proceed normally.

> A number of investigations have found that many women who have given birth to children with Down syndrome have a genetic variation in the way they metabolize folate; in effect, these mothers have an increased need for folate to maintain normal cellular processes.[56] Some studies have found

that homocysteine is elevated and/or folate levels are depressed in mothers of children with Down syndrome.[57] The most recent research, a comprehensive meta-analysis of thirty-seven studies, strongly concludes that the genetic variation known as "MTHFR 677 C>T polymorphism," which results in some degree of impairment of folate metabolism, is associated with a significantly increased risk of Down syndrome. Importantly and hopefully, the authors state that nutrition may reduce this risk: "The high intake of folate may neutralize the metabolic impact of MTHFR polymorphism."[58]

However, it is clear from these studies that genetic variations are not necessary for a woman to have a child with Down syndrome, and that other factors must be involved. It seems probable that a deficiency of dietary folate is a major factor, along with the nutrients that work together with folate. Inadequate folate in a woman prior to conception may result in problems similar to those caused by the metabolic inability to use folate properly.

The research is still ongoing to answer the question as to whether or not folic acid or folate supplements reduce the incidence of Down syndrome. Simply fortifying food with folic acid has not changed the incidence of Down syndrome, according to one study.[59]

What does this mean, practically speaking, given the evidence that Down syndrome occurs more frequently in the children of mothers who cannot use folate as efficiently as others? My strong recommendation is to take supplements of methyl folate in the amounts suggested above *before conception* to reduce the incidence of neural tube defects, and be aware that it may possibly reduce the incidence of Down syndrome. Your childbearing years may be over before all the studies are in.

Folate works together with zinc and vitamin B12, and it requires vitamin C to be properly absorbed. Vitamins do not function in isolation, and taking a good multivitamin/multimineral supplement is an excellent preparation for pregnancy, as suggested in Chapter 11. If you are a woman in your late 30's or in your 40's, or if you have other reasons to be concerned about Down syndrome, I recommend the amounts of vitamins in Chapter 10 under the heading, "Age-Related Infertility/Infertility of Unknown Cause."

A PERSONAL NOTE

When I got pregnant with our eighth child at age 47, it was quite a joyful surprise, since my last baby had been born when I was 41. I had given up hope quite a while before. I had been aware at that time (1999), that research on the link between folic acid and prevention of Down syndrome was in progress, because in 1996 I had attended a national conference on the nutritional treatment of Down syndrome.

There I had the opportunity to meet nutritionally-oriented physician Dr. Julian Whitaker, who in response to my question about preventing

Down syndrome said, without hesitation, "Folic acid. You are going to see research forthcoming on the link between folic acid and prevention of Down syndrome. Right now the evidence is circumstantial. But the biochemical evidence is coming."[60] Almost three years later, when I realized I was pregnant, I was glad that, for general good health, I had been taking 3,000 mcg of folic acid (along with 1,000 mcg of B12 and comprehensive vitamins) for three or four months.[61] I did not request an ultrasound, but I felt very positive that the baby would be normal. Nevertheless, the encouraging information on treatment for children with Down syndrome made me very relaxed throughout the pregnancy.

It was in October of 1999, when I was already three months pregnant, that the original article on the topic of folic acid for prevention of Down syndrome was published. I must admit that I went through that pregnancy much more confident about having a healthy baby then, at age 47, than I did at age 41, when I was six years younger, but not aware of any information linking nutrition to the prevention of Down syndrome.

A DEBT OF GRATITUDE. All of us want the best for our children, and it is a normal maternal instinct to want your children to be as healthy as they can be. For me, the initial research on folic acid and Down syndrome was a huge encouragement when I was pregnant so late in my fertile years, because it gave me great hope and confidence that the baby would be genetically normal. I also felt that if Down syndrome did occur, I would have plenty of nutritional information aimed at helping the baby be as healthy as he or she could possibly be. I also had a firm trust that God knew what we could handle.

As it turned out, Monica was a completely healthy baby and continues to be healthy and happy. Nevertheless, I still consider my attendance at the national conference on treatment of Down syndrome children with nutrition in 1996 as one of the high points of my life. The passion of the health professionals there on behalf of those children was electrifying. The hope that they offered to the many parents of Down syndrome children in attendance was real, as several of them were parents of children with Down syndrome themselves. One presenter had adopted three children with Down syndrome!

I count it a great honor to have met Dr. Lawrence Leichtman there, with his passion for the health of these precious children. Most of all, I loved their recommendation as to when parents should start the nutritional intervention: "Theoretically, they should begin as soon as it is diagnosed, and if not, certainly as soon as they are born."[62]

THE FATHER'S ROLE

The role of the father in miscarriage and birth defects is a factor which is infrequently considered. Damage to a man's sperm may cause infertility, but it is apparently rare for a damaged sperm to survive in the female reproductive tract long enough to fertilize the ovum, especially when millions of healthy sperm are more able to do so.

Older age of the father may be a contributing factor to miscarriage,[63] and researchers estimate that about 5 percent of Down syndrome is related to an extra number 21 chromosome in the sperm involved in conception.[64]

Sperm have a very high need for oxygen because of their high energy use as they swim. Because they are very small cells, they carry few protective antioxidant enzymes with them. **Oxidative stress** is what damages sperm. Exposure to toxins, whether from workplace materials, cigarette smoking, alcohol, or house and garden chemicals, ultimately results in oxidative stress. The effect of aging on sperm is also explained as oxidative stress. The damage that prolonged heat exposure causes to sperm is summarized as oxidative stress.

The all-important DNA, the genetic contribution of the father, is damaged by oxidative stress.[65]

Avoiding exposure to toxins and excessive heat reduces oxidative stress and sperm damage. Improved nutrition provides antioxidants that counteract oxidative stress.[66] These nutrients—vitamins A, C, and E, folate, zinc, and others—are detailed as part of the discussion of male fertility in Chapter 15.

In any type of infertility, including repeated miscarriage, both parents should strive for the best nutrition possible, as outlined in Part 1. Keep in mind that it takes perhaps two months for improved nutrition practices to affect complete sperm development (see Chapter 15). Once conception has occurred, the father's physical contribution to his child is complete, but his continued emphasis on good nutrition will not only enhance his own health; it will also be the best encouragement to excellent nutrition that he can offer to his expectant wife.

SUMMARY—CHAPTER 12

1 While miscarriage is unfortunately common, recurrent (repeating) miscarriage is not. Many of the same factors that cause cycle irregularities or infertility increase the risk of miscarriage, but good diet and taking multivitamins before and during pregnancy can reduce the risk of miscarriage.

2 "Ovum quality" refers to the cell division of the ovum that occurs in the 24 hours before ovulation. When egg quality is good, conception and healthy development are likely to occur. Vitamins and mineral that support cell division are recommended to protect and improve ovum quality.

3 Some of the same factors that cause irregular cycles may contribute to an increased risk of miscarriage. These include short luteal phase, low thyroid function, under weight and obesity. Nutrition directed at improving these may reduce the risk of miscarriage.

4 Supplements of folic acid and/or multivitamins have been shown to significantly reduce the incidence of several types of birth defects, including congenital heart defects and neural tube defects. In addition, supplements of folic acid and multivitamins reduce the occurrence of umbilical defects, limb defects, and urinary tract defects. They decrease the risk of childhood brain cancers and leukemia; taking folic acid throughout pregnancy reduces the risk of childhood brain cancer by 50 percent.

5 Although virtually all of the published research on preventing miscarriage and birth defects have used the synthetic vitamin, folic acid, instead of the natural form, methyl folate, research shows that some individuals have genetic variations that limit their ability to use folate. The natural form, methyl folate, should be preferred to the synthetic form, folic acid, despite the many studies using folic acid and the lack of studies using methyl folate.

6 Folate works together with other B vitamins, especially vitamin B12, to decrease the production of the damaging amino acid homocysteine, which may be the actual culprit in many birth defects.

7 Targeted nutritional support is now available to help children with Down syndrome to compensate for the biochemical problems caused by this genetic disorder.

8 New evidence suggests that supplements of folate and/or multivitamins before pregnancy may decrease the incidence of Down syndrome, as research shows that women who have a genetic inability to use folate properly have increased levels of homocysteine, and an increased incidence of having children with Down syndrome.

9 Sperm cells carry half of the genetic material for a new child, but these cells are tiny, have high energy requirements, and so are prone to oxidative damage. Nutrition to counteract oxidative damage may help prevent miscarriage and birth defects.

10 The father's role in miscarriage and birth defects may be smaller than that of the mother, but good nutrition for overall male fertility is the most prudent course to take when a couple is concerned about pregnancy loss or birth defects.

PERIMENOPAUSE, MENOPAUSE & BEYOND

13

This ancient blessing succinctly reveals the biological purpose of menopause. The normal, natural, and predictable loss of fertility that has been part of womanhood throughout the ages ensures that women have a life span potential well beyond their childbearing years. Menopause makes it possible for women to nurture the children to whom they have given birth. Menopause allows women to live long enough to help their grown children as they become parents, and to enjoy the age-old delight of seeing their "children's children."

Menopause actually refers only to a woman's last period, which typically occurs around ge fifty. A woman in her forties or fifties who has gone for twelve months without a menstrual period is said to have passed menopause. If she does have a period after that, oops! — the twelve-month count begins again! Perimenopause is a much more useful term when dealing with the longer process traditionally called "the change of life." **Perimenopause** is the gradual decline in fertility that ends with menopause. Perimenopause generally begins in the early forties. During this time, the ovaries slowly decrease their output of the reproductive hormone progesterone. You may be surprised to learn that the hormone estrogen may increase during the perimenopause, leading to a hormonal imbalance often called **estrogen dominance**. Before or after menopause, however, estrogen gradually drops to approximately half of what it was during the fertile years.

Women often experience about two years of obvious cycle irregularity before the actual menopause—the last period—occurs. During this time of transition, progesterone drops to very low levels. However, even after menopause, both the ovaries and the adrenal glands continue to secrete sex hormones, and the body fat plays a major role in producing estrogen.

It's important to realize that many of the changes of the perimenopause are completed during the five years that follow menopause.

Good nutrition and other good health habits continue to be the keys to vibrant good health during perimenopause and for long afterward. You'll notice that many of the topics addressed below refer you to previous chapters of this book. Why?

The years of declining fertility are part of a continuum, and the strategies for optimal reproductive health are not essentially different from what they were in your earlier years.

SEEKING OR AVOIDING PREGNANCY

If you are attempting to become pregnant in your forties, you should know that fertility declines significantly during the early forties and sharply after age 45. Yet many women can become pregnant and have children in their early forties. Some women can become pregnant when they are 45 or 46. A few women will be able to conceive during the year that they are 47. Once you have your 48th birthday, there is little basis to hope to become pregnant or to fear that you might.[1] This is true even if you are charting normal-looking cycles indicating ovulation, mainly because the ova have degenerated. The uterine tubes' ability to transport ova also diminishes, and the endometrium loses its ability to nourish a fertilized ovum.

SEEKING PREGNANCY. If desire to have a baby but are having difficulty conceiving in your forties, refer to the section in Chapter 10 entitled "Age-Related Infertility" for specific nutritional recommendations which may be helpful to achieving pregnancy at this age. See also Chapter 12, "Repeated Miscarriage & Birth Defects," because the risk of miscarriage unfortunately climbs as women approach the end of their childbearing years. Nevertheless, there are nutritional strategies to reduce that risk. And consider Chapter 15, "Men's Fertility and Reproductive Health" since your husband is also getting older, and his fertility might also be declining. Please note that the above information relating to age and fertility decline refers to seeking pregnancy *naturally*, but even medical treatment for infertility may not overcome the age-related decline of the forties.

AVOIDING PREGNANCY. If you are avoiding a pregnancy, continue to chart and to follow the Couple to Couple League's guidelines for the perimenopause time, no matter what your age. It is worth reminding you that nutrition to improve your cycle regularity makes NFP easier to use at every stage of life, including during the perimenopause.

Your goal should be a smooth, healthy, and happy transition from the fertile years to menopause and beyond.

NFP will literally help you to "chart the course," giving you insight into what is happening as your hormones change—another wonderful benefit of NFP.

CYCLE IRREGULARITIES

Cycle irregularities are to be expected, especially during the final two years or so before menopause. Your cycles may gradually shorten during your mid-forties, only to become much longer in the transition before menopause. Your menstrual periods may become lighter and shorter than before, but you also might experience a few heavier and longer periods. It's common in perimenopause for the real period to be preceded by one, two, or three days of light spotting, called "irregular shedding." It's also common for the period to end with a brownish color to the menstrual flow, instead of the normal pinkish color.

 Both irregular shedding before the actual period and brownish bleeding at the end of the period are signs of low progesterone.

Your charts might also reveal a pattern of short luteal phases (less than ten or eleven elevated temperatures after ovulation), which are another indication of lower levels of progesterone. Occasional anovulatory cycles ("cycles" without the temperature shift indicating ovulation) may occur, and your last few periods may follow anovulatory cycles. Sometimes spotting will occur between episodes of more typical menstrual bleeding.

However, you should also not be too quick to accept any cycle irregularity as an inevitable part of perimenopause, especially if you are only in your early or mid-forties!

Instead, try to uncover other causes of the irregularity by considering the following:

LUTEAL PHASE DEFICIENCY. Luteal phase deficiency, discussed under that title in Chapter 8, refers to inadequate progesterone in the second half of the cycle. It may be detected with charting, because ovulation followed by less than ten or eleven postovulatory elevated temperatures is typical of this hormonal imbalance. The pattern may repeat, month after month. Luteal phase inadequacy is common in the forties, and may underlie the bothersome mood swings of PMS at any age. Reread Chapter 6, "Premenstrual Syndrome (PMS)," because the nutritional strategies to overcome PMS are very helpful in improving an inadequate luteal phase. In fact, even if you have tried the PMS nutritional plan in the past but have discontinued it, you may be pleasantly surprised at the difference it makes during this stage of life.

THYROID DYSFUNCTION

Despite lab testing for suspected thyroid problems, it's still all too common for the diagnosis of hypothyroidism to be missed.

Undetected low thyroid function can cause cycle problems at any stage of a woman's life, but it can also begin for the first time during the perimenopause and later. Long cycles or anovulatory cycles, if they occur along with very low temperatures on the NFP chart (preovulatory temperatures below 97.3°F), are signs that you most likely have low thyroid function. Or, you may experience short, regular cycles with short luteal phase occurring with low preovulatory temperatures. Often the mucus pattern is that of ongoing less-fertile mucus.

One cause of low thyroid function is the rise in estrogen during the perimenopause years, since excess estrogen (estrogen dominance) interferes with the action of the thyroid hormone.[2] There are other causes, including unmet nutritional needs of the thyroid gland. See "Low Thyroid Function" in Chapter 8 for information on detecting and correcting thyroid problems.

MENOPAUSE AND THYROID DYSFUNCTION

If during the perimenopause or after, the common menopausal complaints such as hot flashes, mood disturbances, and memory problems do not resolve, ask your health care practitioner to check your thyroid. Either hypothyroidism or, less commonly, hyperthyroidism can cause such problems. If self care is not helpful, medical care for thyroid dysfunction can improve the symptoms.[3]

LOW BODY FAT. Being underweight or lacking sufficient body fat (see "Underweight or Inadequate Body Fat" in Chapter 8) can cause long cycles or a total lack of ovulation and periods at any age. However, if you lose too much body fat during your forties, you may believe you are in perimenopause or are past menopause when you are not! If you have doubts as to whether you are truly past menopause, you can have your FSH and LH tested. These two hormones become and remain irreversibly elevated after menopause, making true menopause easy to ascertain via testing. Conversely, inadequate body fat is one common cause of *low* FSH and LH, which also causes irregular or absent periods. Unlike true menopause, loss of cycles due to low body fat is reversible with weight gain.

I have counseled several women in their mid-forties who believed that they were going through menopause, yet the answer to their cycle irregularity or lack of periods was a strenuous exercise program and dieting for weight loss,. If you have begun dieting or vigorous exercise and have developed irregular cycles, anovulatory cycles, or have lost your periods completely, consider this possibility carefully. It's worth regaining some body weight or cutting down on the exercise to restore your normal hormone levels and cycles, as bone loss may accompany the amenorrhea (loss of menstrual cycles) caused by loss of body fat.

EXCESS BODY WEIGHT OR WEIGHT GAIN. Just as low body fat affects the reproductive hormones, so does excess body fat. If you have had fairly regular cycles during your most fertile years, and do not have polycystic ovary syndrome (PCOS), gaining weight during the perimenopause can be both the cause and the effect of estrogen dominance. Excess body fat is a source of estrogen, and estrogen affects several other hormones in such a way as to favor fat storage. High estrogen levels during perimenopause may underlie such problems as fibroid tumors, tender breasts, mood swings, gallbladder disease, anxious depression, weepiness, and foggy thinking.[4] I believe that the best approach to dealing with weight gain in perimenopause is with a diet relatively low in starchy and sugary carbohydrates, along with regular exercise and targeted supplements, as is described in "Overweight without PCOS" in Chapter 9. Dropping even a modest amount of weight can help some women have more regular cycles.

HEAVY OR PROLONGED BLEEDING

Heavy or prolonged bleeding may be caused by uterine fibroid tumors, which are benign (noncancerous) growths within the wall of the uterus. Many women have them without symptoms, but if during this time of life you begin having heavy, painful, or prolonged periods, suspect fibroids and seek a diagnosis by a medical doctor. Estrogen dominance during the perimenopause stimulates the growth of fibroids, sometimes causing them to grow as large as a grapefruit. In such cases you may be able to notice the increase in the size of your abdomen, especially if you are slender. Once estrogen declines significantly after menopause and beyond, fibroids usually shrink.

The most common cause of hysterectomy in the United States and elsewhere is to treat fibroid tumors. Even if you are past childbearing, however, there are compelling reasons to save your uterus rather than to have a hysterectomy. The uterus is a placeholder for the rectum, bladder, and vagina. Equally important, when the uterus is in place, the ovaries function better because their blood supply runs along the uterus and its tubes. That blood supply enables the ovaries to continue to produce their hormones, even for several years after menopause.

If a doctor has confirmed that you do not have fibroid tumors or any other significant medical condition, please refer to Chapter 6, "Shorter, Lighter, & Pain-free Periods." The nutritional suggestions there apply to women of every age.

> **My experience as an NFP counselor is that heavy bleeding not caused by fibroid tumors or other medical conditions is one of the easiest problems to overcome with improved nutrition, no matter what the age of the woman.**

HOT FLASHES AND NIGHT SWEATS

Hot flashes and night sweats are caused by low, fluctuating estrogen levels. They are most likely to occur in the two years before menopause and for variable lengths of time afterward. They are usually a sign that the change of life really is in progress. On the other hand, sometimes much younger women experience hot flashes or night sweats in the weeks after childbirth, when estrogen levels have suddenly dropped sharply. Significant weight loss or loss of body fat due to strenuous exercise can bring them on at younger ages also.

Whatever the cause, hot flashes and night sweats can be slightly to profoundly annoying. It's thought that the low, fluctuating hormones send an erroneous signal to the nervous system, causing it to respond as if your body is overheated. The nervous system then triggers the blood vessels of the skin to dilate and the sweat glands to secrete. As annoying as they can be, hot flashes and night sweats are harmless to your health, unless night sweats significantly disrupt your sleep. They do disappear as your body readjusts to the lower levels of estrogen.

IS IT A HOT FLASH?

How do you know if you are having a hot flash? If you need to ask, you probably have never had one! They are named well—you suddenly feel quite overheated, especially your face, and you may break out in a sweat. You may or may not appear to blush. Hot flashes usually last for just a minute or two. They may occur many times a day or only every few days. They are not usually accompanied by anxiety, as you might suppose, but anxiety, stress, or embarrassment can bring them on. Being too warm is a major cause, but often there is no obvious trigger. The nighttime variety, night sweats, can be mild or severe. If they are mild, you wake up with a sense of being too warm, maybe a little damp or sticky. If they are severe, you wake up drenched in sweat. Fortunately, there are some very effective strategies to reduce the frequency and severity of these "vasomotor symptoms," as researchers call them.

LIFESTYLE STRATEGIES. At night make sure your clothing and bedding are made from lightweight natural fiber that breathes. Keep your sleeping room cool. During the day, dress lightly or in layers, so that you can remove a sweater or jacket if necessary. Avoid hot drinks, which can provoke them. Carrying ice-cold bottled water with you and drinking it as needed can put a stop to an unwelcome hot flash. Caffeine may or may not cause hot flashes, but alcohol is likely to do so. Watch out for spicy-hot foods, which can bring them on. Here's a trick that can help if you want to avoid blushing during a hot flash: exhale and hold your breath as the hot flash comes on. This initiates a reflex that causes the blood vessels in your skin to constrict, counteracting the blood vessel dilation of the hot flash.

OVERWEIGHT OR UNDERWEIGHT. Body weight affects the tendency to have hot flashes. If you are overweight, the extra insulation of the body fat may make you prone to them. Conversely, if you tend to be underweight, you may be susceptible to them because a lack of body fat results in reduced estrogen levels.

VITAMIN E AND FLAX OIL. Vitamin E (400–800 IU/day), together with flax oil (five to ten 1 g capsules per day, or 1–2 teaspoons of the liquid), is very helpful for reducing the incidence and severity of hot flashes and night sweats. Even more flax oil, up to 6 teaspoons or 30 g/day, is safe and healthy for hot flashes.[5] Take vitamin E when you use flax oil, as vitamin E protects the essential fatty acids in the flax oil from oxidative damage.

If your hot flashes are mild and not too frequent, you may experience them as almost amusing, as a minor episode not even significant enough to be called an annoyance. That's how I experienced them during my change of life. I always considered myself to have been "born cold and never warmed up." It was funny for me to find that even using a hair dryer could trigger a mild hot flash!

VITAMIN B6 MAY INCREASE HOT FLASHES

Dr. Guy Abraham, who performed double-blind studies relating vitamin B6 to a decrease in PMS symptoms, has said that large doses of vitamin B6 make hot flashes worse because B6 reduces estrogen.[6] Aware of this, I avoided vitamin B6 for three years during my perimenopause, even though my hot flashes were mild. Eventually I increased it again to about 200–300 mg per day, and wondered why I ever avoided it! Yes, it did bring on a few mild hot flashes, but the energy, mood improvement, and especially the mental sharpness I experienced after resuming vitamin B6 were well worth it. Along with the other supplements discussed in Chapter 3, try to get at least 50–100 mg of vitamin B6 daily,[7] unless you find that it is responsible for increasing hot flashes or night sweats to an annoying level.

VAGINAL DRYNESS

Estrogen is responsible for stimulating vaginal secretions, and a decline in estrogen underlies vaginal dryness, a common symptom that tends to worsen in the years beyond menopause. Dryness in the vagina can cause an uncomfortable sensation of irritation or itchiness; it can make intercourse difficult, and it increases the risk of both vaginal and urinary tract infections. Vitamin A, vitamin D, vitamin E, zinc, flax oil, and cod liver oil in amounts as listed in Table 7, Chapter 3, are all helpful to this condition. Vaginal lubricants can be used during intercourse if necessary.

> According to the late Dr. John Lee, author of *What Your Doctor May Not Tell You about Menopause*, a small amount of prescription cream containing the natural estrogen estriol, without other forms of estrogen, is safe to apply to the vagina twice a week to relieve vaginal dryness.

Vaginal suppositories of estriol can also help overcome bladder incontinence and prevent bladder infections.[8]

LOSS OF SEXUAL DESIRE (LOW LIBIDO)

Interestingly, vaginal dryness at this time of life is not necessarily related to low sexual desire. Why not? As estrogen declines, a woman's natural androgens ("male" hormones) from her ovaries and adrenal glands are no longer overshadowed by estrogen. In effect, the androgens are unmasked. Sometimes this leads to a minor increase in unwanted body hair, but androgens also stimulate female desire. It's quite possible that your sexual desire might increase around the time of menopause. However, if a drop in sexual desire does occur during perimenopause or after menopause, there are several possible explanations. It should not be considered normal or inevitable.

POSSIBLE CAUSES OF LOW DESIRE. One possible cause of low libido is thyroid dysfunction. Refer to "Low Thyroid Function" in Chapter 8 for more information on this topic and ways to correct it. Another is being very thin or lacking enough body fat. The stress of low body fat causes hormonal changes that reduce the output of the sex hormones. Gaining a modest amount of weight may improve desire. Oppositely, overweight or obesity can also cause low sex drive. It's not necessarily due to poor body image, as you might guess. Rather, excess body fat converts the natural androgens from the ovaries and adrenal glands into estrogen. A moderate amount of weight loss—perhaps 10 percent of the total body weight—may help to restore sexual desire.

Because androgens come from the adrenal glands as well as from the ovaries, supporting the adrenal glands through improved nutrition, as discussed in Chapter 4, "Increasing Your Energy & Decreasing Your Stress" is an excellent strategy to increase sexual desire.

NATURAL PROGESTERONE. If, nevertheless, decreased desire is still a problem, natural progesterone cream applied to the skin during the second half of the cycle, after ovulation is confirmed by the sympto-thermal NFP chart, may be helpful. Once you stop having periods, the progesterone cream can be used during the second half of each calendar month. While Dr. Lee recommended over-the-counter natural progesterone cream for women with low desire,[9] in some cases, very small amounts of prescription testosterone cream may be helpful instead.[10] Read *Dr. John Lee's Hormone Balance Made Simple: The Essential How-to Guide to Symptoms, Dosage, Timing, and More* in order to acquaint yourself with the uses of natural progesterone, estrogen, and testosterone (See "Further Reading").

One note of caution: It's prudent to have your health practitioner's counsel before you use progesterone cream, even though it is not under prescriptive control. See "Low Sexual Desire" in Chapter 14 for further information on this topic.

MOOD SWINGS, ANXIETY, AND DEPRESSION

Perimenopause and the years immediately following menopause have the reputation of being times of unstable moods, poor mental focus, and decreased energy levels. There are many self care strategies to avoid or lessen such problems, starting with better nutrition.

If you are troubled by mood swings, meaning short-term changes between normal moods and anxiety, irritability, or "the blues," look first at stabilizing your blood sugar levels.

Proper function of your adrenal glands, which sit atop each kidney toward the back of the waist, is key to accomplishing this task.

ADRENAL GLAND FUNCTION. Drops in blood glucose force the inner part of the adrenal glands, the adrenal medullae, to secrete the stress hormones norepinephrine and epinephrine, formerly called "adrenaline." These hormones raise the blood glucose levels, but they also produce nervousness, irritability, and anxiety. A sugary treat that suddenly elevates blood glucose levels may seem to help out for a while, but other hormones, especially insulin, will soon produce a reactive drop in blood glucose levels. Along with the blood sugar drop come fatigue, brain fog, and another spurt of stress hormones!

 Regular meals and snacks, each a combination of protein, unrefined carbohydrates, and healthy fats, are the best way to get off the blood glucose roller coaster.

See Rule 6 in Chapter 1 for more information on the effects of refined sugar on blood glucose levels.

Mood swings, anxiety, and low energy can also be improved by nutrition aimed at bolstering the function of the adrenal cortices (plural of "cortex"), which are the separate, outer parts of each adrenal gland. Most people are hardly aware of the adrenal cortices, unless they have heard that they produce the stress hormone cortisol. Yet the adrenal cortices do an amazing amount of "behind the scenes" work. They coordinate the physical response to all types of stress, whether the stress is from illness, infection, sleeplessness, pain, low blood glucose, overwork, or emotional causes. They are essential in managing the stress of the changes of perimenopause. Moreover, they produce androgens, the "male" hormones. These hormones promote sexual desire in women; equally as important, some androgens are converted to estrogen by the body fat.

Nourishing the adrenal glands pays off well with calmer nerves, improved sexual desire, and normal levels of estrogen in the body. Among the many tasks they perform, adrenal cortical hormones keep blood glucose levels up between meals. Because low blood glucose can make it difficult to concentrate, healthy adrenals prevent the common complaint of "brain fog" during the change of life.

The adrenal cortices actually produce about fifty different hormones, but they can become exhausted, favoring production of some of their hormones at the expense of the others. Reducing stress in your life is certainly helpful to them, but nutrition aimed at meeting their needs is at least as beneficial as stress reduction.

NUTRITION FOR THE ADRENAL GLANDS

The adrenal glands need a variety of nutrients, literally from A to Zinc: vitamin A, the B vitamins, especially pantothenic acid, plenty of vitamin C, vitamins D and E, and the minerals magnesium, zinc, and manganese. They must have an adequate supply of the essential fatty acids to produce their hormones. Fresh, unheated salad oils and supplements of flax oil (five to ten 1 g capsules or 1–2 teaspoons daily) supply these fatty acids. Cod liver oil, which supplies the ready-made EPA and DHA as well as some vitamin A and D, may be used also. Adequate salt is another nutrient that the adrenal glands require.

Reducing caffeine intake is beneficial to the adrenals. Caffeine acts on them like a whip on a tired horse—short-term stimulation, for sure, but long-term consequences as the adrenal glands become exhausted by the overstimulation. No doubt one of the unhealthy ways that caffeine affects the adrenals' stress response is by causing sleep disruption. You need more sleep at this time of life, and so do your adrenal glands! Sleeping and waking at regular times actually develops a healthy pattern of secretion of the adrenal hormones. Try not to let caffeine interfere with your sleep, and do not let lack of sleep interfere with your adrenal glands. One of the best ways to reduce stress is to get more sleep, and get it on a regular schedule.

IMPROVING SLEEP

Poor sleep is a common complaint of women before and after menopause. The sleep hormone melatonin drops significantly around the transitional time of menopause. You can try supplementing melatonin, about 0.3 to 3 mg half an hour before bedtime, as explained in the section on sleep in Chapter 4, "Increasing Your Energy & Decreasing Your Stress." Another option is the use of supplements of gamma-amino butyric acid (GABA), an amino acid complex that is a neurotransmitter in the body. One hundred mg before bedtime is a typical dose. I personally use a related nonprescription product called Kavinace, by NeuroScience (Osceola, WI; www.neuroscienceinc. com). While the label recommends two capsules one to two times daily, I have found one half or even one quarter capsule right before bed very helpful to immediate and restful sleep. My own experience is that this is not in the least habit forming, and I use it only intermittently. When I have used it at a higher level for three days in a row, I can notice a slight depressive effect. Please discuss this and any related products with your health care practitioner, particularly if you suffer from mood disorders.

For a comprehensive, easy-to-understand book that emphasizes nutrition for perimenopause moods, focus, and energy, read nutritionist Ann Louise Gittleman's *Before the Change: Taking Charge of Your Perimenopause*. (See "Further Reading.") In addition to better diet and supplements, it explains the role of exercise, stress reduction, adrenal support, and natural hormone replacement during this period of life. It recommends supplements and herbs such as black currant oil and borage oil, which may be valuable to some women. Gittleman's book, I believe, is the best available to help y ou make an emotionally smooth, healthy, and happy transition from the fertile years to menopause and beyond. It is also excellent for women already past menopause.

MAINTAINING HEALTHY BONES

With the medical and media spotlight on osteoporosis for the last few decades, many women rank concerns about this disease as their greatest fear of menopause. They are concerned about breaking a hip and becoming disabled. They are concerned about vertebral fractures and becoming stooped. They are equally concerned about the side effects of medications to prevent bone loss.

Good news: There are four effective self care strategies for maintaining healthy bones for life: weight-bearing exercise, bone-building nutrition, healthy body weight, and safety habits to prevent fractures.

WEIGHT-BEARING EXERCISE. Bone is living tissue, and the microscopic bone-laying cells, called osteoblasts, don't like to be squashed! When they "feel the squeeze"—that is, when pressure is put on them by your walking, jogging, running, jumping, or lifting, they respond by laying solid bone material around themselves until they have fortified a microscopic shell and are left safe and still alive within it. Weight-bearing exercise "puts the pressure on" the osteoblasts, and the result is strong bone. Eventually, over a number of years this bone will deteriorate, but bone-dissolving cells called osteoclasts periodically invade worn bone, and like a crew of miniature miners, they clear out a tiny stretch of old bone. That sets the stage for new osteoblasts to come in, get "squashed," and respond by laying solid new bone material around themselves. Pressure on bones is an essential ingredient for new bone formation. By contrast, did you know that astronauts in weightless space suffer rapid and substantial bone loss? Their osteo*clasts* keep removing old bone, but their bone-building osteo*blasts* have no motivation to do their job!

Regular weight-bearing exercise—putting the pressure on your osteoblasts—is not optional if you wish to have strong bones for life. If you are not currently exercising regularly, find some activity that you enjoy, whether it is walking the dog, working out at a gym, or jogging around your neighborhood. That exercise will additionally help to regulate your insulin levels and burn calories, contributing to weight control. It will elevate your mood, especially if you do it in the great outdoors and don't overdo.

MUSCLE STRENGTHENING EXERCISES. Weight-bearing exercise is fundamental for bone health, but don't forget that muscle strengthening exercises do another essential job. They are the key to maintaining the ability to hold, lift, carry, bend, kneel, and take the stairs. If there is only one muscle-strengthening exercise that you are willing to do, it's squats to maintain lower body strength. Just a few sets of squats done several times a week will make a noticeable difference in the ease with which you bend over, genuflect, rise from a sitting position, and stand up after reaching for something on the floor.

BONE-BUILDING NUTRITION

> Exercise alone cannot do the job of building up bone, because bone requires a large number of raw materials to renew itself.

Many people name calcium first when they think of providing the body with the raw materials to make bone, but this is only one aspect of nutrition for healthy bones.

Susan Lark, M.D., offers excellent advice for bone health. She points out that calcium and other minerals from the bones are naturally released to neutralize acid in the blood. A diet that chronically produces excess acid requires the bones to give up extra calcium to buffer that acid. As people age, this constant loss of minerals begins to take its toll, and thinning bones results. Oppositely, a diet that is more alkaline allows the bones to hold on to their calcium, reducing bone loss.[11] The kind of protein you eat affects the acidity of your body.

PROTEIN. About one third of bone is the thread-like protein collagen, which decreases the brittleness of bone. Adequate protein is therefore essential to bone health, but excess animal protein, especially from red meat, poultry, and dairy, causes acidity as it is metabolized within the body. Dr. Lark instead recommends moderate use of protein foods, as well as emphasis on protein sources which produce less acid: whole grains (except wheat), beans, nuts, fish, and eggs. Many fruits are quite acidic, so she believes they should be limited. But most vegetables are somewhat alkaline, and are good sources of magnesium and potassium, both of which she calls **bone-sparing** nutrients.[12] Sugar, caffeine, alcohol, and fizzy soft drinks, even those without sugar, produce excess acid in the body. Plenty of water tends to dilute acid within the body, and she recommends drinking more water—one more benefit of adequate hydration! Her recommendations are consistent with the "Twelve Rules for Better Nutrition" in Chapter 1.

CALCIUM AND VITAMIN D. What about the micronutrients? Calcium is key, but it cannot be absorbed out of the intestines and into the blood unless vitamin D is present. Vitamin D can be made by the action of sunshine on the skin, but for people who work indoors and live in a climate with a cold winter, supplements of vitamin D are essential for optimal health. There are numerous healthy "side effects" to adequate vitamin D intake. A recent review of the research on vitamin D and menopause has revealed that besides its effect on bone strength, this wonderful vitamin is beneficial to cardiovascular health, to moods, mental sharpness, and weight control in menopausal women.[13] Vitamin D also decreases the risk of cancer,[14] including breast cancer.[15]

It has become routine for men and women both to be checked for blood levels of vitamin D, but all too often those levels are below what is ideal. You may wish to supplement 2,000 IU of vitamin D per day, or whatever amount your health practitioner recommends after your blood levels of vitamin D have been evaluated.

CALCIUM AND PHOSPHORUS. If you use dairy products, you not only get the calcium, but you also get the often-overlooked mineral phosphorus. Phosphorus is the second most abundant mineral in bone. It is seldom mentioned by nutritionists because it is considered to be widely available in the diet, but that is not always the case.[16] If you have reason to be concerned about osteoporosis, I recommend supplements that include "MCHC" (microcrystalline hydroxyapatite concentrate), a mix of naturally-occurring bone minerals, including calcium and phosphorus. I personally am very pleased with a supplement called Bone Builder, manufactured by Ethical Nutrients (Aliso Viejo, CA www.ethicalnutrients.com), which contains these nutrients as well as the bone-healthy mineral boron.

CALCIUM AND MAGNESIUM. While calcium and vitamin D are important in preventing osteoporosis in later years, calcium should be balanced with magnesium, which is plentiful in the bone and enables the body to use calcium. You can subtract 250 mg of calcium from your supplemental intake of calcium for each cup of milk or serving of other dairy products in your diet, and you may wish to adjust the ratio of total calcium (dairy plus supplements) to supplemental magnesium to equal 1:1, or approximately 1,000 mg calcium (dairy plus supplements) to 1,000 mg of supplemental magnesium. As noted in Chapter 3, "Supplements to Consider," magnesium in the form of magnesium oxide is too laxative for many people. A mix of magnesium oxide and chelated magnesium in the form of magnesium aspartate, magnesium citrate, or magnesium gluconate is less likely to cause loose bowels.

In addition to calcium, phosphorus, magnesium, and vitamin D, there are a number of other nutrients that enable the bone cells to lay down new bone: zinc, silica, boron, vitamin K, vitamin C, and the essential fatty acids.[17]

HEALTHY BODY WEIGHT. Good nutrition also includes maintaining an adequate body weight. The reproductive hormones estrogen and progesterone stimulate bone health. In the fertile years, including the perimenopause, if enough body fat is lost, these reproductive hormones decrease and lack of ovulation and loss of periods result. As the perimenopause gives way to menopause, progesterone falls essentially to zero, and the body fat becomes the major source of estrogen.

Thin women, with their low estrogen from body fat,
have a well-established increased risk of osteoporosis
compared to women of normal weight.

THAT MID-LIFE WEIGHT GAIN

The modest increase in weight that many if not most women experience during perimenopause and after menopause is a natural and healthy readjustment of the body to the change in its hormonal status. This is not to advocate obesity, but rather, a comfortable weight for your age. It may be 10 or 20 pounds higher than when you were 25, even a bit more if you were quite slender back then. In fact, a body weight of 132 pounds or more offers protection against bone fractures.[18] Did you know that one reason thin women are more prone to bone fractures than heavy women is that thin women have less padding than their heavier sisters?

FRACTURE-PREVENTING SAFETY HABITS. The final key to bone health is preventing fractures through proper safety habits. Gillian Sanson, author of *The Myth of Osteoporosis*, advocates strongly for behavioral changes to decrease the chance for fractures. She correctly points out that it is bone *fractures*, not bone density itself, that will impact your quality of life as you age. (See "Further Reading.")

Hip fracture is a particularly debilitating bone injury, and preventing such a fracture should be a high priority for everyone, including men. Only a small percentage of hip fractures occur spontaneously—that is, the neck of the femur (thigh bone) breaks under the weight of the body without a fall or other accident causing it. The vast majority of hip fractures, about 95 percent, occur in response to falls.[19]

One of the most effective things you can do to prevent bone fractures as you age is to implement safety measures to prevent falls. Now is the time to form the habits of using hand railings on steps, taking extra precautions on wet or icy outdoor decks, and keeping small items and pets from underfoot. Do you walk up and down your household steps with large clothes baskets held in both hands? Do you dash down your stairs in slippery socks? Are you ready to change unsafe habits such as these? It may be a humble concession to age to start safety habits while you feel youthful and vigorous, but good, well-ingrained safety habits now may prevent disaster when you are much older.

Compressive fractures of the vertebrae (backbone) may not cause intense pain, but they can cause deformities of the spine and poor posture, limiting ease of movement. On the other hand, poor posture may just be a bad habit. This is an excellent time to evaluate your posture. How much poor posture is the habitual but reversible failure to "stand tall"?

If osteoporosis is a concern of yours, read *The Myth of Osteoporosis*, with its careful referencing of the medical literature. (Despite the unfortunate title, the author does not consider the serious bone disorder osteoporosis a "myth.") While the author downplays the value of the Dexa Scan test of bone density, I disagree, and I believe that it should be routinely done in women well before the perimenopause years. I urge you to have such a test soon, if you have never had one. If your test lets you know that your bones are dense and strong, keep up the good work!

If your test should come back showing low bone density, *The Myth of Osteoporosis* will be an excellent resource. It will alert you to the possible inaccuracies in your test or in its interpretation. It will reassure small-boned women that in fact their petite body build may contribute to poor test results despite healthy bones. Most of all, it will inform you of the marginal usefulness but major side effects of drugs intended to increase your bone density. Instead, the book recommends the four keys to bone health reviewed above: weight-bearing exercise, bone-building nutrition, adequate body weight, and fracture-preventing safety habits.

PROGESTERONE CREAM. Dr. John Lee advocated natural (**bio-identical**) progesterone cream for prevention of osteoporosis.[20] Even though it is available over the counter, if it is of interest to you, you should look for a medical doctor familiar with its use to assist you. Natural progesterone cream is certainly no substitute for the combination of exercise, improved nutrition, body weight awareness, and fracture prevention, but it may be a useful addition to your bone health approach. It has many other benefits to perimenopausal and menopausal health—especially to sexual desire and overall moods.

BLADDER CONCERNS

During the perimenopause and after menopause, many women become prone to urinary bladder problems. Low estrogen and the aging process together affect the bladder in several ways. While often hot flashes and osteoporosis seem to be the major topics of conversation and research when it comes to menopause, for many women urinary bladder problems are a much greater day-to-day concern. Depending on the nature, frequency, and severity of the bladder problems, they can negatively impact quality of daily life.

URINARY TRACT INFECTIONS. The mucous membranes of the vulva, where the urethra exits, become thinner and drier after menopause due to low estrogen. This gives harmful bacteria a better chance to take hold and cause a urinary tract infection. Prevention and care of these all-too-common bacterial infections at any age is discussed in Chapter 14, "Miscellaneous Problems That Affect Women," under the topic of "Bladder Infections."

URINARY STRESS INCONTINENCE. Leaking urine, or urinary incontinence, is yet another bladder problem related especially to perimenopause. It is also common during pregnancy. If you have been pregnant in the past, you may be aware of **stress incontinence**, which means leakage of urine when you laugh, cough, or sneeze. Stress incontinence occurs because the pressure on the abdomen from your abdominal muscles as you suddenly laugh, cough, or sneeze compresses the bladder. The controllable circular muscle, the urethral valve muscle, is not strong enough to withstand the pressure and leakage results. Researchers are not entirely sure how pregnancy causes stress incontinence, but it subsides after childbirth and fades away for years—until perimenopause. At that time, it may be caused by loss of muscle tissue in the urethral valve, which weakens it. Weight gain may add pressure to the urethral valve. For unknown reasons, this type of urinary incontinence seems to subside after the menopause.[21]

URGE INCONTINENCE. Urge incontinence occurs when you feel a sudden urge to urinate that seemingly just can't wait. It may occur on arising after a night's sleep, or it may surprise you as you enter the bathroom and your bladder seems as if it's automatically ready to empty before you are! This type of incontinence is believed to be related to nerve dysfunction, though its cause is not well understood. It increases with age. A history of daytime wetting in childhood may be a risk factor for urge incontinence.[22]

PREVENTING OR OVERCOMING URINARY INCONTINENCE. The Kegel exercise, the same exercise that is recommended to increase the ability to experience sexual orgasm, was originally developed in order to overcome urinary incontinence. You may have already learned how to perform this exercise during a childbirth class. If not, here's how you do it: When you are on the toilet, you stop a stream of urine for several seconds by consciously contracting the very urethral valve muscle mentioned above. Like a muscle in your arm or leg, it responds to this workout by becoming thicker and stronger. Try performing Kegels five or six times each time you urinate, except don't try it when your bladder is uncomfortably full. For more information on the Kegel exercise, see "Weak Pelvic Floor Muscles" under the topic "Other Factors in Low Desire" in Chapter 14.

If necessary, you can perform a Kegel contraction before you cough or when you feel a sneeze coming on. In doing so, you are consciously increasing the contraction of the urethral muscle that holds the urethra closed. In the case of urge incontinence, you may be able to train your bladder by consciously disregarding its "urgent" signal when you know your bladder is not full and is not irritated. The Kegel contraction may again be helpful. Avoiding the same foods that irritate the bladder and increase the risk of urinary tract infections may also help out with urge incontinence, the type of incontinence that increase with age. Refer to "Bladder Infections" in Chapter 14 for a list of these foods.Overweight after menopause typically includes abdominal fat, which puts pressure on the bladder. Working against obesity is helpful for many reasons, including both stress and urge urinary incontinence. Finally, vaginal suppositories of estriol can help overcome bladder incontinence and prevent bladder infections.[23] Such natural hormone supplements are available only by prescription.

BEAUTIFUL SKIN

The aging process most noticeably affects the skin, of course, but there are natural approaches to maintaining beautiful skin. The first, I think, is to recognize the beauty of age. For example, my husband's Aunt Lorraine lived to be almost 101, and spent the first 100 years of her life in vigorous good health. She was an elementary teacher back in the one-room schoolhouse days, the adoptive mother of a fine son, a grandmother and great-grandmother, an avid gardener, a hard-working farm wife, and the loving caretaker of her husband, whom she outlived by fifteen years. Deeply involved in her small town community and church, she wrote letters regularly to a host of correspondents, was interested in everybody, and was loved by everybody. Her 100th birthday party was hugely crowded with family, friends, and well-wishers. She was a beautiful woman, inside and out, for all the 30 years that I knew her. She had beautiful skin, too. Aged skin? Wrinkled skin? Well, yes, I suppose she did. It wasn't relevant. That's what I mean by recognizing the beauty of age, and accepting it in yourself is the first step to beautiful skin.

However, excellent nutrition is the foundation for healthy, beautiful skin. The outer layer, the epidermis, is particularly helped by the fat soluble nutrients vitamins A, D, E, and K, and the essential fatty acids. Flax oil in particular (about 10 grams or 2 teaspoons daily) or fish oil and other healthy oils such as olive oil condition and moisturize the epidermis "from the inside out."

The deeper layer, the **dermis**, is the connective tissue layer. It has somewhat different needs. It requires vitamin C for the synthesis of its structural proteins, collagen and elastin. It requires sulfur-containing amino acids. These are most plentiful in eggs and the "cruciferous" vegetables—broccoli, cabbage, Brussels sprouts, and other members of the cabbage family. Both the epidermis and dermis require protein.

Holistic dermatologist Dr. Terry Loong of London points out that inflammation is harmful to the skin, as it is to the entire body. Poor gut health results in inflammation that can show up on the skin. Taking probiotics and avoiding personal food sensitivities decreases inflammation. Avoiding sugar, caffeine, alcohol, and gluten promotes gut health and enables the skin to become clearer and brighter. Dr. Loong also recommends a more alkaline than acid diet, including plenty of green foods and sources of the healthy omega-3 fatty acids, such as salmon.[24]

Almost everyone knows that prolonged exposure to the sun damages the skin, but moderate summer sunshine exposure for just ten or fifteen minutes daily to a person in shorts and a T-shirt is very effective in enabling the skin to make vitamin D, with its powerful anti-cancer potential. Exercise is healthy for the skin because it increases the blood flow through it. Conversely, smoking is extremely damaging because it causes the blood vessels of the skin to vasoconstrict, decreasing its blood flow. Using only natural cosmetics with absorbable oils helps to keep the surface of the skin conditioned and healthy.

SUGAR AND YOUR SKIN

If you need one more reason to motivate yourself to cut sugar out of your diet, here it is: According to cosmetic dermatologist Frederic Brandt, M.D., reducing your sugar intake can make your skin look ten years younger, because sugar accelerates the breakdown of the collagen and elastic proteins in the dermis. Elevated blood glucose levels cause glucose to bond with body proteins, resulting in a damaging process called glycation that affects virtually all tissues, including these two skin proteins. Dr. Brandt's thirty-day "detox" diet for beautiful skin is much like the recommendations in this book, particularly the recommendations for those attempting to overcome yeast overgrowth (Chapter 10). That is, he recommends a sugar-free and starch-free diet for thirty days, but non-starchy vegetables, non-dairy animal protein, and a few fruits are allowed. As a side effect, he mentions how much more energetic and clearer-thinking eliminating sugar makes you![25] You will no doubt be hearing more about the damaging molecules caused by glycation, which are called **advanced glycation end products**—AGEs for short. They are serious factors in blood vessel disease, age-related brain dysfunctions, as well as skin aging.

May I close with just one more anecdote about my dear Aunt Lorraine? She gardened avidly until she was 100, and she ate what she grew. She always had a row of vitamin bottles on her neat kitchen counter. But perhaps as significant, she was well known for how she dealt with dessert. If there was party or a potluck, someone would usually bring an angel food cake, without icing. Aunt Lorraine would have just one thin slice. Everyone knew that that was the way she liked it, and one piece was all she would eat!

SOMETHING TO SMILE ABOUT

If you are absolutely committed to avoiding facial wrinkles, here are a couple of facts and four guidelines that really work. First, you already know that overexposure to the sun ages the skin. But equally as important, the muscles of facial expression are the culprits for much of the wrinkling of the face, because they insert into the skin and gradually pull it into predictable creases. Year after year, that movement adds up.

The four guidelines:

1. Stay out of the sun!

2. Don't frown!

3. Don't talk!

4. Don't smile!

(See, life really is worth a few wrinkles! :-))

SUMMARY—CHAPTER 13

1 Menopause is part of the natural life transition designed to enable women to live long enough to rear their children.

2 The transition from the fertile years to infertility begins with **perimenopause** in the early 40's, and is completed a few years after **menopause**, the last period, which ocurs sometime around age fifty.

3 Some women may hope to become pregnant during the perimenopause, while others will avoid pregnancy. Fertility declines in the forties, and by age forty-eight almost all women will be unable to become pregnant.

3 A number of changes take place during the perimenopause and in the years following menopause, mostly relating to the decline in progesterone and the rise and then decline of estrogen.

4 As the body readjusts, NFP charts are a great aid to understanding what is happening and when.

5 Thyroid problems affect the cycle at any age, but often begin in the perimenopause.

6 Improved nutrition, the same as during the fertile years, is still the best way to maintain vibrant good health. Nutrition can help with some cycle irregularities, irregular bleeding, hot flashes, vaginal dryness, sexual desire, and mood changes.

7 Long-term bone health is promoted by weight-bearing exercise, bone-building nutrition, healthy body weight, and fracture-reducing safety habits.

8 Bladder problems increase during the perimenopause and after menopause. Urinary tract infections, stress incontinence, and urge incontinence are the most common such problems. Nutrition and other self care practices, especially the Kegel exercise, are helpful strategies to avoid them.

9 Beautiful skin is promoted by a variety of vitamins and minerals, adequate protein, attention to gut health, and avoidance of sugary foods.

MISCELLANEOUS PROBLEMS THAT AFFECT WOMEN

14

Natural family planning users are truly the most health-conscious women I know. They are interested in all aspects of reproductive health, and are diligent in seeking out and using self-help options if they exist. Using NFP in itself reduces a number of reproductive health risks, which is one reason women are drawn to natural means of family planning. But there are a few miscellaneous problems that may occur anyway. Self-care strategies for preventing or overcoming them are offered below. (This chapter excludes sexually transmitted diseases, which must be dealt with medically and are not covered in this book.)

VAGINAL INFECTIONS

There are two major types of vaginal infections—yeast infections and the less common bacterial infections. NFP is a great help in avoiding them since it does not decrease the protective mucus, as hormonal birth control often does, and it does not irritate the vagina, as barriers and spermicides do. In addition, by practicing NFP, you become aware of the ordinary, healthy cervical mucus discharge and therefore have the benefit of early recognition should infection occur.

YEAST INFECTIONS

Vaginal yeast infections occur all too frequently in women. The yeast organism *Candida albicans* is normally found in the healthy vagina, but several factors can make it get out of balance and cause infection. The decreased acidity and increased production of glycogen, a natural carbohydrate, that occur during pregnancy or the use of hormonal birth control can trigger yeast infections. Since yeast thrives on sugar, overconsumption of sugars and refined starches is a major risk factor. Antibiotics are an important contributor to yeast infections because they destroy the "friendly" bacteria that inhabit the vagina and naturally inhibit yeast organisms. Irritations in or around the vagina can also trigger outbreaks of yeast. Tight clothing, damp clothing, synthetic underwear, douches and feminine hygiene sprays are sources of such irritation.

How do you know if you have a yeast infection? Yeast causes a discharge that tends to be whitish, thick and caked. The discharge does not have a bad odor; it may smell a little bit like baking bread. There is often itching of the vulva or vagina, and there may be reddening of the labia and even of the upper thighs.

As usual, an ounce of prevention is worth a pound of cure. With reference to the role of sugar, one hundred women with chronic vaginal yeast infections were found to have "…excessive oral ingestion of dairy products, artificial sweeteners and sucrose. Eliminating excessive use of these foods brought about a dramatic reduction in the incidence and severity of Candida vulvovaginitis."[1] Translation: Cutting out sweet junk foods, including artificial sweeteners, is the first step to avoiding yeast infections. One of my NFP clients ended twenty years of recurring yeast infections by limiting sugar and caffeine and taking supplements similar to those in Chapter 3.

If antibiotics are truly necessary, eating yogurt daily during and following treatment will help restore normal intestinal bacteria.

 Instead of or in addition to yogurt, good quality probiotics are a useful tool to help prevent vaginal yeast infections.[2]

Probiotics differ, so try to obtain a high quality brand with a variety of different friendly bacteria, as discussed in Chapter 3. Vitamins A and E and the essential fatty acids in flax oil (five to ten 1 g capsules or 1–2 teaspoons daily) are generally healing to all mucus membranes. Zinc works along with vitamin A to support the immune system, as does vitamin C.

Cotton underwear and loose-fitting, natural-fiber clothing that "breathes" are helpful to preventing yeast infections. Don't wear pantiliners if you are not having a period; cotton-crotch underwear, carefully washed with bleach and well rinsed, is a better choice. Frequently-changed sanitary napkins are preferable to tampons. If you swim regularly, change into dry clothing immediately afterward, as yeast organisms thrive in a warm, damp environment.

If you choose to use a menstrual cup, make sure you change it frequently and wash it carefully. If you get a yeast infection while using it, discontinue it, at least for a while. Consider whether or not it might be causing irritation that allows yeast organisms to take hold. If you have a bacterial infection, discontinue using it.

Intercourse should be avoided during yeast infections in order not to spread the yeast cells. The penis may also become infected with yeast, so that yeast infections may be passed between the spouses. In one study, semen of the spouses of some women with recurrent yeast infections was found to contain yeast organisms thought to infect the seminal vesicles of the man. Yeast was also found to colonize the mouths of husbands of some women with recurrent yeast vaginitis, suggesting that oral-genital contact might be a source of reinfection in such women.

Treating the husbands systemically for yeast in these cases greatly reduced the incidence of vaginal infections in the wives.[3]

Over-the-counter anti-yeast medications have made these annoying outbreaks treatable with self care, but recurrent yeast infections are a prime symptom of general candidiasis, or yeast overgrowth. This topic is discussed in detail in Chapter 10, under the heading "Yeast Overgrowth/Gut Disbiosis." *The Yeast Connection and Women's Health*, by William Crook, M.D., contains a wealth of information on yeast-related problems, including vaginal infections and a related condition, vulvodynia, or genital pain in women. (See "Further Reading.")

BACTERIAL VAGINOSIS

Bacterial infection of the vagina is less common than yeast infection. Bacterial vaginosis, as it is called, typically causes a gray or yellowish discharge that has a foul or fishy-smelling odor. It may cause itching, general pelvic pain, pain on intercourse, cramps, pain on urination, or low back pain. Intrauterine devices (IUDs) and diaphragms may contribute to these infections, again illustrating the value of NFP.

Prevention of such infections is of course the primary goal. Wiping from front to back is a usual recommendation for preventing bacterial contamination from the feces. The same irritating substances mentioned relative to yeast infections (feminine hygiene sprays, tight clothing, and so forth) should be avoided in order to prevent bacterial infections. Sanitary napkins, frequently changed, are preferable to tampons and menstrual cups when bacterial infections are a problem.

Since cervical mucus helps protect against infection, you should be especially careful during the "dry" times of the month if you are prone to bacterial infection. Consider nutritional aids, particularly flax oil and vitamin A, if scant mucus is a problem.

For postmenopausal women who experience vaginal irritation due to dryness, flax oil is very helpful (5–10 g/day), as are vitamins A, D, and E, and zinc. (See Table 7, Chapter 3, for amounts.) All of these are very healing to the vaginal membranes. There is some evidence that probiotics ("friendly" bacteria taken by capsule) may help prevent bacterial vaginosis, since friendly bacteria tend to crowd out the wrong kind of bacteria in the colon, where the infective bacteria originate.[4]

As with yeast infections, abstinence is advisable when bacterial infections are present. If antibiotic treatment is necessary, be careful to avoid getting a yeast infection, as discussed above. Husbands of women who are troubled by frequent bacterial infections of the vagina should be examined also and treated if infection of the penis or prostate is present, though most prostate infections are not communicated to the woman.

Accurate diagnosis is essential for vaginal infections that do not quickly respond to home remedies. For those with reason to believe that their infection could be sexually transmitted, medical diagnosis and treatment of both spouses by a physician is a must.

BLADDER INFECTIONS

Differences in anatomy explain why women are far more prone to bladder infections than are men. Since the urethra of the female is shorter and infective bacteria come from the outside, it is a shorter trip to the bladder for such bacteria in women than in men. The female urethra is also closer to the anus, where the infective bacteria usually originate. Sexual activity is the most important risk factor for urinary tract infections,[5] as the urethral opening lies close to the vagina.

Urinating within thirty minutes after intercourse is a useful practice for women who are prone to bladder infections, as is emptying the bladder every two hours or so during the day.

This flushes away bacteria and prevents overstretch of the bladder wall, which reduces its blood supply. If you are prone to urinary tract infections, be sure that you empty your bladder as completely as possible each time you urinate, leaning forward a bit and not rushing. Making sure that you do not sit in one place for long periods of time is another helpful habit, especially if you have had past urinary tract infections after long hours of travel. Drink plenty of pure water to dilute the urine and encourage emptying.

Certain foods may cause inflammation of the bladder. Consider whether any of the foods listed under the topic below might contribute to your tendency to bladder infections.

INTERSTITIAL CYSTITIS/PAINFUL BLADDER SYNDROME

Some women are bothered by chronic or recurrent episodes of bladder pain and inflammation, termed interstitial cystitis and painful bladder syndrome. Certain foods may increase these symptoms, according to a study based on the experience of people who have such interstitial cystitis. The most commonly reported foods that resulted in bladder pain were as follows: caffeinated foods and beverages, with coffee being the worst, followed by cola drinks, tea, decaffeinated coffee, dark chocolate, and milk chocolate candy; carbonated drinks and alcoholic beverages; foods containing hot peppers, such as burritos; other spicy foods; artificial sweeteners, including aspartame and saccharin; juices, including cranberry juice and pineapple juice; tomato products; horseradish and vinegar. Conversely, using baking soda to produce less acidic urine has been reported to be the most helpful self care.[6]

Note that the commonly-recommended cranberry juice is on the list of bladder irritants! Yes, it somewhat inhibits bacteria, but most cranberry drinks are loaded with sugar, and any acid or spicy food can irritate the urinary tract in women who are prone to bladder infections, allowing the bacteria to take over.

Bladder infections are more easily prevented than cured through self-help strategies, and you may need an antibiotic if you develop one. Here is a final tip if you ever find yourself with a urinary tract infection which makes it painful to empty your bladder: Pour a large glass of warm water slowly over the vulva as you urinate. Those who have had such infections report that this is a tremendous help.

LOW SEXUAL DESIRE

A young woman once wrote a letter to Couple to Couple League's *Family Foundations* magazine, asking for help because her sexual desire was high only at mid-cycle, the fertile time. Since the couple was avoiding a pregnancy, this led to a frustrating situation—by the time infertile days were available after ovulation, the wife's desire had faded. The letters from the readers who responded to the writer were insightful, sensitive and mature. One writer dealt with communication between the spouses regarding the problem, its possible causes and its resolution. All the respondents charitably encouraged the woman to face this difficulty with graciousness and prayer, and some shared their own similar struggles.

I would like to discuss this issue from the physical aspect, because there is a very good chance that women like the original letter writer experience low libido (low sexual desire) because of physical factors involving overall health and, in particular, hormonal balance. This is not to dismiss other possibilities—the interpersonal, emotional or spiritual. Nor do I intend to equate the level of desire of a woman to the overall happiness of her marriage. I think that most people would agree, though, that it is easier for a husband to please his wife, and for a wife to please her husband, when her libido naturally makes her appreciative of and responsive to his attention.

LOW DESIRE IN THE POSTOVULATORY INFERTILE TIME

When a woman experiences desire only during the fertile time and loses all desire during the rest of the month, she is experiencing a form of low sexual desire that should be recognized as such.

Even if she were seeking a pregnancy and not abstaining during the fertile time, this would be a frustrating problem. Women are sexually receptive at all times of the month, and it is the norm for women to be able to respond sexually whether or not they are in the fertile time. Some studies have shown that women have two peaks of desire: one during the fertile time, and one during the premenstrual days. Some have even written that many women find the infertile premenstrual days a time of higher libido than the actual fertile time.

The late John Lee, M.D., author of *What Your Doctor May Not Tell You about Menopause*, stated that libido depends more on levels of progesterone than on estrogen or androgens ("male hormones") in women. His experience is that women who use nonprescription natural progesterone cream during the second half of their cycle (the luteal phase, or postovulatory phase) report a noticeable increase in desire.[7] This makes sense, because progesterone stimulates thyroid function and also serves as the precursor for some adrenal hormones. Both glands are involved in libido.

If you are in your fertile years, however, you should first attempt to improve your own progesterone levels naturally with diet and nutritional supplements, rather than with hormone supplements. (See "Luteal Phase Deficiency" in Chapter 8). If you do choose to use progesterone cream, always wait until the third day of elevated temperatures that confirm ovulation before doing so. Once you are past menopause, if you wish to use over-the-counter natural progesterone cream, you can do so for two or three weeks of each calendar month. In any case, even though it is nonprescription, you should consult with a knowledgeable physician first.

Guy Abraham, M.D., developed and tested a diet and supplement plan for over-coming premenstrual syndrome (PMS), which is often caused by low progesterone levels in the luteal phase. He created Optivite, a complete multivitamin/multimineral supplement which, under double-blind conditions has relieved the symptoms of PMS. Vitamin B6 and vitamin C, major nutrients in Optivite, have been shown to raise the levels of progesterone, at least in some women. (See Chapter 6 for details.)

I spoke by telephone with Dr. Abraham about the effect of Optivite on womanly desire. "Yes, that has been unexpected, but we have received many reports of increased desire in women using Optivite. Husbands will say, 'This is the woman I married again.' Not all women, but some women report that they are more receptive, even more interested in initiating relations during the premenstrual days."[8]

If you are experiencing low desire during the luteal phase, first try to improve your nutritional (and indirectly, hormonal) status with Optivite or the similar ProCycle PMS and improved diet, as outlined in Chapter 6. Equally as important, five to ten 1 g capsules of flax oil a day may make a noticeable difference in desire. When the ovaries have the nutritional building blocks they need, they are more likely to produce optimal amounts of their hormones. This is also true of the thyroid gland and adrenal glands, whose hormones also affect libido.

OVERALL LOW DESIRE

LOW THYROID FUNCTION

For many years it has been known that low thyroid function (hypothyroidism) is a major contributor to low sexual desire.

Low thyroid function is common, and many women have been tested for it. But Mary Shomon, author of *The Thyroid Hormone Breakthrough*, points out that thyroid tests are notoriously unreliable, and the understanding that "subclinical hypothyroidism" exists has gained acceptance. Thyroid function affects basal body temperature, and if your preovulatory basal temperatures are in the range of 97.3°F or below, you have good reason to suspect that low thyroid function might be your problem, even if you have been tested and the tests have been normal. See "Low Thyroid Function" in Chapter 8 for information on nutrition and other help for low thyroid function. Mary Shomon's book is an excellent resource as well. (See "Further Reading.")

POOR ADRENAL FUNCTION. The adrenal glands, which sit atop each kidney, have a major role in the physical response to stress.

Consider poor adrenal function if your sexual desire is low, especially if you have been under prolonged stress.

Why? Among the many roles they play, the adrenals produce androgens that increase libido in women. Besides coordinating the response to stress and producing these "male" hormones, they regulate the immune response, they are vital for salt balance in the body, and they keep the blood glucose levels up between meals. Stress of any type, whether physical or emotional, increases the workload of the adrenals. In addition to emotional stress, low blood glucose, underweight, excess exercise, pain, allergy, illness, and sleeplessness can all affect the adrenal glands, increasing their need for nutrients. In order to make their hormones, the adrenals need many nutrients, including vitamin

C, the essential fatty acids (five to ten 1 g capsules of flax oil daily) zinc, manganese, and B vitamins, especially pantothenic acid. Attention to the nutrients the adrenals require can improve libido. See Chapter 4 for more information on the adrenal glands.

OVERWEIGHT. Overweight or obesity may be related to low desire in some women. This is not necessarily due to the "body image" that an overweight woman in our weight-obsessed society may be burdened with, but simply due to the hormonal situation. Overweight results in elevated estrogen levels and lowered androgens, because body fat converts androgens from the adrenals and ovaries into estrogens. High levels of estrogen lower progesterone, and both androgens and progesterone are involved in female libido. Pullout: A modest, gradual weight loss, coupled with moderate exercise and good nutrition, is helpful to regaining a better balance of hormones and improving desire. (See Chapter 9 for more information on overweight.)

UNDERWEIGHT OR INSUFFICIENT BODY FAT. Dropping too much weight can cause a drop in desire because estrogen and progesterone levels drop. A woman who lacks adequate body fat will ultimately experience delayed ovulation, and even complete amenorrhea if the weight loss is great enough. How much weight is enough? If you are ovulating more or less regularly—by day 18 or so—probably the underweight is just on the border. Even if you are not ovulating at all, usually a gain of just a few pounds, or a decrease in vigorous exercise, will bring back the cycles. The decrease in stress and the increase in sex hormones will very likely improve desire. (See Chapter 8, "Underweight or Inadequate Body Fat.")

YEAST OVERGROWTH. Dr. William Crook, author of *The Yeast Connection and Women's Health*, was a proponent of the theory that some people have abnormal amounts of yeast organisms in their bodies. These organisms, according to this viewpoint, disrupt many systems of the body, including the immune system and the hormone glands. When the hormones are disrupted, loss of sexual desire is one of many possible effects.

Yeast may get out of hand when sugar intake is excessive, when antibiotics are taken for long periods, or when cortisone drugs or birth control pills are used. Avoiding yeast-containing foods, eating good quality yogurt, and maintaining a healthy, low-sugar diet with supplements as listed in Table 7 (Chapter 3) helps the body to keep yeast in balance. When yeast organisms are under control, the function of the thyroid gland, adrenal glands and ovaries improves, and so will sexual desire, according to Dr. Crook. If you are bothered by yeast infections or overall poor health, refer to "Yeast Overgrowth/Gut Dysbiosis" in Chapter 10 of this book and to Dr. Crook's book also. (See "Further Reading.")

MENOPAUSE. As fertility declines in the 40s, the adrenals' production of androgens contributes importantly to women's sexual desire. Desire may in fact increase in the 40s and afterward because as estrogen declines, the androgens produced by the adrenals are "unmasked." That is, their effects are more obvious because they are not overshadowed by estrogen. Let me state it clearly:

> **Do not accept the common belief that desire inevitably drops as menopause approaches. If your desire does drop at that time, look to low thyroid function or poor adrenal function, and work to correct the problem.**

In some cases, small amounts of testosterone can restore desire in women, especially during the perimenopause and beyond. Dr. John Lee recommends that women try natural progesterone cream for six months, and if desire is still not restored, that they talk with their doctor about natural testosterone, which is available only by prescription.[9]

The amino acid L-arginine increases the blood flow to the genitals, increasing sexual sensitivity in some women. A proprietary blend of L-arginine, Panax ginseng, Ginkgo biloba and damiana leaf, along with several vitamins and minerals, was formulated and tested under double-blind conditions for its effect on sexual desire, sexual satisfaction and satisfaction with the overall relationship. Taken daily for four weeks, this supplement, called ArginMax for Women, was shown to be most helpful to women in the perimenopausal transition, but was also moderately helpful to overall sexual satisfaction in postmenopausal women.[10] ArginMax for Women is available at www.arginmax.com, and is recommended by women's health writer Susan Lark, M.D. Alternatively, Dr. Lark recommends 500 mg of arginine one to three times daily.[11] Be aware, however, that arginine can cause flare-ups of genital herpes, as well as the herpes virus that causes cold sores in the mouth.

LOW DESIRE POSTPARTUM

The high hormone levels of pregnancy contribute to the increased desire that many women experience if they stay rested and healthy throughout the pregnancy. But the steep drop in hormones after the birth may produce the opposite effect, especially during the first few months of breastfeeding. All of this is quite natural, and recognizing it as a temporary situation gives perspective.

> **Nevertheless, desire can pick up long before fertility returns after childbirth, even as a woman continues breastfeeding.**

I have frequently noticed very low temperatures when counseling women who are naturally infertile while breastfeeding. These reflect low thyroid function, called "postpartum thyroiditis." (See Chapter 11 for a discussion of this topic.)

Poor adrenal function is another possibility; the stress of pregnancy, childbirth and a new baby can increase the needs of the adrenal glands, and their hormones are also involved in milk production. I suggest that you practice nutrition aimed at meeting the needs of both the thyroid and adrenal glands, starting with flax oil (five to ten 1 g capsules/day) and including the other vitamins and minerals listed in Table 7, Chapter 3. The book *A Natural Guide to Pregnancy and Postpartum Health*, by Dean Raffelock, D.C., and Robert Rountree, M.D., is an excellent source of information that you may wish to review. (See "Further Reading.")

Women who have difficulty keeping their weight up while breastfeeding may not realize that underweight is the cause of their low desire, not the actual breastfeeding. Attention to taking in more good foods to increase body fat may be helpful overall. Some of the information that follows may also apply to postpartum mothers.

OTHER FACTORS IN LOW DESIRE

HORMONAL BIRTH CONTROL. I've heard this line a number of times: "I got on the pill so I could have sex any time I wanted it, but it made me so I didn't want it." If this sounds like you, getting off the pill or other forms of hormonal birth control is the first step to improved desire, as well as improved overall health. But work hard to improve your nutrition so that your body "bounces back" and produces its own hormones in the right amounts. See the topic in Chapter 10, "Discontinuing Birth Control Pills or Other Hormonal Birth Control" for nutritional strategies to help out. Should the problem of low desire continue, refer to the other subtopics in this chapter. More than one factor could be involved.

OTHER MEDICATIONS. A number of medications may adversely affect desire in women: statins for cholesterol, antidepressants, blood pressure medicines, stimulants, and antihistamines.[12] In some cases you may be able to decrease or discontinue such medications by improving your diet, your body weight or your exercise level. Working with a nutritionally-oriented doctor in such a situation is the best way to discontinue such medications.

WEAK PELVIC FLOOR MUSCLES. Having poor tone in the skeletal muscles that support the bladder, uterus and rectum does not cause low desire, but it can interfere with sexual climax. Strengthening the pelvic floor muscles, technically called the pubococcygeal muscles, can enable a woman to experience orgasm more readily. First, it's useful to think of these muscles as a sort of round, flat floor to the pelvis's wide, bony opening. There are three openings in this pelvic floor: first, the urethra; second, the vagina; and third, the rectum. Skeletal muscles of the pelvic floor wrap around these openings in a figure "8" pattern. When these muscles are consciously contracted, they can stop a stream of urine, tighten the entrance of the vagina, or close the anus against the passage of gas or feces.

It does not take much time or effort to strengthen all of the pelvic floor muscles, but it does take know-how and a commitment of just a few minutes a day. First, practice stopping a stream of urine while you are on the toilet by strongly contracting the external urethral sphincter, the ring of muscle that closes the urethra. Second, practice strongly contracting the external anal sphincter, the ring of muscle around the anus that allows you to consciously stop the passage of gas. When you do these exercises you will automatically tighten the muscles around the vagina.

Once you are familiar with both muscles, you can practice strengthening them at a convenient time. Strongly contract and hold each muscle, one at a time, or both together, for several seconds. Repeat about twenty times a day to increase their strength and tone.

The benefits of strong pelvic floor muscles are several: better support for the bladder and uterus; better control of the bladder, especially during pregnancy and later in life after menopause; and better ability to achieve sexual climax, as these muscles are the ones that are consciously contracted during intercourse to produce the female orgasm. If you have difficulty experiencing orgasm, don't look for psychological counseling first, but rather counseling explaining the *physical* components of the sexual response.

PAIN DURING INTERCOURSE. If you feel pain during sexual relations, you should certainly discuss it with a compassionate physician. Sometimes a woman may be injured during childbirth; for example, an episiotomy may be poorly repaired.

> **Sometimes estrogen levels are low—from postpartum changes, from menopauseor from underweight—and in response the vaginal tissues become thin and vulnerable to injury.**

If this seems to be the case for you, see "Vaginal Dryness" and "Loss of Sexual Desire (Low Libido)" in Chapter 13. If the problem is endometriosis, please refer to that topic in Chapter 7 for nutritional strategies that can reduce endometriosis pain. Whatever the cause, it is surely worth serious effort to find the source of the trouble and to follow through with appropriate treatment.

DAY-TO-DAY HELP WITH LOW DESIRE

INADEQUATE SLEEP

Cheating the need for sleep is a sure way to lower sexual desire. I've never seen any research that substantiates it, but I believe that most women need more sleep than most men. It's been written many times before, but it is worth repeating: How can a husband and wife have satisfying times of intimacy if both are exhausted from the day's activities? When a couple using NFP is abstaining periodically, they usually have a fairly good idea of when the time of abstinence will end. Planning ahead for time together, taking a nap in the afternoon, or spending time together in the morning are all possibilities. How do we get more rest? When are we both most rested? Can we make time in the morning or early evening? These are questions that spouses should discuss with each other if fatigue is involved with low desire. (See "Adequate Sleep: Quantity and Quality," in Chapter 4.)

TOO FREQUENT INTERCOURSE. Yes, too much of a good thing can dull desire. Part of the heightened libido typically experienced by women who abstain during the fertile time results from the abstinence itself. By contrast, when relations are had more frequently than your natural level of desire, you may find yourself believing the problem is lack of desire, when it is at least partly caused by sexual satiety. This is a topic best discussed between the two of you, so that both understand that the out-of-sync desire is not a lack of love on your part, nor a lack of consideration on his part. For couples with no reason to abstain, sexual satiety might also contribute to seeming low desire, and a decrease in "quantity" may make for an increase in "quality."

"FOR THE MOMENT" SENSORY STRATEGIES. All of five senses are involved with womanly (and male) desire. For example, dark chocolate has the reputation as the food of lovers. It pleases the taste buds, but it also contains caffeine-like compounds that help overcome the original enemy, fatigue. Likewise, the sense of smell is related to desire. Aromatherapy, or the use of essential oils such as cedarwood oil, sandalwood oil, jasmine oil, and many others, may be worth trying during those special times. If you are interested in more information on this topic, you can safely Google the word "aromatherapy" without accidentally accessing immoral websites.

Some women are tempted to view sexy movies in an attempt to increase their libido. Please, don't be seduced by such images of other people.

> **Instead, a wonderful way of using the sense of vision for sexual desire is to spend a little time looking at photos of your wedding, of family outings, or of other fun and meaningful family events that rekindle the memories of why you are so much in love with your husband.**

Talking and cuddling outside the bedroom about your past and future together combines the senses of hearing and touch. Deep communication resolves petty annoyances and strengthens your bond. For most women, the emotional simply cannot be separated from the physical.

A SENSE OF HUMOR. C.S. Lewis wrote in his classic book, *The Fours Loves*, that Venus, as he termed sexual desire, is nothing if not fickle. If you are dealing with low sexual desire, see if you identify with his spot-on perspective, published in 1971:

> [Venus] herself is a mocking, mischievous spirit, far more elf than deity, and makes game of us. When all external circumstances are fittest for her service she will leave one or both the lovers totally indisposed for it. When every overt act is impossible and even glances cannot be exchanged—in trains, in shops, and at interminable parties—she will assail them with all her force. An hour later, when time and place agree, she will have mysteriously withdrawn, perhaps from only one of them. But sensible lovers laugh. It is all part of the game...[13]

SUMMARY—CHAPTER 14

1 Vaginal infections, whether from yeast organisms or from bacteria, are unpleasant in themselves, but they also can interfere with the mucus sign of fertility.

2 A sugary diet, hormonal birth control and antibiotics are all risk factors for vaginal yeast infections. Eliminating all of these, except for essential antibiotics, can help reduce the incidence of yeast infections. Using yogurt or probiotic supplements crowds out yeast organisms.

3 Bacterial vaginosis may be prevented by good hygiene and nutrients aimed at healing the vaginal wall and promoting normal cervical mucus. There is some evidence that probiotics may also reduce the occurrence of vaginal bacterial infections.

4 Bladder infections may be prevented with hygienic practices aimed at keeping harmful bacteria away from the urethra. Certain foods and drinks, such as those that contain caffeine, spices and acid, have been found to contribute to inflammation of the bladder (interstitial cystitis) in some people. Reducing consumption of these may help reduce the risk of bladder infections as well.

5 Low sexual desire may have a number of causes. When it occurs only in the postovulatory phase, low levels of progesterone may be involved, and natural nutritional strategies aimed at raising progesterone may be helpful.

6 Overall low desire can be caused by low thyroid function, poor adrenal gland function, overweight, underweight and yeast overgrowth (gut dysbiosis). Loss of libido during menopause may relate to low thyroid function, poor adrenal function or lack of sleep, rather than to menopause in itself.

7 Postpartum changes, including breastfeeding, may cause a temporary drop in libido, which usually returns even as the mother continues nursing.

8 Certain medications, including the pill, may reduce sexual desire. Weak pelvic floor muscles are not a cause of low desire, but learning exercises to strengthen them can improve a woman's ability to experience orgasm. Pain during intercourse can certainly inhibit desire, and help from a compassionate physician is recommended.

9 Day to day strategies to improve womanly desire include, first and foremost, adequate sleep. Too frequent sexual relations can seemingly result in a lack of desire. Waking up all the senses with natural sensory stimuli can improve libido.

10 As C.S. Lewis has pointed out in *The Four Loves*, having a sense of humor can help lovers have perspective as they deal with low libido.

MEN'S FERTILITY & REPRODUCTIVE HEALTH

Enjoy life with the
wife you love, all the
days of the fleeting
life granted you
under the sun.
— Ecclesiastes 9:9

How gratifying it is to see so much new research investigating the role of food choices, body weight, vitamins, minerals and other supplements for improving male fertility! For far too long, the contribution of nutrition to male fertility has been overlooked. Yet when it comes to fertility, the man's reproductive function is equally as important as the woman's. While estimates vary, recent data suggest that about 40 percent of infertility is due to male factors.[1] The spinoff of this new research not only will help many couples to achieve pregnancy, but it also offers insight into other reproductive problems that affect men, from sexual desire to prostate health.

Recognizing that the husband is equally involved in conception, the Couple to Couple League recommends that both spouses work as a team to improve their nutrition and other lifestyle factors as part of their self care to overcome infertility. This is true even if charting or medical diagnosis indicates a problem only with the woman's fertility. Let me restate this vital point:

**If you are having difficulty conceiving, both husband and wife
should strive to systematically improve your nutrition and overall health,
whether or not you have reason to believe the infertility is due only to one of you.**

The infertility could involve both of you, but even if it does not, improved nutrition by one spouse can help compensate for subfertility in the other.

MALE FERTILITY

"Quality and quantity" is the expression used by reproductive physiologists to summarize the two absolute essentials of male fertility. It refers to the male reproductive cells, the sperm. The quality of the sperm refers to their ability to move forward, to digest away the tissue surrounding the ovum, and to engage in actual fertilization. Quality can be judged by microscopically observing the shape (**morphology**) of the sperm as well as their forward movement (**motility**). Normal sperm have an oval head, a mid-piece that acts like a power pack, and a long, single tail; abnormalities such as double heads or short, twisted tails should be relatively few. Sperm should be capable of forward movement by the whipping motion of the tail, and clumping of the sperm, called **sperm agglutination**, should not occur in more than a fourth of the sperm cells.

 Recent research affirms that sperm quality also includes the genetic material in the head of the sperm, the all-important DNA.

The quantity of sperm necessary for normal fertility is amazing: Each of the three to five milliliters of ejaculated semen typically contains from 60–120 *million* sperm. When the sperm count drops to "only" 15-20 million per milliliter, the man is usually infertile. These numbers seem to be necessary to overcome the acidic environment of the vagina, to compensate for loss as sperm migrate through the female reproductive tract, and to provide for adequate numbers if ovulation occurs two or three days after intercourse. Dozens of sperm must arrive in the vicinity of the ovum to chemically digest its covering before the nucleus of a single sperm can fuse to the nucleus of the ovum, the event that begins the life of a new individual.

LIFE HISTORY OF THE SPERM

The testes develop in the abdomen of a male embryo by eight weeks of gestation. About a month before birth, they are drawn down into the scrotum by a coordinated array of ongoing processes. Throughout babyhood and childhood, the testes remain small, producing only minimal amounts of testosterone. Why? Early in life, tiny amounts of testosterone signal the hypothalamus of the brain to reduce the hormones capable of stimulating both testosterone and sperm production. At puberty, the hypothalamus changes. For the first time, it stimulates the pituitary hormones LH and FSH—the exact hormones that are secreted by the female's pituitary. In the adolescent male, LH causes the testes to produce increasing amounts of testosterone, and as a result, the profound changes of puberty begin: growth spurt in height, enlargement of the muscles, drop in the pitch of the voice, growth of the beard, and increase in the size of the genital organs themselves.

Beginning at puberty and continuing throughout adulthood, FSH, along with testosterone, causes the microscopic tubules within the testes to produce sperm. The very walls of these tubules are lined with so-called **diploid** cells; that is, these cells contain the 46 chromosomes typical of most human cells. By the process of cell division called **meiosis**, these cells divide in such a way as to produce sperm cells with the **haploid** number of chromosomes—23 in the human being. Thus, 23-chromosome sperm are formed which potentially can fertilize a 23-chromosome ovum, resulting in the conception of a unique new offspring with 46 chromosomes.

A final point: This cell division (meiosis) occurs extremely rapidly, and so requires many nutrients that are known to allow the genetic material to replicate and the cells to divide. In addition, once the cell division is completed, the sperm undergo maturation, losing much of the protective cytoplasm around the nucleus, and gaining a tail as well as the energy-producing mid-piece to power the tail for the forward movement. Nutrients that enable energy production are also needed by sperm.

You may be aware that for more than a generation, average sperm counts in men have been falling significantly throughout the world.[2] Among the probable culprits in this decline are exposure to environmental estrogens, pesticides, industrial chemicals, and heavy metals such as lead and cadmium.[3] Smoking, alcohol overuse, overweight, and poor nutrition also contribute. Anabolic steroids and some prescription medications can cause sperm counts to drop. High body temperature caused by hot workplaces or from sitting for long hours is yet another factor.

OXIDATIVE STRESS. Research has led to the conclusion that oxidative stress is at the root of many if not most factors that reduce male fertility. What is **oxidative stress**? In laymen's terms, it refers to damage to cells by reactive by-products of their normal oxygen usage. These by-products can be neutralized by cellular enzymes and by non-enzyme antioxidant vitamins, minerals, and other food molecules. For several reasons, sperm are more susceptible to oxidative stress than are most other cells. For example, they have a high rate of oxygen usage, but they have almost no cellular material around their nuclei to offer protective antioxidant activity.

The negative effects of heat exposure, smoking, infection, excess exercise, and aging are all related to oxidative stress. Even functions of sperm that cannot be easily measured are harmed by oxidative stress. Their ability to digest away the covering of an ovum and to fuse with the ovum is reduced by oxidative stress. The DNA itself is damaged by oxidative stress.[4]

Oxidative stress decreases to the extent that exposure to high temperatures, extremes of exercise, industrial chemicals, cigarette smoke, pesticides, heavy metals, and even household chemicals can be avoided. Meanwhile, improved nutrition provides antioxidants that counteract oxidative stress, as well as other nutrients needed for sperm production and for the production of male hormones.

DIET FOR MALE FERTILITY

OVERALL NUTRITION FOR MALE FERTILITY. Only recently have research studies begun to focus on a healthy diet as the foundation for male fertility. The large Rochester Young Men's Study (2009-2010) divided young, presumably fertile college-age men into two groups based on their general diet: "prudent" or "Western." "Prudent" diet included a high intake of fish, chicken, fruit, vegetables, beans, and whole grains. "Western" diet was defined as a high intake of red and processed meat, refined grains, pizza, snacks, high-energy drinks, and sweets. Compared to young men who ate the "Western" diet, men who ate the prudent diet had significantly better sperm motility.[5] A Polish study published in *Urology* in 2016 evaluated the overall diet of a large number of men who were actually dealing with infertility. Men who ate the same "prudent" diet described above had a significantly lower incidence of DNA damage to their sperm compared to men who ate the "Western" diet described above.[6] It is worth mentioning that DNA damage cannot be measured by the usual methods of sperm evaluation, so it is possible for a man with normal sperm counts and motility to have such damage.[7]

PROCESSED MEAT VERSUS FISH. The Rochester Young Men's Study also reported that consumption of processed red meat was related to a lower total sperm count.[8]

 Another large dietary study, this time of infertile men, found that intake of processed red meat correlated with poor sperm morphology, but that high intake of fish correlated with higher sperm counts and more normally-shaped sperm.[9]

One explanation: Sperm cells have a higher percentage of the unsaturated fats, such as those found in fish, compared to most other body cells.

DAIRY FOODS. The Rochester Young Men's Study found that men who consumed three daily servings of full-fat dairy foods, notably cheese, showed significantly more problems in sperm morphology (shape, an aspect of sperm quality) and in sperm motility than men who consumed less dairy.[10] Milk, especially full-fat milk, is a source of natural cow estrogen, though the authors suggested that "dairy may be implicated in direct testicular damage."[11]

SATURATED FATS. The finding that processed meat and dairy foods negatively affect semen quality may be related to a large Danish study that found that young men with a high intake of saturated fats were more likely to have a reduced semen quality.[12] Both red meat and full fat dairy contain saturated fats. A more focused study of men with sperm with low motility reported that consumption of saturated fats correlated with poor sperm motility, while higher intake of the beneficial omega-3 unsaturated fats was associated with better sperm motility.[13]

***TRANS* FATS.** The same study just referred to above also found that intake of *trans* fats was associated with a higher incidence of poor sperm motility.[14] In addition, the Murcia Young Men's Study, done in Spain (2010-2011), found that college-age men of presumably normal fertility who ate significant amounts of *trans* fats had lower sperm counts compared to men who avoided such fats.[15] The Murcia researchers reported that French fried potatoes and commercial baked goods were the main sources of *trans* fats. Everyone, of both sexes and all ages, should avoid artificially produced *trans* fats. Fortunately, it is much easier to do so now than in the past, since the awareness of the cardiovascular harm done by *trans* fats has been well publicized.

SOY FOODS. Soy foods such as soy milk, soy nuts, and tofu contain weak estrogens called isoflavones. Eating significant amounts of such foods has been implicated in reduced sperm concentrations, according to Harvard School of Public Health researchers, who studied ninety-nine men who were the male members of infertile couples. Soy foods reduced sperm concentrations in a "dose-related" fashion. That is, higher soy food intake lowered sperm concentrations more, and men with the very highest intake of soy foods actually had 41 million fewer sperm per millimeter than men who did not use soy foods. The effect of soy foods on sperm concentrations was especially pronounced in overweight and obese men. (Total sperm counts were not reduced, however, as semen volume increased slightly among soy users.)[16] If you consume soy foods or soy milk frequently, you should consider cutting back. However, consumption of soy oil, such as is commonly found in salad dressings, was not investigated in this study, as it is not a protein food rich in isoflavones.[17]

SUGAR-SWEETENED BEVERAGES. Investigating the effect of intake of sugar-sweetened beverages, the Rochester Young Men's Study reported that men who consumed more than 1.3 servings of sugar-sweetened beverages per day had lower sperm motility compared to men who drank very little of such beverages. This effect was seen only in lean men, not in overweight men, and was not related to caffeine consumption. The majority of the sugar-sweetened drinks were reported to be non-carbonated drinks such as sports drinks, not carbonated beverages, as you might assume.[18]

CAFFEINE. Despite the fact that a number of studies exist linking caffeine consumption in women to delays in achieving pregnancy and to increased risk of miscarriage, caffeine has not been shown to be strongly linked to infertility in men.[19] However, stress and poor diet are linked to oxidative stress in sperm,[20] so it seems prudent to use caffeine in pleasant moderation, and to rely more on adequate sleep and improved nutrition for a natural, overall boost in energy.

PUTTING IT ALL TOGETHER: DIET FOR MALE FERTILITY

How do we summarize this new dietary research? For protein, fresh fish is number one, and chicken and lean natural red meat are better choices than processed red meats, whole fat dairy foods such as whole milk and cheese, and soy-based foods. Completely avoiding *trans* fats, generally avoiding sugary drinks, sugary treats, and refined grains is good for everyone, including those who are dealing with infertility. Emphasizing the "prudent" diet as described above—abundant in fruits, vegetables, beans, and whole grains--will naturally increase the intake of the valuable antioxidants so necessary to sperm function. While eggs were not mentioned in these studies, they are a rich source of true vitamin A and are definitely on the list of healthy foods. The dietary recommendations in Part 1 of this book, as modified here, are a sensible starting point for improved diet.

LIFESTYLE

ALCOHOL AND NICOTINE. Excess alcohol intake reduces testosterone levels and depletes protective antioxidants.[21] Smoking causes negative effects on all aspects of sperm health—motility, morphology, and the DNA.[22] It also contributes to erectile dysfunction and loss of libido.

ANABOLIC STEROIDS. Use of anabolic or androgenizing steroids by young men to enhance muscle-building results in a decrease of LH and FSH, which in turn results in less natural testosterone and lowered sperm production. This may or may not be reversible once these hormones are discontinued, but certainly the wisest course is not to use them. The higher the doses and the longer they are used, the more likely are deleterious effects to overall health and fertility.

What if you have used anabolic or androgenizing steroids in the past or are using them now? Discontinue the drugs and allow about six months for hormones and fertility to recover, making sure that you are not taking body-building food supplements that may contain unlabeled anabolic steroids.[23]

The best self care approach to regain the natural functions of the testes is to follow the sensible dietary and supplement recommendations discussed in this chapter, which are aimed at increasing sperm quality and counts.

The role of the temperature of the testes in fertility should also be considered, as discussed in the section on the next page. If after six to twelve months you are still dealing with low semen quality, be aware that there are injectable natural hormones that a doctor can use to help you overcome this type of infertility.

PRESCRIPTION DRUGS. A number of prescription medications can interfere with male fertility. Anti-cancer drugs often have as a side effect a decrease in sperm production, as do immune-suppressants used after organ transplants. Anti-inflammatory agents, opiates, anti-androgen drugs used for prostate enlargement, anti-depressants, and a number of others can reduce semen quality.[24] Again, the best self care either during or after medication use is to implement all of the dietary and supplement recommendations in this chapter, and also consider the role of body temperature as it relates to the function of the testes.

CELL PHONES. Cell phones emit radiofrequency electromagnetic waves, a low-level energy source that rapidly dies away with distance.

Yet in several studies, frequent cell phone use has been related to lowered sperm counts and abnormal sperm shape and movement.[25]

Cell phone use is so widespread and so variable that it is difficult to design studies comparing a group of men who use cell phones to a group of men who do not, but the effect seems to be "dose-related"—more cell phone use has a greater impact than lesser use. If infertility is a problem with either spouse, storing the cell phone away from your body—not in your pants pocket—is the best compromise for this seemingly indispensable device.

TEMPERATURE AND MALE FERTILITY

Sperm production occurs because original sperm cells within the testes constantly divide at a very fast pace. This cell division is dependent on enzymes which are highly sensitive to elevated surrounding temperature. The location of the testes outside the body, the sweat glands on the scrotum, and the muscles which allow the testes to fall away from the pelvis when the temperature rises all show the remarkable design of the body to regulate the temperature of the testes to about 3°F (2 °C) below core body temperature.

When a husband and wife are having difficulty conceiving, one of the first self-care strategies that they should implement is to take measures to keep the temperature of the testes within their normal range: boxer shorts rather than briefs to allow the testes to fall away from the warm core; loss of some excess body fat if obesity is a problem; replacing hot outdoor endurance exercises with swimming or less strenuous activities; and standing up and walking around at least hourly if you have a desk job where you must sit for hours.

Note: High temperatures in the testes, which can put a stop to sperm production, do not affect testosterone production. If high temperatures have been the problem, it will be about two months before sperm production rises, since it takes that long for sperm to mature.

BODY WEIGHT

OVERWEIGHT. Overweight and especially obesity can reduce fertility in men. Body fat produces estrogen in both sexes. Excess estrogen interferes with the function of testosterone, and estrogen signals the man's hypothalamus to decrease LH and FSH, which normally stimulate testosterone and sperm production.[26] Obesity leads to a higher risk of damage to the DNA, even when sperm counts remain normal.[27] The effect of excess body fat is proportional to the amount; morbid obesity (BMI over 40) increases the risk of low sperm count more than obesity.[28] Some of this effect may be attributed to the higher temperature of the testes within the scrotum when infertility occurs with obesity.[29] Losing weight is a challenge, but finding a diet and exercise plan that suits your lifestyle and attempting to lose at least a moderate amount of weight can improve the levels of male hormones.[30] You of course will reap many other health benefits as well.

UNDERWEIGHT. Extreme weight loss in men progressively reduces sexual libido, testosterone levels, sperm motility, and sperm production, all of which can be restored when the man regains his weight.[31] Men's fertility is far less sensitive to underweight than to overweight or obesity,[32] but very vigorous exercise does increase oxidative stress on the body.[33] If you are a man who really does push the limits with strength or endurance training, consider reducing your exercise to a more moderate level if you and your wife are experiencing a delay in conceiving.

VITAMIN, MINERAL AND FATTY ACID SUPPLEMENTS FOR MALE FERTILITY

Should you take vitamin/mineral supplements to improve your fertility? The following paragraph, remarkable for the simplicity of its suggestions and the compassion of its authors, completed a review article on male fertility and nutrition:

> The concept of subfertility is evolving, especially as it relates to males. Whereas in the past men may have been classified as infertile when they were unable to father a child, it currently is recognized that many such individuals indeed are capable of becoming fathers. Among the factors that may temporarily prevent a given man from impregnating his partner is some form of **micronutrient/mineral insufficiency**. Several micronutrients have been shown to improve reproductive outcome when administered to subfertile men, but it is not clear whether such deficiencies act alone or in synergy with other factors. To date, questions on best therapeutic practice regarding vitamin supplementation have been addressed insufficiently. Considering the extent of subfertility on a worldwide basis and the stress it places on couples desiring a child, it seems prudent to at least consider multivitamin supplementation as an early and essential broad-based therapeutic intervention for both males and females. Such a benign intervention is less expensive and more accessible in many areas of the world where specialist medical care for infertility is out of reach for the vast majority of the population.[34]

OMEGA-3 FATTY ACIDS

DHA AND EPA. Sperm cells concentrate far more unsaturated fatty acids than do most other cells of the human body. The omega-3 fatty acids, especially DHA (docosahexaenoic acid), which is found along with EPA (eicosapentaenoic acid), add flexibility to the cell membrane. That membrane flexibility ultimately enables the head of the sperm to digest away the covering of an ovum and to fuse with it in fertilization.

A number of studies have shown that low DHA is related to poor sperm quality and fertility in men, and some studies have shown that supplementing DHA in the form of fish oil improves semen quality.[35]

FLAX OIL. Yet DHA and EPA are not truly essential nutrients. They are derivatives of the hard-to-get omega-3 essential fatty acid, alpha-linolenic acid. Long-time male fertility researcher Frank Comhaire of Belgium recommends supplements of flax oil, noting that it is a rich source of alpha-linolenic acid, which is low in subfertile men. Alpha-linolenic acid is converted to the healthy fatty acids EPA and DHA, so necessary for fertilization. According to Dr. Comhaire, flax oil also contains several plant phytonutrients called lignans, which in the intestines are converted to weak, short-lived estrogens. These weak estrogens actually act opposite to what the name implies. They inhibit the conversion of male hormone into estrogen, thus decreasing the amount of estrogen in men, which has a beneficial effect on sperm production.[36]

WALNUTS AS A SOURCE OF ALPHA-LINOLENIC ACID

In an amazing practical application of the benefit of alpha-linolenic acid to male fertility, researchers provided walnuts (75 g per day, about one-half cup shelled, raw walnuts) to presumably fertile young men eating a "Western-style" diet. Walnuts are a significant source of alpha-linolenic acid, though flax oil is a considerably richer source. After three months, sperm motility and morphology significantly improved in these men, and DNA damage to their sperm decreased.[37]

Several B vitamins, vitamin C, and zinc are required to convert the alpha-linolenic acid of flax oil into the active fatty acids EPA and DHA. As an alternative to flax oil, Dr. Comhaire does recommend fish oil, with its abundant EPA and DHA. Because EPA and DHA are so highly unsaturated, he notes that it is mandatory to provide antioxidants [for example, vitamin E] along with fish oil.[38]

FLAX OIL OR FISH OIL? How much fish oil or flax oil should you supplement? The ideal amount for male fertility has not been determined.[39] About 5–10 grams (1-2 teaspoons) daily of fish oil, preferably cod liver oil, and/or 5-10 grams (1-2 teaspoon) of flax oil is my recommendation for male infertility. Cod liver oil and other fish oils have ready-made DHA and EPA, though they do not provide the lignans mentioned above. Supplemental vitamin E in the range of 400 IU protects fish oil and flax oil from oxidative damage, and is valuable to male fertility in itself.

VITAMINS AND MINERALS

ANDROVITE FOR MEN. A diet rich in antioxidants and other nutrients is essential for optimal sperm production.[40] But before detailing the benefits that various vitamins and minerals have on male fertility, I would like to jump ahead to the conclusion, and recommend the multivitamin/multimineral Androvite for Men. (See "Resources.") It "covers all the bases" so well that most men who are hoping to overcome infertility or other reproductive problems need only to supplement with Androvite to meet the majority of their vitamin and mineral needs. Androvite contains 1,000 mg of vitamin C, 50 mg of zinc, 400 mcg of folic acid, 400 IU of vitamin E, and 200 mcg of selenium per full dose. See Appendix A, "Labeled Contents of Recommended Supplements," for the complete vitamin and mineral amounts in Androvite. Research that supports the ingredients in this supplement is summarized below.

VITAMIN C. In one of the most dramatic studies ever published on the effect of nutrition on reproductive function, twenty-seven men with infertility apparently due to sperm agglutination (sperm which stick together and thus cannot move forward) were divided into two groups. Twenty received supplemental vitamin C (1,000 mg/day) plus calcium, magnesium, and manganese. At the end of two months, the wives of each of the twenty men who received supplemental vitamin C had become pregnant. In contrast, no wife of any subject in the group which did not receive supplemental doses had become pregnant. This program of supplementation significantly improved sperm quantity, morphology, and motility, and reduced spermagglutination.[41]

A follow-up study used pure vitamin C (200 or 1,000 mg/day) and confirmed the beneficial effect of this nutrient on the same measures of fertility in men with spermagglutination. In only one week, sperm counts for those receiving 1,000 mg/day of vitamin C rose an average of 140 percent.[42] Similar results have been found when vitamin C has been supplemented in men who smoke.[43]

> Vitamin C is ten times more concentrated in semen than in blood, and testosterone production also depends on adequate vitamin C.

This powerful antioxidant vitamin also plays a major role in preventing damage to the DNA of the sperm. Importantly, damaged sperm DNA can be responsible for male infertility even when sperm count, motility and morphology are normal.[44]

A newer study on presumably fertile young men showed again the value of vitamin C to semen quality; a higher intake of vitamin C correlated with better sperm motility and increased semen volume. The authors noted that "the reference daily intake or recommended daily intake (RDI) for vitamin C is 60 mg per day…. Our study raises doubts about whether the current RDI may underestimate vitamin C requirements needed with regard to semen quality."[45] A 2017 review article notes that 1 g/day (1,000 mg) is the amount used in the majority of studies on male infertility.[46]

ZINC AND FOLATE. Zinc is another nutrient which is absolutely essential for sperm production and for synthesis of testosterone by the testes. The highest concentrations of zinc in the body are found in the sperm cells and in the prostate gland, and the prostate contributes importantly to male reproductive capability. Zinc works together with the B vitamin folate (folic acid is the synthetic form) in the synthesis of DNA molecules, which dividing sperm cells produce at a rapid rate.

Low folate in men is associated with damage to the sperm's DNA.[47]

In a controlled, double-blind study, both fertile and infertile men were given supplements of zinc (66 mg) and folic acid (5,000 mcg) daily for six months. After six months, infertile men with low sperm counts had a 74 percent increase in sperm quantity.[48] The richest source of zinc is red meat; fish, poultry, and dairy products do not contain as much, and a strictly vegetarian diet may lead to zinc deficiency.[49] Folate is plentiful in dark green leafy vegetables. Supplements which include both are valuable to male as well as to female fertility. While Androvite for Men has 50 mg of zinc per full dose, it has only 400 mcg of folic acid. Increase your folate by supplementing methyl folate (the natural form of this B vitamin) in amounts of 2,000-3,000 mcg/day. Research has shown that men with a common genetic variation that affects their use of synthetic folic acid have lower sperm concentration compared to others.[50] Natural methyl folate can overcome this genetic variation.

SELENIUM AND VITAMIN E. Selenium has a number of roles in the body, and it is highly concentrated in the testes. It is needed by the sperm to make their mid-pieces,[51] which is the part between head and tail where energy production takes place to allow for their forward movement. Vitamin E is a major antioxidant that works together with selenium. Infertile men who supplemented both of these nutrients (225 mcg selenium and 400 mg vitamin E daily) for three months had improved sperm motility.[52]

More important, selenium, either alone or with other antioxidants (vitamins A, C, and E), given to infertile men with poor sperm motility resulted in an 11 percent pregnancy rate within three months of taking the supplements, as compared to no pregnancies in the control group.[53] Vitamin E supplemented along with other nutrients, including vitamin A and essential fatty acids, has resulted in increased pregnancy rates among men with very low sperm counts.[54] Vitamin E alone (300 mg twice daily) resulted in a 21 percent rate of pregnancy achievement within six months in men with poor sperm mobility compared to no pregnancies in control subjects.[55]

VITAMIN A. Vitamin A, which aids the lining membranes throughout the body, similarly benefits the cells lining the testes' tubules—and these cells are the developing sperm! Men have a higher need than women for vitamin A, and it affects men's reproductive organs significantly. Vitamin A deficiency results in shrinkage of the epididymides (ducts through which sperm pass to the vas deferens), seminal vesicles, and prostate gland. Severe deficiency causes degeneration of the seminiferous tubules (site of the germination, maturation and transportation of sperm within the testes), resulting in decrease of semen volume, sperm count, and sperm motility.[56] Vitamin A, a major antioxidant, is found in cod liver oil, butter, eggs, and meat. The related form, beta-carotene, which is abundant in orange, red, and yellow vegetables and can also be supplemented, has been related to higher sperm motility.[57] Along with other antioxidants (vitamins C and E), higher intake of beta carotene correlated with higher sperm counts and motility in presumably fertile men between ages 20 through 80.[58]

B VITAMINS. A damaging metabolite, **homocysteine**, creates oxidative stress on the body. Homocysteine levels are decreased by the three "big B's": folate, B6, and B12. Australian infertility researcher Kelton Tremellen recommends daily supplements of 5,000 mcg folic acid, 100 mg B6, and 100 mcg of B12 to reduce the oxidative stress caused by homocysteine in infertile men.[59] The B vitamins are also involved in producing LH and FSH from the pituitary gland, and these two hormones stimulate sperm production and testosterone secretion in men.

MULTIVITAMINS/MULTIMINERALS. The ordinary protocol for scientific inquiry is to vary one factor at a time in controlled experiments. But because nutrients work together, a recent review article points out that "Combination therapies potentially are more beneficial in managing subfertility because antioxidants act by different mechanisms... If a complex formulation is selected, however, there is no accepted means to disentangle specific effects of the individual components upon semen parameters...."[60] For individual couples, though, the goal is not to design a controlled study, but to improve infertility and to have a baby. That's why a good multivitamin/multimineral is basic to improved fertility. Let me quote the same authors again, as I did at the beginning of this section:

> Considering the extent of subfertility on a worldwide basis and the stress it places on couples desiring a child, it seems prudent to at least consider multivitamin supplementation as an early and essential broad-based therapeutic intervention for both males and females. Such a benign intervention is less expensive and more accessible in many areas of the world where specialist medical care for infertility is out of reach for the vast majority of the population.[61]

OTHER SUPPLEMENTS FOR MALE FERTILITY. In addition to fish oil and/or flax oil, and vitamins and minerals, as detailed above, a number of other supplements are valuable for improving male fertility.

COENZYME Q10. Coenzyme Q10 (CoQ10), also called ubiquinone, is neither a vitamin nor a mineral, but rather, a complex fat-soluble molecule that releases energy in cells and also acts as an antioxidant. About half of it is made by the body, and the other half is obtained in the diet. Because sperm must produce much energy to move forward, their "power-pack" mid-pieces concentrate CoQ10. Recognizing this fact, a number of researchers have investigated the role of CoQ10 in male fertility. For example, 106 infertile men with poor sperm counts, motility, and morphology received 300 mg of CoQ10 as a supplement for six months. Their sperm counts and motility improved significantly compared to controls who received a placebo.[62] In a similar study, 287 infertile men with poor semen quality were given 300 mg CoQ10 twice daily for twelve months.

> **During this one-year study of Coenzyme Q10, sperm counts, motility, and morphology all improved significantly, and most heartening of all, one third of the men were able to impregnate their wives.[63]**

Can diet alone provide enough CoQ10 to cause such effects in subfertile men? Researchers studying infertile couples at Massachusetts General Hospital evaluated the overall diets of the men. They calculated that average dietary CoQ10 intake was only 19 mg/day, about ten times less than amount used in many clinical trials. The authors concluded that "CoQ10 intake from food alone may be insufficient to optimize semen parameters."[64] That said, the Young Men's Rochester Study noted that even though very few of the presumably fertile young men studied ate organ meats [liver, heart, kidney], which are especially rich in CoQ10, those who did had significantly higher sperm quantity and quality than the majority who did not eat organ meats.[65]

Along with the vitamins and minerals suggested above, consider 200-300 mg/day of CoQ10 to improve sperm counts, motility, and morphology.

> **Even though CoQ10 in the form of ubiquinone has been well studied, the form of CoQ10 called "ubiquinol" is a stronger antioxidant. It can be used in the amount of 150-200 mg/day for at least four months.[66]**

As an aside, CoQ10 (200 mg/day) is also valuable for female fertility.

L-CARNITINE AND ACETYL-L-CARNITINE. These two related nutrients are co-factors that can be made by cells and used to produce energy. They act as powerful antioxidants as well. Still, most of them come from the diet, mainly meat, poultry, and fish. In the male, they are abundant in the fluid of the epididymides, where sperm maturation takes place. Studies of the effect of these on male fertility have been performed using a proprietary product called Proxeed, which contains both of these as well as CoQ10. (Available at www.proxeed.com.) In the case of the carnitines, doses in the range of 2 g/day of L-carnitine plus 1 g/day of acetyl-L-carnitine have improved sperm quality and modestly increased pregnancy rates to 6.7 percent in three months.[67] A more recent review of the literature showed that carnitines resulted in a very significant increase in pregnancy rate compared to placebos, and also greatly reduced the percentage of abnormally shaped sperm.[68]

ASTAXANTHIN. In a promising pilot study, a potent antioxidant found in algae, **astaxanthin**, was given in amounts of 16 mg daily to Swedish men being treated medically for infertility. This resulted in an amazing 54 percent pregnancy rate in three months, compared to an 11 percent pregnancy rate among untreated controls.[69] The astaxanthin was in a proprietary preparation called Astacarox, (AstaReal AB, Sweden). There are several proprietary preparations of astaxanthin available. If you chose to try it, and I suggest that you do, use the same amount as in this study (16 mg/day).

TABLE 13
SUPPLEMENTS FOR MALE FERTILITY (IN ORDER OF LIKELY BENEFIT)

Fish oil, preferably cod liver oil, certified contaminant-free	5-10 g (1-2 teaspoons/day) and/or flax oil, 5-10 g (1-2 teaspoons/day) Total of the two oils up to 10 g/day

Vitamin A*	25,000 IU, 80% as beta-carotene
Vitamin C*	1,000 mg
Folic Acid*	400 mcg (0.4 mg)
Vitamin E*	400 IU
Zinc*	50 mg
Selenium*	200 mcg (0.2 mg)

* These are found in Androvite for Men. See Appendix A.

Coenzyme Q10, preferably in the form ubiquinol	150-200 mg/day (if ubiquinone, 200-300 mg.day)
L-carnitine or acetyl-L-carnitine	2 g/day of the first and 1 g/day of the second
Additional folate	2,000-3,000 mcg/day
Additional vitamin B12	100-1,000 mcg/day
Astaxanthin	16 mg/day

WORKING TOGETHER TO IMPROVE MALE FERTILITY

Sperm require over two months to mature from start to finish. Improvement of male fertility through nutrition may not occur immediately, except possibly in the case of sperm agglutination. Please remember that whenever infertility is a problem, the first step is for both of you to improve your nutrition and to employ all the fertility techniques taught by the Couple to Couple League. You may incorrectly assume that one spouse's subfertility is the cause, but often it is both spouses'. Give yourselves six to nine months for self care to make a difference.

HELPING ONE ANOTHER

Timing of intercourse based on the NFP chart, following a few days of abstinence, can help to compensate for a low sperm count in the husband as well as for poor mucus patterns in the wife. Attempting to optimize reproductive health through nutrition may also enable one spouse to compensate for the other's subfertility. For example, the wife's attempting to increase her cervical mucus with vitamin A may help to overcome infertility due to low sperm count or low sperm motility in the husband, and if excellent nutrition raises a man's sperm count to higher levels or better motility, it could aid the problem of partially blocked uterine tubes in the wife. But most of all, when the two of you form a team, in the kitchen as well as in the bedroom, you encourage each other.

MALE REPRODUCTIVE HEALTH

LOW LIBIDO OR ERECTILE DYSFUNCTION. These two topics are not the same, and they may or may not be related. Low libido refers to low sexual desire, and the term erectile dysfunction has replaced the older term "impotence."

> The hormone testosterone is responsible for the physical basis of male libido, but actual sexual function depends not only on the levels of testosterone but also on other factors.

NUTRITIONAL FACTORS

 Dietary imbalances that affect fertility may also affect libido and erectile function.

Obesity and overweight can cause loss of libido, since excess body fat reduces the levels of testosterone.[70] Both zinc and vitamin C raise testosterone levels. Some medical doctors recommend as much as 80 mg of zinc daily to improve testosterone levels and sexual libido in men. One thousand mg/day of vitamin C is a usual recommendation for male fertility.[71] I suspect that all of the above-mentioned vitamins, minerals, and essential fatty acids that improve semen quality (**Table 13**) would also be helpful to male desire and performance. Since nutrients work together, it's better to supplement all of them rather than to rely on just one or two.

In men, erection depends on the release of the signal molecule nitric oxide (NO). There are self care strategies to increase NO. First is exercise, which is a natural NO booster. Leafy greens and beets are foods that increase NO; berries, citrus fruits, green tea, red wine, and dark chocolate decrease erectile dysfunction.[72] The herb pycnogenol, taken along with the amino acids arginine and citrulline and the oak tree extract, roburin, improved erectile function.[73] A proprietary combination of pycnogenol, arginine, and citrulline, called Prelox Plus, is available at www.drwhitaker.com.

LOW THYROID FUNCTION. Low thyroid function (hypothyroidism) is several times more common in women, but it does occur in men. When it does, it can cause a decrease in testosterone levels. Not surprisingly, erectile dysfunction and loss of libido may result; however, the effect of hypothyroidism on actual male fertility is not well established.[74] The more subtle situation, called **subclinical hypothyroidism**, may also result in low levels of testosterone.[75]

SELF-TEST FOR THYROID FUNCTION

If you are interested in judging your own thyroid function, you can try the "Barnes basal temperature test" discussed in Chapter 8 under the topic "Low Thyroid Function." In brief, you take your oral or underarm waking (basal) body temperature for several days, and then consider the results. According to Dr. Barnes, a man's underarm (equivalent to oral) basal temperature should be in the range of 97.8°F to 98.2°F. While I have noted in Chapter 8 that I consider this standard somewhat too high for women, I have no reason to doubt its accuracy for men.

The multivitamin/multimineral Androvite for Men contains nutrients that are ideal to support thyroid function—iodine, zinc, selenium, B vitamins, and vitamins C, A, and E. In addition, flax oil and/or fish oil should be supplemented to nourish the thyroid gland. As in women, not all low thyroid function responds to nutrition. If you believe that low thyroid function might be the cause of low libido, sexual dysfunction, or infertility, medical diagnosis and treatment is the next step if nutrition does not make a difference within about six months. Again, refer to "Low Thyroid Function" in Chapter 8 for further information.

The health of the prostate gland importantly affects the ability to maintain an erection. Therefore, the following sections should also be considered.

PROSTATITIS

A large number of urologists' patients are men with acute or chronic **prostatitis**.

Prostatitis refers to infection or inflammation of the prostate gland, which is a disorder completely different from the benign prostatic hypertrophy (enlargement) that commonly causes problems in men over age fifty.

The symptoms of prostatitis include pain between the legs or in the rectal area and sometimes pain with intercourse. More severe infection or inflammation causes pain in the urethra and frequency of urination. Flare-ups can cause temporary erectile dysfunction. It is also possible for a man to have a chronic low-level prostate infection or inflammation without being aware of it.

The usual medical treatment for prostatitis is antibiotic therapy. However, the infective microorganisms are notoriously difficult to eradicate and long-term treatment is often necessary. Many urologists routinely advise increased frequency of intercourse to "flush out" the gland, which empties its secretions into the urethra during intercourse. This obviously poses a problem to couples practicing chaste periodic abstinence as part of NFP. Fortunately, a number of natural strategies can immensely help the prostatitis-prone man to prevent the troublesome flare-ups.

AVOID FOODS THAT PRODUCE AN IRRITATING URINE. Spicy or acid foods can cause intense attacks of prostatitis within hours. Condiments such as mayonnaise, ketchup, mustard, relish and so forth should be avoided. Tomatoes, raw onions, sausages, pizza, tacos, soft drinks, tea, coffee and alcohol are other culprits. Sometimes food additives in processed items cause reactions that home-cooked equivalent dishes do not.

DRINK PLENTY OF WATER. Water dilutes the urine, and helps to avoid irritation to the prostate gland.

AVOID URINE BACKFLOW INTO THE PROSTATIC DUCTS. The bladder should be emptied regularly and not allowed to become overfull. "Shy bladder" is common among men with prostatitis, and relaxation, not straining, should be practiced when urine is voided.

IMPROVE BLOOD FLOW TO THE PROSTATE GLAND. Exercise such as running, boxer shorts instead of briefs, and hot baths all aid circulation to this gland. Conversely, cigarette smoking, prolonged sitting, and constipation impede its blood flow. Avoid nasal sprays and other cold or allergy remedies which constrict nasal tissues—they do the same to prostate vessels, and infections thrive where blood flow is poor.[76]

NOURISH THE PROSTATE PROPERLY. Zinc is highly concentrated in this gland, and up 80 mg per day of supplemental zinc may be helpful, if it is balanced with 3 mg of copper.[77] Vitamin A, B vitamins, including B6 (50 mg twice daily), vitamin C, and selenium also contribute to prostate health.[78] Selenium is important to all of the male reproductive organs. The prostate gland also has a high need for the essential fatty acids.

CONSIDER WHETHER YEAST OVERGROWTH MAY BE INVOLVED. See "Yeast Overgrowth/Gut Dysbiosis" in Chapter 10 for further information on this subject. The anecdote below illustrates this possibility.

SELF HELP FOR PROSTATITIS

An otherwise healthy 35-year-old man developed chronic prostatitis, and had taken "ten different courses of antibiotics within two and a half years." The bouts were occurring more and more frequently; longer treatment with antibiotics was required, and finally, a course of antibiotics did no good at all. During this time he gradually realized that certain foods triggered these attacks—soda pop, alcohol, processed meats, condiments, and most other processed foods. By strictly avoiding these, he could control the prostatitis, but he felt he was "always on the razor's edge" if he ate the wrong food.

He learned from Dr. William Crook's *The Yeast Connection* that chronic prostatitis is a possible symptom of yeast overgrowth, and he recalled that during his final few flare-ups his urologist could not culture bacteria from his prostatic fluid. He tried eating plain yogurt and noticed that it somewhat reduced the constant inflammation that troubled him. Reasoning that yogurt bacteria are largely killed off by the stomach's acid, he tried capsules of acidophilus, which are designed to release friendly bacteria into the intestine, where they combat yeast. They helped immensely.

He has not had a major recurrence nor used antibiotics for three years, and he considers the low-level inflammation virtually gone. Along with capsules of probiotics daily, he takes vitamins and minerals and eats only low-sugar, unprocessed foods, except for occasional treats. Testing has confirmed that he is highly allergic to yeast, but he believes that medical treatment is unnecessary at this time. He reports that he feels better now than before the prostatitis started, and jokes that he is "forced to eat only healthy food," though his sensitivity to many of his former trigger foods has decreased markedly. One can only speculate about how his problem would have progressed had he not on his own found the yeast connection.

BENIGN PROSTATE ENLARGEMENT

Enlargement of the prostate gland (**benign prostate hypertrophy** or **BHP**) is a common condition in men over age fifty. Its symptoms include annoying frequency of urination and a poor stream of urine when voiding, and it can interfere with sexual functioning. Left untreated, it can ultimately damage the entire urinary system. Diet, vitamins, minerals, and particularly herbal remedies are helpful to this problem.

DIET. Eating fruits and vegetables that are rich in antioxidants, including the phytonutrients beta-carotene, lutein and vitamin C, decreases the risk of benign prostate hypertrophy, according to a very large study of American men.[79] Beta-carotene is found in orange and yellow plant foods such as carrots, and lutein is found abundantly in kale, collard greens, spinach, zucchini, and pumpkin. This is not to imply that a vegetarian diet is recommended for prostate health, but that the wonderful phytonutrients in plant foods truly should be eaten in abundance.

VITAMIN/MINERAL SUPPLEMENTS. The hormone prolactin rises as men age, and it contributes to prostate hypertrophy. The prolactin-inhibiting factor is the same in men as in women. This factor is dopamine, and levels of dopamine are increased by vitamin B6 and magnesium. These can be taken in the range of 50–100 mg B6 and 500–1,000 mg magnesium daily. Zinc also helps to reduce prolactin levels. Androvite for Men, as mentioned previously, is an excellent multivitamin/multimineral supplement for all aspects of male reproductive health.

ESSENTIAL FATTY ACIDS. Flax oil (5-10 1 g capsules, or 1–2 teaspoons of the liquid daily) and/or cod liver oil (5-10 g/day or 1-2 teaspoons daily) provide fatty acids that are beneficial to the prostate gland. Androvite contains the vitamin E required as an antioxidant to protect these fatty acids.

HERBS. Extracts of the herb saw palmetto have been used successfully to reduce prostate enlargement, poor urine flow, and sexual dysfunction.[80]

Saw palmetto is a source of the compound beta-sitosterol, which works by reducing the activity of an enzyme that changes testosterone into a more potent compound called dihydrotestosterone (abbreviated as DHT). DHT stimulates the growth of the prostate. There are many brands of saw palmetto available, and often they contain additional ingredients such as the herbs *Pygeum africanum*, stinging nettle, and pumpkin seed oil. All of these contain beta-sitosterol. Beta-sitosterol is also available in purified, more potent forms. The extract in the study cited above is called Permixon, and the men in the study used it in 160 mg amounts twice daily for two years. The positive results occurred within the first six months of use, except for the improvement of sexual function, which occurred after a year of use.[81]

You may also wish to visit a health food shop to compare various supplements of saw palmetto in terms of the amount of beta-sitosterol and for the addition of other herbs. Or, see www.drwhitaker.com for information on supplements for prostate health formulated by nutritionally-oriented medical doctor Julian Whitaker, M.D. Dr. Whitaker has updated and altered his formulations as new research or new products become available. (See "Resources.")

PREVENTING PROSTATE CANCER

Prostate cancer is a leading cancer killer among American men. Reducing the risk of this type of cancer is a topic of great research interest, and several large, long-term studies are underway to shed light on the link between nutrition and prostate cancer. Both diet and supplements are being investigated for their role in preventing this disease, and there is much reason for optimism.

DIET. The incidence of prostate cancer is notably low in Asian countries, a fact that has been attributed to diet and lifestyle rather than to genetics. This is so because when Asian men move to North America, after a few years their risk of prostate cancer approaches that of Caucasian Americans.[82] Because of this, certain foods that are commonly used in Asia are being tested for their value in preventing prostate cancer. Such foods include soy products and green tea. Because of their effect on other aspects of male reproductive function, discussed previously, it is best to limit soy foods. Green tea, however, is very high in antioxidants, and new studies are adding evidence that drinking green tea frequently may reduce the incidence of prostate cancer.[83]

Intake of the phytonutrient lycopene, abundant in tomatoes, especially cooked tomatoes, has been found to reduce the risk of prostate cancer.[84] Other sources of this potent antioxidant include watermelon, pink grapefruit, apricots, and papaya.[85]

Consuming *trans* fats, which are found in hydrogenated and overheated vegetable oils, is a risk factor for the most common type of prostate cancer.[86]

FRESH FISH FOR MEN WITH PROSTATE CANCER

Analysis of studies on fish consumption and prostate cancer indicates that eating fish does not reduce the incidence of prostate cancer. However, for those who already have prostate cancer, fish consumption seems to reduce metastasis (spreading of cancer) by 44 percent and death from prostate cancer by 63 percent. The omega-3 fatty acids in fish are known to be anti-inflammatory, which may be the link to decreased aggression of the prostate cancers. Fresh fish, not preserved [canned or dried] fish, were responsible for this beneficial effect.[87]

Chapter 1 of this book, "Twelve Rules for Better Nutrition," suggests eating more plant foods, especially the brightly-colored ones, and avoiding *trans* fats. These rules also encourage eating a greater variety of whole natural foods and avoiding sugary treats and refined starches. While the latter have not been examined in reference to prostate cancer, poor food choices certainly crowd out the healthy foods.

VITAMIN AND MINERAL SUPPLEMENTS. In a major placebo-controlled, long-term study, selenium supplements (200 mcg/day) reduced the death rate of many types of cancer by approximately half, and similarly reduced the risk of prostate cancer.[88] (Androvite for Men contains 200 mcg of selenium per full dose.) Supplementation with vitamin E and beta-carotene also significantly reduced the incidence of prostate cancer in a large study.[89]

OTHER CONCERNS. Four large studies conducted in the 1990s showed that, for unknown reasons, the occurrence of prostate cancer is approximately doubled in vasectomized men.[90] Avoiding vasectomy is one sure way to reduce this risk.

AGE-RELATED CHANGES IN MEN

What can the two of you expect as time passes on? In men, there is no obvious "change of life" as there is in women. Whereas you can state confidently that all women become naturally infertile at menopause, no such statement can be made about men, and many older men with younger wives have fathered children. However, the male hormone testosterone gradually but steadily declines with age, which can affect both sexual desire and sexual function. Sperm quality and quantity on average decrease after age 55. Other changes in the function of the various reproductive organs can affect erection and ejaculation, even when sexual desire remains normal. The media have made us all too aware that there are drugs which can improve the age-related decline in sexual ability. Good diet, good supplements, exercise, and weight control, as well as the remedies for prostate health just discussed, can naturally help with these issues while improving every other aspect of a man's overall health.

SUMMARY—CHAPTER 15

1 Male infertility should be considered even when a couple has reason to believe that it is the woman who is infertile, and all aspects of self care should include both members of the couple.

2 The two essentials of male fertility are quality of the sperm—meaning proper shape, ability to move forward, and healthy DNA—and quantity of sperm i n the semen.

3 Oxidative stress from metabolites of the high energy use of sperm is thought to underlie many if not most factors that reduce male fertility. Antioxidants are vitamins and minerals and other food molecules that counteract oxidative stress. They are valuable to male fertility. Attention to all of the following will reduce oxidative stress and improve male fertility:

> **DIET:** New research shows that dietary choices affect sperm quality and quantity. Most helpful are fish and chicken, beans, whole grains, fruits, and vegetables. Most harmful is consumption of *trans* fats. Sweets, refined treats, sugar-sweetened beverages, and soy foods are also to be avoided, along with processed red meat and full fat dairy foods (milk and cheese).

> **BODY TEMPERATURE:** Sperm are sensitive to elevated temperature. A man's fertility can be improved by avoiding or reducing exposure to high temperatures from workplace heat, constant sitting, excess endurance exercise, or overweight.

> **LIFESTYLE:** To be avoided are excess alcohol, nicotine, anabolic steroids, frequent cell phone use, non-essential prescription medications, industrial or household chemicals or pollutants.

> **BODY WEIGHT:** Obesity, particularly morbid obesity (BMI over 40), affects all aspects of male fertility. A sensible diet of your choice to reduce your weight is recommended. Conversely, if you are extremely underweight, try to gain a few pounds.

> **ESSENTIAL FATTY ACIDS SUPPLEMENTS:** Fish oil, preferably cod liver oil, and/or flax oil increase the valuable omega-3 fatty acids, which are essential to male fertility

VITAMINS AND MINERAL SUPPLEMENTS: "A through Zinc," including vitamin A; the B vitamins, especially folate, B6, and B12; vitamins C and E; and the minerals selenium and zinc. All have been shown in studies to improve sperm quality or quantity, and in some studies have increased pregnancy rates. The multivitamin/multimineral Androvite for Men is a good source of most of these nutrients.

OTHER SUPPLEMENTS: The energy-releasing cofactor coenzyme Q10 in the form of ubiquinol and the powerful antioxidant astaxanthin are also recommended, along with L-carnitine or L-acetyl carnitine, which also release cellular energy. All have been studied for their effect on male fertility.

4 Male sexual desire and sexual function can be decreased by nutrient deficiencies, especially deficiencies of zinc and vitamin C, and by obesity. Nitric oxide (NO) is a necessary signal molecule for erection; leafy greens and beets are among the foods that allow NO to be made. Some herbal preparations also raise the levels of NO.

5 Low thyroid function may be involved in low desire and erectile dysfunction.

6 Prostatitis is a common infection or inflammation in men of all ages. Fortunately, a number of self-help strategies can reduce the incidence of prostatitis.

7 Benign prostate hypertrophy (BPH), which increases as men age, causes annoying symptoms with urination and can impair sexual function. Antioxidant-rich plant foods reduce the incidence of BPH, and extracts of the herb saw palmetto provide beta-sitosterol, which can reduce the symptoms of BHT and improve sexual function.

8 Diet and supplements can reduce the incidence of prostate cancer, which is a leading cancer killer of men.

9 For unknown reasons, vasectomy is linked to a near doubling of the occurrence of prostate cancer.

QUESTIONS & ANSWERS, PART 2:
OVERCOMING REPRODUCTIVE PROBLEMS & CHALLENGES

16

For I know well the plans I have in mind for you, says the Lord, plans for your welfare, not for woe! Plans to give you a future full of hope. —Jeremiah 29:11

Q: My breasts hurt so much sometimes that I can't even hug my husband. Other times they feel uncomfortably full, but I'm not nursing. Please don't tell me it's my coffee—I'll give up anything else!

It probably is caffeine, as you have no doubt suspected by the correlation between your coffee habit and your symptoms. Cutting down on caffeine is the primary dietary change that will help you. Flax oil (5–10 g/day; 1–2 teaspoons if you use the oil rather than capsules) and vitamin E (400–800 IU/day) are also useful for painful breasts. You may notice that binging on sugar, salt or starchy foods causes water retention in a day or two, and retained fluid further aggravates breast tenderness.

Since **mastalgia**, as breast pain is technically called, is a common PMS symptom, the PMS nutritional strategy is well worth considering. If fact, new research shows that chasteberry (*Vitex agnus castus*), which helps some women with PMS, may also help with breast pain.[1] If you choose to try chasteberry extract, I suggest you use it in the form Fertility Blend, as recommended in Chapter 6.

Q: I am prone to migraine headaches. Is there a way of handling them without medication?

Not all headaches are migraines, but migraine headaches are often throbbing headaches on only one side of the head. In about 10 percent of people who are prone to them, they begin with odd symptoms such as visual disturbances, speech disturbances, and sensitivity to light. The best approach is to prevent them, and diet and supplements are valuable for doing so. First, look for triggers and eliminate them whenever possible. Low blood sugar (hypoglycemia) is a major trigger for migraines in susceptible people, and avoiding blood sugar swings is a key strategy. Eat protein, fiber-rich plant foods, and natural fats at every meal and snack. Avoid alcohol and limit sugary treats. Even sweet fruits can cause a migraine, so all sweets should be eaten cautiously and on a full stomach only. Chapter 4 has further information about maintaining blood sugar levels.

The B vitamins and magnesium are helpful to maintaining normal blood glucose levels. Folic acid (2,000–4,000 mcg/day) is particularly valuable when taken with general supplements as suggested in Table 7 (Chapter 3).

Bright lights, chemical odors such as those from cleaning agents, gas stations, new carpets or cigarette smoke can trigger migraines. Foods that contain the amino acid tyramine—aged cheeses, wine, beer—are possible culprits for precipitating migraines. So is MSG (monosodium glutamate), found in soy sauce. Reducing your caffeine intake is helpful, but do so gradually since sudden withdrawal may trigger a migraine.

If you feel that a migraine is coming on, there are things you can do to prevent it completely, or at least moderate the pain. First, get out of bright light and into dim light. Then, if you can, eat a hearty snack of protein, carbohydrate, and fat, such as cheese and crackers, or a hamburger on a bun. Take about 800–2,000 mcg of folic acid with it.

Most valuable of all, though, is to get uncomfortably cold for a little while. If it is winter, go outside without your coat on for five or ten minutes, but watch out if bright sunlight is reflecting off the snow. If it is warm out, take a cool shower in a dimly lit bathroom. The water does not have to be icy cold, and you can alternate with warm water so that you are not miserably cold. Or, if you are caught where you cannot do either, try soaking your hands and feet in very cold water, or putting icy cold wash cloths on your forehead or the back of your neck. The chill causes blood vessels in your skin and elsewhere to constrict, rerouting more blood to your brain. That's why this is so helpful. When you are cold enough to get goose bumps, you are probably cold enough to make this very effective trick work for you. Just remember to stay in dim light while you do so.

Q: I have PMS, and my doctor recommended Optivite three times a day. But when I feel good I forget to take them, and when I feel bad, it's too late! Any suggestions?

Today it is easy to set reminders in our phones. But I also have another idea that works wonderfully. If you are married, ask your husband to take sincere responsibility for getting your vitamins out and reminding you to take them. If you are single, ask your mother, sister or roommate to help you in this way. This situation is very common among PMS sufferers, and those who live with you will probably be glad to help! For your part, respond maturely to their support.

If you live alone, place your vitamins where you will remember to take them—for example, in the bathroom so you can make them part of your after breakfast teeth-brushing routine. If you work outside the home, put them in your purse, and ask a trusted friend to remind you. Then, try not to let her down.

Q: Can I use ProCycle PMS and Fertility Blend together? I am hoping to get pregnant.

Yes, use a three-fourths dose of ProCycle PMS (three tablets daily) plus the full dose of Fertility Blend. You could also use a two-thirds dose of Optivite with Fertility Blend, or two-thirds dose of Professional Pre-Natal Formula with Fertility Blend. Check with your doctor, of course. I recommend that you continue these if you get pregnant using them.

Q: I have been having trouble getting pregnant, but my charts look pretty normal, like I am ovulating. I have not had any fertility testing, but my doctor said that I

probably am having a luteinized unruptured follicle every month, and that is why I am not getting pregnant. Could you explain what this is?

A luteinized unruptured follicle is a rare event. It means that the follicle fails to release the ovum at the time when ovulation would normally occur, but then it begins to secrete progesterone, as if it were a corpus luteum. It can make the luteal phase longer than normal, but often with a weak temperature rise. Usually the cycle ends with a period. With no ovum released, the cycle is infertile, though you would not know it while you were in such a cycle.[2]

I suggest you look for other explanations for your infertility, as there are many more likely reasons that a woman can ovulate and still not get pregnant. Carefully evaluating your own charts with reference to the information in this book is a basic starting point. Refer to the Introduction to Part 2, especially the information under "Maturation of the Ovum" which explains how ovulation can occur regularly without pregnancy following. Also see Appendix B, "Focus on Infertility." In the event that fertility evaluation and ultrasounds confirm that you do in fact have luteinized unruptured follicles, hormonal treatment administered by a physician can be used to stimulate the release of the ovum.

Q: **We are postponing a pregnancy for now using NFP. But I've got mucus from the time my period ends until I ovulate on day 25 or so. We would need to abstain a lot less if I didn't have such a long patch of mucus every month.**

Improved nutrition can very possibly help you, and either a shorter mucus patch or a shorter cycle length will make a difference. I would like to provide you with a checklist to help you identify possible underlying causes of the long cycles or prolonged mucus. Then, you can refer to the appropriate sections of this book for specific nutritional aids. Keep in mind that more than one cause could apply to your situation. If so, do not "double up" on the suggested supplements. Just cover all the bases using Table 7 (Chapter 3) as a guide. Check into all of the following that might apply.

> 1. Are you nursing a baby? Have you discontinued nursing within your last three cycles? The cycle characteristics you describe are normal for cycling, nursing mothers, but classic cycle patterns are equally normal if you are nursing only a little. You can encourage your reproductive hormones to complete the transition from breastfeeding subfertility to full fertility with excellent diet and supplements. Table 13 (Chapter 11), "Suggested Food Goals for Pregnant and Nursing Women," will be helpful if you are nursing a great deal; see Table 1 (Chapter 1), "Suggested Daily Food Goals," if you are nursing very little or have weaned. Supplements as in Table 7 (Chapter 3) should be considered, and be very sure that vitamins A and E, the B vitamins, iodine and essential fatty acids are well-supplied. Professional Pre-Natal Formula by Life Time is excellent for both pregnant and nursing women, along with flax oil or fish oil supplements. (See "Resources" and "Appendix A".)

2. Have you recently discontinued birth control pills or other hormonal birth control? If so, it is possible that their residual effects are still affecting you. It may take up to four cycles for mucus patterns to become normal after discontinuing hormonal birth control, and I have talked to women who believe that various negative effects have persisted for years after they went off the pill. (See "Discontinuing Birth Control Pills or Other Hormonal Birth Control" in Chapter 10.)

3. Are you in your late 40s? Perimenopausal cycle changes could account for this pattern. See Chapter 13, "Premenopause, Perimenopause, & Menopause" for nutritional suggestions for this time of life. If you are younger, look for other explanations besides age.

4. Are you slender or underweight, even a little bit? Do you exercise vigorously? Have you dieted recently, even if you are still overweight? (See "Underweight or Inadequate Body Fat" in Chapter 8.)

5. Are your preovulatory basal temperatures around 97.3°F or lower? You may have a tendency to low thyroid function—maybe not enough to cause major symptoms, but enough to explain your prolonged mucus and delayed ovulation. (See "Low Thyroid Function" in Chapter 8.)

6. Could you be deficient in vitamin A? Another sign of this is heavy or prolonged menses. (See "Diet for Better Healing and Normal Blood Clotting" and "Supplements for Better Healing and Normal Blood Clotting" in Chapter 7). The recommendations to lighten heavy periods are helpful to prolonged mucus.

7. Is your luteal phase usually less than twelve days from the first day of the temperature shift up to and including the last day before your period begins? (See "Luteal Phase Deficiency" in Chapter 8.)

8. Are you obese or substantially overweight? (See Chapter 9.)

9. Is there any light at all in your bedroom at night? Some women's mucus patterns improve when night lighting in their bedrooms is eliminated or controlled. (See "Sensitivity to Night Lighting" in Chapter 10.)

10. Do you drink more than two or three cups of coffee a day, or the equivalent in caffeinated soda? Are you eating chocolate almost daily? (See "Caffeine Consumption" in Chapter 10.) Do you use NutraSweet or other artificial sweeteners daily? (See the question and answer on this topic in Chapter 5.)

11. If none of the above applies, I recommend that you try the PMS nutritional plan as outlined in Chapter 6. If you are slender but not really underweight, try gaining just two or three pounds. Make sure that you are getting sufficient iodine (150 mcg/day) and vitamin E (400–800 IU/day). And finally, review the suggestions in Chapter 10 under the heading "Yeast Overgrowth/Gut Dysbiosis."

If these suggestions will make a difference, they will do so within about three months.

Q: **Do you have any advice about acne? I wish I could say I'm interested in it for my teenage daughter, but I actually have a problem with it myself, especially before my period.**

Yes, there is nutritional help for **acne vulgaris**, as pimples and blackheads are called. Acne vulgaris is caused by infection of the oil glands of the skin, the sebaceous glands. It is not the same as **acne rosacea**, or "adult acne," which has to do with excess proliferation of blood vessels in the skin of the face and neck. (I comment on rosacea below.)

Acne vulgaris may be related to high insulin levels, which in women trigger the production of male hormones and other factors that stimulate the skin to overproduce skin cells and sebum, the natural oil from the sebaceous glands. Really cutting down on foods that are sugary or high in refined starches (white flour) is very helpful.[3] *Trans* fats are also to be avoided, but the healthy oils such as olive oil and canola oil are beneficial. Milk is controversial when it comes to acne; some studies have found whole milk helpful, whereas some authors strongly advise against it. Chocolate is another controversial food; it is probably the sugar in it, not the chocolate itself, that makes so many teenagers reluctantly agree that yes, it is bad for their skin.

Fish oil (5 grams or 1 teaspoon daily) and/or flax oil (five to ten 1 g capsules or 1–2 teaspoons daily) are both beneficial when it comes to acne, as they have significant anti-inflammatory effects and also promote production of a more liquid sebum that is less likely to clog the sebaceous glands. You can use either or both together in the amounts just listed. The fat-soluble vitamins are also good for acne prevention: vitamin A, (8,000 IU of true vitamin A if pregnancy is a possibility; up to 25,000 if it is not; your doctor may prescribe higher levels); vitamin E (400–800 IU); and vitamin D (400–1,000 IU). Zinc works along with vitamin A, and 25–50 mg is helpful. Some nutritionally-oriented doctors specifically recommend higher amounts of zinc for acne, in the range of 100 mg, but you should certainly have your doctor's approval before using more than 25–50 mg. Acne vulgaris responds quite rapidly to improved nutrition, within a couple of weeks or a month.

If you are having symptoms that are consistent with polycystic ovary syndrome (PCOS), such as long, irregular cycles or evidence of elevated male hormones, please see Chapter 9, which deals with this topic. Chapter 9 discusses nutritional ways to decrease elevated insulin levels, which has many benefits, including benefits to acne vulgaris.

With reference to acne rosacea, the difficult-to-treat, progressive reddening of the skin of the face and neck, I believe that the same recommendations given here for acne vulgaris are advisable; that is, keep the sugary and starchy foods that increase insulin levels to a minimum. In addition, increasing the amount of acid in the stomach and increasing the digestive enzymes may help out with rosacea. It may be worth purchasing digestive enzyme tablets designed to supplement both stomach and small intestinal secretions. These are available in health food shops. Other self care includes avoiding very cold or very hot environments, and wash your face very gently with cool water and milk soap.

Q: **I quit nursing my baby eighteen months ago, but my breasts have still not completely dried up, and my luteal phase is still short.**

Galactorrhea, or milk in the breasts of non-nursing women, is not uncommon among those who have been pregnant. It most often indicates excessive prolactin secretion, or it can be a symptom of hypothyroidism, or, more rarely, hyperthyroidism. These topics are discussed in Chapter 8 under the headings "Luteal Phase Deficiency," "Low Thyroid Function," and "Hyperthyroidism." An evaluation by a doctor can and should be made to determine the cause of galactorrhea, but the temperature chart itself contributes to the diagnosis. Very low or very elevated waking temperatures suggest, respectively, low or elevated levels of thyroid hormone. A short luteal phase suggests evidence of high prolactin levels when there is milk in your breasts.

The nutritional suggestions for lowering prolactin are listed as the subtopic "Abnormal Luteal Function (Luteal Phase Deficiency)" in Chapter 6. Vitamin B6 alone, in amounts of 300–600 mg/day, has eliminated both galactorrhea and amenorrhea caused by prolactin excess.[4] I once counseled a woman with secondary infertility who had a leakage of milk from one breast, even though her youngest child was six years old. She had received medical treatment for infertility without success. She tried the full dose of Optivite (300 mg vitamin B6; see Appendix A for complete contents), and within only a few days the leakage of milk stopped. In addition, she got pregnant without fertility treatment during her next cycle.

Fairly high amounts of vitamin B6 (200–300 mg/day) may be necessary to lower prolactin levels significantly, but magnesium in generous amounts (800–1,000 mg/day) may make less B6 necessary. Vitamins and minerals are natural substances that will get at the underlying cause, and are far preferable to the synthetic drug bromocriptine (Parlodel), which specifically lowers prolactin.

NutraSweet can raise prolactin levels and cause long cycles. Make sure you avoid it, and avoid other artificial sweeteners as well. (See the question and answer on this topic in Chapter 5.)

> **You may be surprised to learn that galactorrhea is frequently undetected by women who have this condition.[5]**

Careful expression of each breast, from edge to nipple, should be part your routine breast self-examination. While usually the explanation is hormonal imbalances, even a single drop of fluid should be reported to a doctor, unless you are pregnant or nursing has been discontinued recently.

Q: Is carpal tunnel syndrome treatable by nutrition?

Carpal tunnel syndrome refers to pain, weakness, and numbness of the hands, wrists, and sometimes elbows and shoulders. The usual advice it to avoid hyperextending the wrists by using removable splints. However, there is some evidence that vitamin B6 may be helpful for carpal tunnel syndrome, but it is not conclusive.[6] Dr. John Ellis noted that vitamin B6 and magnesium, which work together, were helpful for such symptoms in pregnant women. (See the subtitle, "Vitamin B6 and Magnesium for Edema" in Chapter 11 for more information.) If you wish to try nutrition for carpal tunnel syndrome, instead of vitamin B6 and magnesium only, use ProCycle PMS as your multivitamin/multimineral. It contains both of these, as well as a good balance of other nutrients which enable vitamin B6 to work more effectively. (See Appendix A.) The omega-3 fatty acids in flax oil or fish oil may be helpful, also, because of their strong anti-inflammatory effect.

Q: Is there any evidence that nutrition can help prevent premature rupture of membranes?

Yes, there is. **Premature rupture of membranes** (PROM) means that the "bag of waters" breaks long before a woman is due to have the baby. It is one cause of premature delivery, because it may trigger premature labor, or labor may be induced because of the ruptured membranes. Smoking is a risk factor for PROM and for other causes of premature delivery. Good nutrition, especially enough dietary protein, generally helps to prevent prematurity, but there is evidence that vitamin C is low in women who have had PROM.[7] This makes sense, because the membranes are strengthened by **collagen**, a thread-like structural protein, and collagen cannot be made without vitamin C. The bioflavinoids, which are nutrients found in the whitish rinds of citrus fruits, work along with vitamin C to do this job.

Q: Is there any way to decrease the risk of getting fibroid tumors? My mother, who is 47, just got diagnosed with one, and I know they run in families.

Fibroid tumors are stimulated by high levels of estrogen, and it is true that they may run in families. Avoiding overweight is perhaps the most effective way of preventing high estrogen levels, and overweight is a risk factor for fibroids. Nutrition aimed at raising progesterone and lowering estrogen is the next step. Vitamins and minerals that work together to do so are vitamin B6, other B vitamins, vitamin C, and magnesium. Optivite or ProCycle PMS, each made to overcome PMS, contain these nutrients and others to help normalize your estrogen and progesterone. See Chapter 6 for complete information on PMS nutrition, which will be helpful to you.

Q: **I am only in my 30s, but I am very concerned about osteoporosis. Yet from what I read, calcium alone doesn't seem to be the answer.**

You are correct; studies on the effects of calcium supplementation on the bone loss disorder **osteoporosis** have not been especially promising. Both vitamin D and magnesium are necessary for the body to use calcium, and it is good to remember that sugar increases the loss of magnesium.

Interestingly, correcting certain cycle irregularities may reduce your risk of osteo-porosis. A study of athletic women published in the *New England Journal of Medicine* established that athletic women who experienced only one or more short luteal phase cycles or anovulatory cycles per year were losing bone mass at a time of life when other women were gaining bone. In this study, luteal phase was determined by basal temperatures, and elevated temperatures of less than ten days were considered a short luteal phase. The authors expressed concern that short luteal phase is a silent risk factor for osteoporosis, because women with short luteal phases usually have very regular menstrual periods.[8] It is certainly an obvious factor to women who chart, and based on research discussed in this book, a reversible one. The anovulatory cycles referred to above are less common than short luteal phase cycles. They may be an extreme form of the short luteal phase cycle, a consequence of underweight, or a manifestation of low thyroid function. These cycle irregularities often respond to proper nutrition; see the appropriate subtitles in Chapter 8 ("Luteal Phase Deficiency," "Underweight or Inadequate Body Fat," or "Low Thyroid Function") for nutrition to overcome them.

Incidentally, I believe that the short luteal phases seen during breastfeeding and during the perimenopause are natural fertility transitions and are not a cause for special concern.

Q: **I am 35 years old and have had six children. I have breastfed them all. I am small-boned, and my grandmother broke her hip when she was seventy. Does having many children increase the risk of osteoporosis?**

This is a question that has interested a number of researchers, and some of the answers are coming from an ongoing study of women from the Old Order Amish religion. They are very family-oriented and have a tradition of large families and of breastfeeding their babies. Results of these studies actually show the reverse of what you might think: Bone mineral density is higher, and therefore risk of bone fracture of the hip is lower, in women who have had large numbers of children. Some of this effect, however, is due to the modest increase in weight that is common as women have many babies, and as women age the benefit is lost. However, having many children (and in this large study five to ten children was most common) had no negative effect on bone density whatever.[9] It might be worth adding that Amish communities are usually farming communities in which milk cows are kept and milk is a major food.

You are probably aware that being small-boned and having a relative with a bone fracture are risk factors for osteoporosis. I encourage you to get a bone density test now, while you are still in your thirties. Diet, exercise, and vitamin and mineral supplements can enable you to maintain or restore your bone health at your age, and finding out what your bone status is now is a great motivator should you find your bones are less dense than you would like. See Chapter 13's topic "Maintaining Bone Health" for more information.

Q: How do you see the role of stress in infertility?

In general, I think that the role of stress as most people understand it is overrated as a cause of infertility. The emphasis on daily life stresses, such as constant deadlines, constant chauffeuring, or the constant need to have the house clean and the garden weeded, misses the point. I do not think that those stresses are the ones that contribute to infertility, at least not directly. It is *physical* stress, which many people seem to overlook completely, that truly can contribute to infertility.

The physical stresses that affect fertility are the chronic stress of poor nutrition, lack of sleep, and in some women, too much physical exertion, even if they enjoy their exercise routines or sports activities.

All of these stresses can be involved even with cycles that show ovulation. The kind of modern stresses that we talk about so much—being too busy or striving for perfection—in my opinion affect fertility mostly insofar as they cause women to miss out on good nutrition and adequate sleep, or make them feel that they must exercise excessively. Improved nutrition, enough sleep, and moderate exercise are what I mean when I write about stress reduction.

That's why I take issue with that unsolicited advice to infertile couples, "Relax!" Yes, an episode of severe emotional stress, such as the death of a loved one, a major financial reversal, or an unwelcome, untimely move across country, can cause a delay in ovulation, sometimes for weeks. But once ovulation resumes, fertility will be restored. Please, if you are not infertile, do not suggest that your infertile friends relax. I have never spoken to a woman anxious to conceive who was not hurt and worried by that counterproductive advice. I facetiously encourage our infertility clients to "go ahead and be uptight!" Knowing that it does not matter is good for their peace of mind.

Q: Can women take Androvite for Men? I don't have PMS, and it looks like three or four tablets would be a good general vitamin.

Yes, you can. You can take the full dose, which is six tablets, even if you become pregnant, assuming your doctor's approval. The labeling of the vitamin A confuses people, but if you read the label carefully you will see that it contains only 5,000 IU of retinyl palmitate (true vitamin A) per full dose; the rest is beta-carotene. Only true vitamin A, not beta-carotene, has been related to birth defects, in amounts beginning at 10,000 IU.[10]

The full dose of Androvite for Men is especially good, I think, for women who need adrenal support, as the adrenals produce steroid hormones and therefore have nutritional needs much like the testes'. I also consider it helpful for thyroid support, due to its substantial mix of minerals along with the vitamins. Because of this, it may be beneficial for hair loss,[11] especially when taken along with flax oil.

With my doctor's approval, I used the full dose of Androvite for Men as part of my prenatal supplementation when I was pregnant with our eighth child, but nevertheless, she turned out to be a girl!

Q: How can I find a good nutritional counselor?

You might be expecting me to give you a website as my response, but I think that the best way to find someone right in your community is to visit your local food co-op or health food shop and ask there for recommendations. Food co-ops in particular are often the unofficial local clearinghouse for information on every variety of alternative health care, including the names and reputations of nutritionally-oriented medical doctors, osteopaths, chiropractors, birth attendants, and so forth. Keep in mind that co-op employees are often members who work only a few hours per week, so if one person cannot help you, perhaps the next day's employees can!

Q: What should I look for in selecting my nutritional counselor?

Here are some traits that I think form the ideal.

1. He or she is a qualified health professional, educated in the functions of the human body. He or she could be a medical doctor, an osteopathic doctor, a chiropractor, a nutritionist, or one of the less familiar naturopathic or homeopathic doctors. If you have serious health problems such as cardiovascular disease, kidney disease, or diabetes, make every effort to find a medical or osteopathic doctor who is aware of the benefits of nutrition for your particular condition.

2. He or she is enthusiastically interested in the role of nutrition in health and disease, and stays informed about new research involving nutrition and health.

3. He or she directs you to appropriate laboratory tests of your nutritional status, and can prescribe nutrients in potencies and chemical forms that are not available over the counter.

4. He or she not only is open to your input, but also considers your awareness and participation in your health care indispensable. The ideal nutritional counselor sees health care as an equal partnership with you, and recognizes that ultimate decision-making rests with you. He or she directs you to websites, asks you to read pamphlets, and recommends whole books. This person is unafraid to say, "I don't know," and appreciates published information or anecdotes that you provide to help make your counseling more effective.

5. He or she recognizes the role of the emotions in health and healing, and is genuinely encouraging and uplifting about the healing power of the human body.

6. He or she is available by telephone or e-mail. After an initial visit or two, and any necessary laboratory assessments, an ideal nutritional counselor is prompt and gracious about answering brief questions by e-mail or phone.

Q: **My doctor is okay with my vitamins and minerals, but he is not really that knowledgeable. Do you think that I would be better off looking for another one?**

Not necessarily. If you have established a good relationship of mutual respect, it is absolutely worth keeping that relationship. If you have no serious health disorders and if you are willing to read in the field of nutrition, you may get along very well by simply letting your doctor know what you are doing. Your good health probably contributes to his openness to nutrition. If on the other hand you have serious health problems to deal with, you may have more to gain if you have the input of another nutritional advisor along with a supportive primary doctor. My experience is that this is a very workable situation as long as the doctor isn't "down on it because he's not up on it!"

Q: **Would you help me understand how you see the difference between artificial birth control and natural family planning? Don't explain the pill or sterilization—what I want to know is what is the difference between NFP and using a condom. In both cases the couple is avoiding a pregnancy, and no early abortion is involved.**

Practically speaking, NFP differs from contraception in the use of abstinence. Those who use NFP abstain, giving up the pleasure of marital relations during the fertile time, since they are choosing to avoid conception. In the case of contraception, the pleasure of the act is taken, deliberately disjoined from the potential for pregnancy.

The abstinence of NFP is a kind of sacrifice. In properly used NFP, a good and pleasing thing (marital relations), is given up for a greater good (ideally, the good of the entire family). I submit that this real difference, this sacrifice, is indeed part of the moral difference.

Sacrifices are often hard to make. Yet God is wonderfully provident to have created us so that the abstinence of NFP is not extreme. Women are fertile only for a few days of each month, and even with the inevitable delays in arriving at the infertile time, each cycle provides several days for the warmth, bonding, and release of the marital embrace.

It could have been different. Our Creator God made us a certain way, but other possibilities exist in nature. Some mammals ovulate only after mating, so that each mating typically results in a pregnancy. Rabbits and llamas are examples of this strategy, which if true of humans would make NFP impossible. Other female mammals cycle regularly, but are only sexually receptive around the time they ovulate. Many grazing animals—horses, cows, sheep and goats—are like this, only mating when fertile. By such comparisons, it seems clear that God created sexuality in humans just as the Catholic Church teaches: marital relations serve the purpose of conception of children as well as the purpose of bonding the couple. God is good!

FURTHER READING

The Adrenal Reset Diet: Strategically Cycle Carbs and Proteins to Lose Weight, Balance Hormones, and Move from Stressed to Thriving, by Alan Christianson, NMD (Harmony Press: 2014). The adrenal glands maintain a normal cortisol rhythm and when this rhythm is off, we can become overwhelmed more quickly, fatigued, gain weight, and eventually, develop even more severe health issues such as heart disease or diabetes. Dr. Christianson provides a pioneering plan for optimal function of these small but powerful organs.

The Art of Breastfeeding: Empowering Women to Give Their Babies the Best Start, by Linda Kracht and Jackie Hilgert (The Couple to Couple League, 2008). A good source of information on introducing solid foods to breastfed babies. Beyond that, however, this is an excellent resource to learn why extended breastfeeding is best for not only for babies, but for mothers, fathers, and families as well. Learn how to get breastfeeding off to a good start, how to navigate common obstacles, and how nursing will impact your fertility cycles.

Aspartame (NutraSweet): Is It Safe? by H.J. Roberts, M.D. (Philadephia: The Charles Press, 1990). Dr. Roberts wrote this book because of the unexpected challenges to his specialty, difficult diagnoses, that occurred after NutraSweet became popular. While the book is not focused on women's health, it nevertheless covers a number of menstrual cycle irregularities that may relate to use of this artificial sweetener. It explains the mechanisms by which it does so; for example, by increasing insulin levels and prolactin levels. It discusses the biochemistry of aspartame and facts regarding its testing for safety.

Beat Sugar Addiction Now!: The Cutting-Edge Program That Cures Your Type of Sugar Addiction and Puts You on the Road to Feeling Great - and Losing Weight, by Jacob Teitelbaum, M.D. (Fair Winds Press, 2010). Uncovers four types of sugar addiction and gives a step-by-step plan for resolving the underlying causes, breaking sugar cravings, and achieving improved health and energy levels.

Before the Change: Taking Charge of Your Perimenopause, 2nd ed., by Ann Louise Gittleman (San Francisco: HarperSanFrancisco, 2004). Here is the book that will be your most thorough yet readable guide to the changes in your hormones and moods as your fertile years pass. It emphasizes improved diet, vitamins, minerals, healthy oils, natural progesterone, exercise, stress reduction, and adrenal gland support. I consider this the best book available on premenopause, perimenopause, and menopause. It is much easier and more enjoyable to use than the late Dr. Lee's book, *What Your Doctor May Not Tell You about Menopause*, but Ms. Gittleman refers to and includes Dr. Lee's recommendations.

Breastfeeding and Natural Child Spacing: The Ecology of Natural Mothering, Classic Edition, by Sheila Kippley (2008). This book has the best information I know of on how to breastfeed, including long-term breastfeeding, and on feeding solids during later babyhood. I am very grateful to my dear friend, Sheila, that I read the original edition of this book before my first child was born. It has helped me with the next eight as well!

Chronic Candidiasis: Your Natural Guide to Healing with Diet, Vitamins, Minerals, Herbs, Exercise, and Other Natural Methods, by Michael T. Murray, N.D. (Roseville, CA: Prima, 1997). The voracious researcher Dr. Murray has provided an excellent resource for men, women, or children with yeast overgrowth, also called candidiasis. Despite the biology involved with this topic, it is clearly and concisely explained. Among the many helpful features of this book is information on natural alternatives to antibiotics for various infections. Dr. Murray's dietary approach emphasizes an overall vegetarian approach, though it does not completely exclude animal products.

Depression-free, Naturally: 7 Weeks to Eliminating Anxiety, Despair, Fatigue, and Anger from Your Life, by Joan Mathews Larson, Ph.D., (New York: Ballantine Wellspring, 2001). Dr. Larson works from the hypothesis that the disorders listed in the title result from biochemical imbalances that are correctable through targeted nutrition. She presents a large amount of information which can be somewhat confusing. However, used as a reference, this book can help you to identify what might be out of balance in your body. It has many specific suggestions for help. In addition to recommending vitamins and minerals, Dr. Larson is a proponent of the use of free amino acids to provide the body with the building blocks to make beneficial neurotransmitters—for example, serotonin.

Dr. Atkins' New Diet Revolution: The Low-Carb Approach That Has Helped Millions Lose Weight and Keep It Off, by Robert C. Atkins, M.D. (New York: Quill, an imprint of HarperCollins, 2002). This is the update of Dr. Atkins' famous book, published shortly before his death in 2003. It is a valuable reference for anyone with polycystic ovary syndrome (PCOS). If you are interested in losing weight, you may find it far too strict, but it is full of many good ideas regarding weight loss. For example, his contention that protein and fat satisfy the appetite, while low fat, high carbohydrate diets promote cravings rings true with many women. It contains an excellent chapter on "vita-nutrients" to supplement while you are trying to lose weight or keep it off. The book is actually fun to read; Dr. Atkins' style is witty and often endearing.

Dr. David Reuben's Quick Weight-Gain Program: Safe, Easy Weight Gain for Every Age and Situation, by David Reuben, M.D. (New York: Crown Publishers, 1996). As far as I can tell, there is no other book available like this one, perhaps because so many people are trying to do exactly the opposite of Dr. Reuben's topic! Most underweight women do not need a book to explain to them how to exercise less and eat more, but if you are having a hard time gaining weight, this book will show you strategies that work. The chatty style is very motivational, though the book emphasizes a sexy body more than a healthy body. It is a good book for men, women, or children, the elderly, and the chronically ill.

Dr. John Lee's Hormone Balance Made Simple: The Essential How-to Guide to Symptoms, Dosage, Timing, and More, by John R. Lee, M.D., and Virginia Hopkins (New York: Warner Wellness, 2006). Finally, here is a relatively short handbook that guides you (and ideally, your health care professional) in the use of natural hormones, especially progesterone, but also estrogen and testosterone. Why, when, which one, and how much are all easily answered.

However, there is one important correction: The sidebar, "The Best Way to Calculate When to Use Progesterone Cream if You're Having Periods," (p. 129–130) is flawed. It uses an outdated "rhythm" approach, recommending that women start using progesterone cream two weeks before they expect their next period. No! Women with cycles who choose to use natural progesterone cream should start it after ovulation is confirmed by the third day of temperature rise, so that the progesterone does not interfere with the preovulatory hormones. In many women who have estrogen dominance, the luteal phase is so short that this recommendation will result in progesterone usage well before ovulation, interfering with the natural hormone processes at that time. According to the Foreword of the book, one of the three major causes of poor results with natural hormones is using them at the wrong time (p. xii). The underlying assumption that women cannot or will not ascertain their ovulation time through NFP charting is simply that—an assumption.

The author frequently refers the reader to the late Dr. Lee's previous books, *What Your Doctor May Not Tell You about Menopause*, and *What Your Doctor May Not Tell You About Premenopause*. These two books have much more information about nutrition, but if you need only the practical help of using hormone creams, they are entirely optional.

While Dr. Lee's *Hormone Balance* points out that estrogen dominance may cause low thyroid function, the book is not particularly aimed at assisting women with low thyroid function from other causes. And with reference to polycystic ovary syndrome, it states that "PCOS disappears rapidly in most women when they cut sugar and refined carbohydrates from their diets," an optimistic assertion that defies the experience of the many women who have struggled with this ongoing metabolic imbalance. Still, it is a worthwhile book for those interested in natural hormone replacement.

The Effects of Light on the Menstrual Cycle: Also Infertility, Clinical Observations, by Joy DeFelice, R.N. (Spokane, WA: The Natural Family Planning Program of the Sacred Heart Medical Center, 2003). Mrs. DeFelice, a natural family planning professional, observed the effect of eliminating night lighting on the regularity of the menstrual cycle beginning in 1976. The research community is now able to explain this phenomenon through the effect of light on the pineal gland and its secretion of melatonin, which affects reproductive hormones. This booklet is a practical guide that explains why and how to eliminate night lighting in order to have more regular cycles and improved fertility. Her advice is no substitute for improved nutrition, but she herself reminds the reader of the necessity of good nutrition, exercise, and stress reduction. If you are having difficulty sleeping, this booklet will help you also.

The Encyclopedia of Natural Medicine, 3rd edition, by Michael Murray, N.D. and Joseph Pizzorno, N.D. (Atria Books, 2012). Focuses on promoting health and treating disease with nontoxic, natural therapies. This groundbreaking book—the leader in its field—shows you how to improve your health through a positive mental attitude, a healthy lifestyle, a health-promoting diet, and supplements, along with plenty of practical tips.

Endometriosis: A Key to Healing and Fertility through Nutrition, by Dian Shepperson Mills, M.A., and Michael Vernon, Ph.D. (London: Thorsons, 2002). A thick book with small print, Endometriosis is like a Bible—open it to any page and you will learn, be encouraged, and be motivated. It contains an amazing array of detailed recommendations for improved nutrition, and always includes the rationale behind the recommendations. It proposes a diet that includes animal products but emphasizes whole fresh fruits, vegetables, grains, and legumes, with moderate use of dairy products. Its recommendation to find and eliminate food intolerances, such as wheat products, is very valuable. Though scientific at its core, it is compassionate in its tone. Recommended by Mary Lou Ballweg, president of the International Endometriosis Association.

Female Fertility and the Body Fat Connection, by Rose E. Frisch, Ph.D. (Chicago: University of Chicago Press, 2002). As a Harvard School of Public Health professor, Dr. Frisch did the groundbreaking research on the link between women's athletic endeavor, body weight, body fat, and menstrual cycles. In this book, she approaches the topic autobiographically rather than through a strictly scientific approach. Yet the science is always present, as she explains the physiology behind the phenomenon of amenorrhea caused by excessive exercise. *Female Fertility and the Body Fat Connection* is not written as a self-help book, but it is fascinating reading about how scientific inquiry progresses once the basic scientific tool—the questioning mind—is engaged.

The Fertility Diet: Groundbreaking Research Reveals Natural Ways to Boost Ovulation and Improve Your Chances of Getting Pregnant, by Jorge E. Chavarro, M.D., Sc.D.; Walter C. Willett, M.D., D.P.H.; and Patrick J. Skerrett (New York: McGraw-Hill, 2009). An important book based on the huge Nurses' Health Study, particularly involving nurses who were trying to get pregnant during the study. Based on analysis of thousands of nurses' reports of diet, exercise, body weight, and so forth, the authors make numerous recommendations for improved diet. It covers the problems with sugary foods and trans fats. It has a chapter on celiac disease. It covers ovulatory infertility, including polycystic ovary syndrome (PCOS). A very nice feature related to PCOS is a chapter that includes evaluation of various weight-loss diets. Please note that *The Fertility Diet* is not a resource for those looking for help with endometriosis, male infertility, PMS, menopause, or cycle irregularities related to low thyroid function, short luteal phase, or age.

Gardening Without Work: For the Aging, the Busy and the Indolent, by Ruth Stout (Echo Point Books, 2013). Describes the easiest way imaginable to garden organically. You need enough fall leaves, grass clippings, spoiled hay or straw to cover your garden deeply—and this book.

Get the Sugar Out: 501 Simple Ways to Cut the Sugar Out of Any Diet, 2nd ed., by Ann Louise Gittleman (New York: Harmony Press, 2008). Here is a book that will explain the problems with sweet additives to our foods. Sugar is only one of the additives that are discussed; high fructose corn syrup, sugar alcohols, aspartame, sucralose, and Stevia are also covered. It contains quite a bit of practical information on reading labels, and offers many tips and recipes to "get the sugar out!"

Hashimoto's Thyroiditis: Lifestyle Interventions for Finding and Treating the Root Cause, by Isabella Wentz, PharmD, and Marta Nowosadzka, M.D. (Wentz LLC: 2013). Includes lifestyle interventions aimed to dismantle the cycle of symptoms. Starts with simple modifications and the removal of triggers, then follows with strategies to repair and allow the body to heal itself.

Health and Healing, by Julian Whitaker, M.D. This popular e-newsletter can be found at drwhitaker.com.

Hypothyroidism: The Unsuspected Illness, by Broda O. Barnes, M.D. and Lawrence Galton (Harper: 1976). Explains what the thyroid gland is, how it works, and the problems its dysfunction can induce. Details case histories of patients, often thought hopeless, whose problems were discovered to be related to hypothyroidism and were cured by Dr. Barnes's simple effective techniques.

Let's Have Healthy Children, by Adelle Davis, revised by Marshall Mandell, M.D.

(New York: Signet Books, 1981). This is the last edition of the original book on diet and supplements for pregnancy. Adelle Davis was far ahead of her time on this topic, though she drew her conclusions and recommendations from the available research literature. The book is still an immense help both for pregnancy and for nutritional care of babies and children. Adelle Davis strongly believed that even the minor complaints of pregnancy — nausea, headache, fatigue, varicose veins, "mask" of pregnancy—are abnormalities that can be prevented or reversed with proper diet and supplements. The book is out of print, but is available via the Internet.

Living Well with Graves' Disease and Hyperthyroidism: What Your Doctor Doesn't Tell You…That You Need to Know, by Mary J. Shomon (William Morrow, 2005). This resource uniquely highlights holistic treatments, and through case studies and testimonials from patients and doctors, presents an honest look at the lifestyles and choices of people living with these conditions.

Managing Morning Sickness, 2nd ed., by Marilyn M. Shannon (Cincinnati: The Couple to Couple League, 1998). This short booklet promotes the hypothesis that overcoming low blood sugar is an important factor in overcoming morning sickness. It includes practical dietary strategies aimed at stabilizing your blood glucose, settling your tender stomach, and preventing low blood pressure. There are suggestions for supplements to discuss with your doctor. As you can guess, I seldom disagree with the author.

The Myth of Osteoporosis: What Every Woman Should Know about Creating Bone Health, by Gillian Sanson (Ann Arbor, MI: MCD Century, 2003). The unfortunate title of this book might discourage a sensible person from opening it, but I have found it to be helpful and reassuring. Mrs. Sanson is part of a family that has a genetic disorder that causes the bone loss disease osteoporosis at a young age, and so she has lived with the information gathering and decision making that such a serious problem requires. She recommends good nutrition, maintenance of normal weight (as opposed to underweight), exercise, and—very important—prevention of fractures as the basis of bone health. She explains the problems with the drug therapies for osteoporosis. She is critical of bone density measurement, a point on which I disagree. Nevertheless, you will learn more practical information about maintaining bone health through this book than through many longer ones.

A Natural Guide to Pregnancy and Postpartum Health, by Dean Raffelock, D.C., Robert Rountree, M.D., and Virginia Hopkins (New York: Avery, 2003). Here is an excellent book with information to help you have a wonderfully healthy pregnancy, and equally as important, a wonderfully healthy and joyous postpartum time with your new baby. As the authors point out, many women are overstressed, anxious or depressed during the postpartum time, and much of that can be helped by better nutrition. The authors note again and again that your baby is made from the food you eat, and nutritional deficiencies often catch up with mothers after the birth. They propose good, preferably organic, whole plant and animal foods. Moreover, they make the case that nutritional deficiencies are very difficult to overcome with improved diet alone, and they are strong proponents of supplementing.

When it comes to the supplements that they recommend, the authors give the amounts that are safe for pregnant women and their unborn babies, and for mothers with nursing babies (though in some cases higher amounts are known to be safe, as in the case of folic acid).

In no other book have I seen the role of supplements in overcoming the toxins in the body or in the environment so well explained. That in itself is very encouraging, as it is easy to get discouraged when you find out about "indoor air pollution," pesticide residues on your fresh produce, and so forth. The book also includes an easy-to-understand chapter on the digestive system, explaining leaky gut syndrome and offering practical solutions for it. I highly recommend this book.

Nutrition Almanac, 6th ed., by John D. Kirschman and Nutrition Search, Inc. (New York: McGraw-Hill, 2007). The best use of this book is as a reference to find out what is in your food. How many calories are in a cup of almonds? How much fiber is in a cup of kidney beans? Are sunflowers a good source of protein? It contains useful information on every vitamin and mineral, and features many charts of the nutrients found in particular foods. It even has a section on phytonutrients, including names and functions of a dozen or so of these newly discovered plant nutrients.

Optivite PMT® and Gynovite® Plus Total Dietary Programs for Women With Answers to the Most Commonly Asked Questions, by Susan A. Beck, B.S.N., R.N., M.A., and Guy Abraham, M.D., (Torrance, CA: Optimox Corp., 1992). This booklet is primarily a guide to taking the vitamin supplement Optivite, which is the multivitamin/multimineral supplement that Dr. Abraham formulated and tested for PMS. In the first few pages, the book summarizes the symptoms and risk factors of PMS. It explains how much Optivite to take based on the Menstrual Symptom Diary, which is included as the centerfold in the booklet. Depending on the improvement in symptoms, it advises adjustment in the total dosage. It also explains the possible side effects of upset stomach, nausea, and loose stools that occasionally occur in women taking Optivite.

The most useful part is the third section, "Common Questions Asked by Our Customers about Optivite." Can you take it when pregnant? (Yes, with your physician's approval.) Can a teenage girl take it? (Yes, the full dose if she is over 100 pounds and menstruating regularly.) Is it okay for men to take Optivite? (Yes, but Optimox Corporation has a product available for men called Androvite for Men.) All in all, there are sixty questions and answers. One question and answer even covers the topic of Optivite and luteal phase deficiency and infertility.

By the way, this pamphlet, as the title implies, devotes a couple of pages to the postmenopausal time and the supplement Gynovite Plus, which is aimed at protecting women's bone health in the time after the fertile years.

Often when I write about vitamin and mineral supplements, I remind the reader to discuss the topic with a nutritionally-aware physician. This little booklet is an excellent resource to have in hand when you do so.

Prescription for Nutritional Healing: A Practical A-Z Reference to Drug-free Remedies Using Vitamins, Minerals, Herbs & Food Supplements, 4th ed., by Phyllis A. Balch, C.N.C. (New York: Avery Press, 2006). This is a thick but easy-to-use reference which lives up to its name. Use it as the family "medical" guide. It is a comprehensive book that contains descriptions of the ailments you are interested in, followed by priority lists of vitamins, minerals, essential fatty acids, amino acids, herbs, and other supplements particular to that ailment.

Preventing Eclampsia: An Interview with Tom Brewer, M.D. by C.J. Puotinen (Townsend Letter for Doctors and Patients, Nov., 2004). This article, easily available through the Internet, concisely summarizes Dr. Brewer's life work, which involved clinical experience with thousands of pregnant women. It details the diet he developed, and compares the medical approach to eclampsia to the nutritional approach. It is completely referenced with 83 citations, all of them annotated by the author. In addition to preventing eclampsia, Dr. Brewer relates his pregnancy diet to better birth weights, more full-term births, and better mental development in children born to mothers who followed his diet.

Saving Dinner: The Menus, Recipes, and Shopping Lists to Bring Your Family Back to the Table: A Cookbook, by Leanne Ely (New York: Ballantine Books, 2009). If you are having trouble getting started with better nutrition, *Saving Dinner* has already anticipated what you need to be successful. The author knows that you need quick-to-cook dishes. She knows that shopping lists will save you time and frustration. She knows that your family wants everything to taste delicious. She even knows that you prefer not to use your oven during the summer! This cookbook contains no dessert menus, but with all the tasty foods to start with and the spices for added flavor, you won't miss dessert. You may wish to follow the menu plans closely, or you may just enjoy browsing through this book, picking up some good ideas to bring the family back to the table. Leanne Ely's website is www.savingdinner.com.

The Schwarzbein Principle II, by Diana Schwarzbein, M.D., with Marilyn Brown (Deerfield Beach, FL: Health Communications, Inc., 2002). The unwieldy name makes it difficult to recommend this book friend to friend, especially when you go to write down the title, but it is a very good book! Dr. Schwarzbein is a nutritionally-aware endocrinologist. Her book covers adrenal burnout, thyroid problems, and elevated insulin levels, always with a nutritional approach. Unlike so many health books written for women by medical doctors, she does not ignore "the elephant in the living room"—birth control pills. She is firmly against these artificial steroid hormones. In Chapter 13, "Step Three: Tapering Off or Avoiding Toxic Chemicals," she includes birth control pills, stating that "....you can never achieve complete hormonal balance while taking BCPs because they disrupt the sex hormone system, and, because all hormones are connected, the body's entire hormone system is disrupted, too." My favorite chapter in the book, however, is Chapter 12: "Step 2: Managing Stress and Getting Enough Sleep." She is right as rain about the need for sleep.

The Supplement Pyramid: How to Build Your Personalized Nutrition Regimen, by Michael A. Smith, M.D. with Sara Lovelady and a foreword by Suzanne Somers (Basic Health Publications, 2014). Comprehensive information on why supplementation is important, which supplements to take for your personalized needs, how to take them, and where to find quality products.

The Thyroid Hormone Breakthrough: Overcoming Sexual and Hormonal Problems at Every Age, by Mary J. Shomon (New York: Collins, 2006). Mary Shomon is herself a woman who has low thyroid function. Spurred on originally by her own search for effective treatment, she has become a patient advocate and tireless writer on the topic of thyroid dysfunction. In this book, she looks particularly at the effects that both hypothyroidism and hyperthyroidism have on all aspects of female reproduction: menstrual pain, heavy menses, PMS, postpartum thyroiditis, infertility, and perimenopausal symptoms. The book is very comprehensive, covering medications for hypothyroidism, treatment for hyperthyroidism, and the link between other hormone dysfunctions and thyroid disorders. If you are troubled by symptoms that may fit thyroid disease, you will get far better medical care if you are informed by this book. While it covers technical topics, it is divided into easy-to-find subtopics, and is written for an intelligent layperson. It recommends charting your cycle to better understand it.

What Every Pregnant Woman Should Know: The Truth About Diet and Drugs in Pregnancy, by Gail Sforza Brewer and Tom Brewer, M.D. (New York: Penguin Books, 1985). Extensively researched but built on Dr. Tom Brewer's experience with several thousand pregnant women, this is the classic book that describes the details of pregnancy nutrition, especially the role of diet in preventing metabolic toxemia of late pregnancy. Though it explains the consequences of poor diet to mother and baby, it is a very reassuring book that shows how a good diet dramatically reduces the incidence of a number of pregnancy-related problems, not just toxemia of pregnancy. There are more than enough books that have been written on pregnancy, but this is the one I place at the top of the list.

What Your Doctor May Not Tell You about Menopause: The Breakthrough Book on Natural Hormone Balance, by John R. Lee, M.D., and Virginia Hopkins (New York: Warner Wellness, 2004). This is the update of the book that made the phrase "estrogen dominance" a household term, and through it Dr. Lee popularized the use of over-the-counter natural progesterone cream. The book is thick and covers many other hormonal problems and hormone interactions that affect women's health. It is not a page-by-page read, but is a reference that takes some time to absorb. In addition to his advocacy for natural hormones, Dr. Lee was a firm advocate of holistic nutrition and comprehensive supplements.

What Your Doctor May Not Tell You About Premenopause: Balance Your Hormones and Your Life from Thirty to Fifty, by John R. Lee, M.D., Jesse Hanley, M.D., and Virginia Hopkins (New York: Warner Books, 1999). There is considerable overlap between Dr. Lee's premenopause book and the other one on menopause. I personally prefer the *Menopause* book, but this one covers infertility and contains sobering information about the health risks associated with oral contraceptives.

Whole Foods for the Whole Family, by Roberta Bishop Johnson, ed. (Franklin Park, IL: La Leche League International, 1993). A user-friendly cookbook for those attempting to improve their home cooking using all natural ingredients. This book contains detailed sections on sprouting and bread baking, and even has a children's section. Many recipes offer options to improve nutrition, accommodate food allergies, add variety, or make meals "quick-n-easy!" I consider this an ideal cookbook, at least for those who are trying to improve their diet while still "cooking American." Out of print, but currently available on Amazon from third-party sellers.

The Yeast Connection and Women's Health, by William G. Crook, M.D., with Carolyn Dean, M.D., N.D.; and Elizabeth B. Crook (Square One, 2007). This book is the latest edition of the original, The Yeast Connection. Part 2, "Yeast Related Problems That Affect Women," includes chapters entitled "PMS," "Vaginitis," "Endometriosis," and "Vulvodynia." Other chapters for both men and women include "Interstitial Cystitis," "Infertility," and "Sexual Dysfunction." Even if you do not have yeast overgrowth, the whole foods, low sugar diet that Dr. Crook advocates will certainly improve your health.

RESOURCES

AMERICAN PRO-LIFE ENTERPRISE

P.O. Box 1281
Powell, OH 43065
1-800-227-8359
www.kuhar.com
order@kuhar.com
Bogomir M. Kuhar, Pharm.D.

The vitamin and mineral supplements recommended in this book are available from American Pro-Life Enterprise, which will send your order anywhere in the continental U.S. for a nominal shipping charge. Besides stocking Optivite, Androvite, ProCycle PMS, Professional Pre-Natal Formula, and other food supplements, American Pro-Life Enterprise stocks a complete line of prescription drugs, health and beauty aids. For an extra "Group Discount" identify yourself as a reader of this book. American Pro-Life Enterprise does not sell any contraceptives or abortifacient drugs or devices. It also donates a portion of the proceeds of pro-life generated sales back to the movement. For information or to place your order for any item mentioned above, call the above toll-free number.

APEX MEDICAL TECHNOLOGIES, INC.

10064 Mesa Ridge Court, Suite 202
San Diego, CA 92121
1-800-345-3208
apexfertility.com

This company sells special kits to ethically obtain a semen sample for analysis.

BLUE RIBBON BABY

www.blueribbonbaby.org

This is the website for those hoping to become pregnant soon, or those already expecting. It is dedicated to continuing the work of obstetrician Tom Brewer, M.D., whose long career centered on promoting healthy, adequate nutrition as the means of preventing pre-eclampsia, or metabolic toxemia of late pregnancy, as it is also called. The website contains detailed charts on what foods and how much of them to eat, and also contains alternatives for expectant mothers who are vegetarians, are intolerant of milk, or need other alternative recommendations. If you have had pre-eclampsia or a premature baby, please get acquainted with this website — especially if you have been told that your situation is not explainable. This is the best on the web for how to eat during pregnancy.

THE BRODA O. BARNES, M.D., RESEARCH FOUNDATION, INC.

P.O Box 110098
Trumbull, CT 06611
1-203-261-2101
www.brodabarnes.org

The Broda O. Barnes, M.D., Research Foundation, Inc., is a not-for-profit organization dedicated to education, research and training in the field of thyroid and metabolic balance. They have been longtime advocates for better testing for thyroid function, including the use of the basal temperature chart, and they also advocate for natural thyroid replacement rather than synthetic thyroid hormone. They carry the late Dr. Barnes' original book, Hypothyroidism: The Unsuspected Illness, and also recommend books on other hormonal dysfunctions, including one on replacement of testosterone in men.

CELIAC DISEASE FOUNDATION

13251 Ventura Blvd. #1
Studio City, CA 91604
1-818-990-2354
www.celiac.org

The Celiac Disease Foundation (CDF) is an organization recognized throughout the world. CDF strives to promote awareness and build a supportive community for patients, families and health care professionals. CDF is actively involved in advocating for patient concerns and networking with other national and international organizations.

The Celiac Disease Foundation's website is a good way to get better acquainted with this disease of gluten intolerance, but it is not a substitute for the care of a doctor and dietitian.

COUPLE TO COUPLE LEAGUE INTERNATIONAL

5440 Moeller Ave, Suite 149
Norwood, OH 45212
513-471-2000, 800-745-8252
www.ccli.org
info@ccli.org

As a volunteer instructor for this organization, along with my husband, I am very partial to it. But I think that I am being completely objective to call it the world's best organization for learning the world's best method of birth control. CCL currently has over 400 teaching couples in the United States and in several foreign countries; find the ones nearest you by checking their website or calling the office.

The professionally trained teaching couples hold classes at local hospitals or churches, or live online. Video classes are also available self-paced online. They cover all aspects of modern "sympto-thermal" natural family planning (NFP):

- Health benefits of NFP
- Effectiveness of NFP in preventing pregnancy, NFP during breastfeeding, and cycle irregularity
- Achieving pregnancy through fertility awareness and other natural fertility aids
- NFP as a way of love and life.

Supplemental classes on how to use NFP during the transition times of postpartum and premenopause are also available.

Teaching couples also provide telephone counseling if cycle irregularities occur, or for any additional questions or consultation needed by new users. Whether you are having difficulty achieving pregnancy or are attempting to act in harmony with your body as you avoid a pregnancy, you will gain much from these professionally prepared, practical classes.

THE ENDOMETRIOSIS ASSOCIATION

8585 N. 76th Place
Milwaukee, Wisconsin 53223
1-414-355-2200
www.endometriosisassn.org

Founded in 1980 by Mary Lou Ballweg, who herself has endometriosis, and Carolyn Keith, the purpose of The Endometriosis Association is to assist women with endometriosis to find the best and most current answers to their particular situation. They cover all aspects of this disease, and are not particularly focused on nutritional approaches.

FERTILITY BLEND FOR WOMEN/FERTILITY BLEND FOR MEN

The Daily Wellness Company
1946 Young Street Suite 360
Honolulu, HI 96826
1-866-222-9862
www.fertilityblend.com

Learn more about Fertility Blend, the supplement which has been tested under double-blind conditions for its effect in increasing the pregnancy rate for women, especially those with low progesterone levels. This supplement has also significantly increased the number of days of elevated temperatures in women who have charted their basal temperatures. It contains chasteberry extract, green tea extract, and a number of vitamins and minerals. This is the wave of the future — compounding several nutrients, not just one, and testing them in a scientifically acceptable way.

FERTILITYCARE CENTERS OF AMERICA

6901 Mercy Road
Omaha, NE 68106-2621
Telephone: 402-505-8917
Website: www.fertilitycare.org

NaProTechnology (Natural Procreative Technology) is a women's health science which has, as its main principle, the ability to work cooperatively with the woman's menstrual and fertility cycle. NaProTechnology relies on the Creighton Model FertilityCare System (CrMS) biomarkers to monitor easily and objectively the occurrence of various hormonal events during the menstrual cycle. CrMS provides valid information that can be interpreted by a woman and by physicians who are specifically trained in this system. You can search for NaproTechnology medical consultants at www.fertilitycare.org/find-a-mc.

GENETICS & DISABILITIES DIAGNOSTIC CARE CENTER

P.O Box 4548
Virginia Beach, VA 23454
Telephone: 1-757-425-1969
Website: www.lleichtman.org

To gain a fuller understanding of the metabolic challenges that people with Down syndrome face, as well as the promising possibility for improving their health through nutrition, see the website of pediatrician and geneticist Lawrence Leichtman, M.D., of Virginia Beach, Virginia. He treats children with Down syndrome using targeted nutritional therapy as well as other approaches. The article titled "Targeted Nutritional Intervention (TNI) in the Treatment of Children and Adults with Down Syndrome" is of particular interest (www.lleichtman.org/tni).

HEALTH AND HEALING

Julian Whitaker, M.D.
1-800-539-8219
www.drwhitaker.com

This newsletter is excellent for keeping up on new research related to general nutrition and health. It is not written specifically for men, but nevertheless, Dr. Whitaker has a great interest in the problems of men as they age. Heart disease, hypertension, cancer, diabetes, arthritis, depression, prostate problems, vision problems and many other common health concerns are topics that he addresses regularly. Dr. Whitaker also comments on the political aspects of nutrition and nutritional supplementation, a particularly enlightening topic.

The website provides much information, links to research publications, and provides access to his multivitamin/multimineral, named Forward, which is an excellent supplement that covers all the bases quite well. Other supplements which he has formulated for particular problems, such as prostate health, joint health, or vision health, are also available by phone or via the website.

LA LECHE LEAGUE INTERNATIONAL

P.O. Box 4079
Schaumburg, IL 60168-4079
1-800-525-3243
www.lalecheleague.org

Breastfeeding involves your baby's nutrition as well as your own. This wonderful organization is dedicated to helping mothers breastfeed successfully, no matter what adverse circumstances may be present. A series of four meetings is held at a leader's home to instruct and encourage you, and your leader provides non-medical telephone counseling also. By all means take the class before your baby is born if possible. You will also meet other like-minded mothers through "The League." If you cannot locate a League leader through your food co-op or white pages of the telephone directory, check their website or contact the central office above.

LIFETIME / NUTRITIONAL SPECIALTIES, INC.

1967 N. Glassell St.
Orange, CA 92865
1-800-333-6168
www.lifetimevitamins.com

LifeTime produces Professional Pre-Natal Formula, an excellent nonprescription supplement which contains vitamins and minerals in amounts very similar to Table 7 (Chapter 3). It is ideal for pregnant and breastfeeding women and for women preparing to conceive. Professional Pre-Natal Formula is far better balanced and far more potent than prescription prenatal vitamins — I suggest you compare labels. Women (or men) who are attempting to overcome anemia or fatigue will also find it an excellent supplement. If your local health food shop does not stock these vitamins, you can order them through American Pro-Life Enterprise, listed above. See www.iHerb.com for listed ingredients.

LOCAL HARVEST

www.localharvest.org

Another browser's delight, localharvest.org puts you in touch with your local organic farms and farmers. More than that, it shows you how to get started eating local. For example, their February 2009 newsletter makes the point that many families are convinced of the why, but are uncertain as to the how when it comes to improved nutrition. Here's the summary of that article, just to give you the flavor of this top-notch website:

> Start with whole foods. Don't make it too hard. Study your region's agricultural strengths and play up to them. Look for ways to be creative with your budget. Be gentle with yourself and your family as you try out new habits. Do these things, and you will set yourself up for a highly satisfying adventure in local eating, and a deeper connection to your food.

THE NATIONAL CELIAC ASSOCIATION

20 Pickering St
Needham, MA 02492
1-888-4-CELIAC
www.nationalceliac.org

The National Celiac Association represents and serves individuals with celiac disease and gluten sensitivities.

OPTIMOX CORPORATION

P.O. Box 3378
Torrance, CA 90510
1-800-223-1601
www.optimox.com

Optimox Corporation developed Optivite PMT, the multivitamin/multimineral supplement which has been shown to alleviate PMS symptoms even under double-blind conditions. Some physicians also support the use of Optivite for pregnant women (six tablets/day plus 500 mg magnesium/day plus folic acid) and for breastfeeding women (four tablets/day plus 500 mg magnesium).

Optimox Corporation also makes a complete vitamin/mineral supplement, Androvite for Men. I consider Androvite an excellent supplement for men who are trying to overcome infertility or other reproductive health problems.

You can phone or visit the website for more information on these supplements or PMS. These supplements may also be ordered from your local pharmacy or from American Pro Life Enterprise, listed above.

SAVING DINNER

Website: www.savingdinner.com

Practical, warm-hearted, and health-oriented, this is a delightful website if you are trying to improve your home cooking. It covers topics such as snack foods, freezer foods, preparing meals with a tight budget, and packing your kids' school lunches. It provides lists to help you to shop and cook for your family. You can select from the low carbohydrate diet, the gluten-free diet, the vegetarian diet, or just the family-friendly healthy diet. It is a browser's delight, but you need to subscribe to get the weekly Menu-Mailer, with its detailed shopping list, menus, and recipes for the week.

TRISOMY 21 RESEARCH FOUNDATION

1-800-899-3413
www.nutrivene.com

Pediatrician and geneticist Dr. Lawrence Leichtman, is the founder of Trisomy 21 Research Foundation. This website provides information about Nutrivene-D, the targeted supplement for children and adults with Down syndrome. If you learn that you are going to have a child with Down syndrome, or if you already have a child with DS, you will find this website full of encouragement and practical suggestions.

APPENDIX A:
LABELED CONTENTS OF RECOMMENDED SUPPLEMENTS

ANDROVITE FOR MEN (OPTIVITE)

INGREDIENT	AMOUNT PER 6 TABLETS	%DV
Vitamin A (as retinyl palmitate and 80% as beta-carotene)	25,000 IU	500%
Vitamin C (as ascorbic acid)	1000 mg	1667%
Vitamin D (as cholecalciferol)	400 IU	100%
Vitamin E (as d-alpha tocopheryl succinate)	400 IU	1333%
Vitamin B1 (thiamine mononitrate)	50 mg	3333%
Vitamin B2 (riboflavin)	50 mg	2941%
Niacin (as niacinamide)	50 mg	250%
Vitamin B6 (as pyridoxine HCl)	100 mg	5000%
Folic Acid	400 mcg	100%
Vitamin B12 (as hydroxocobalamin)	125 mcg	2084%
Biotin	125 mcg	42%
Pantothenic Acid (as calcium pantothenate)	100 mg	1000%
Iron (as amino acid chelate)	18 mg	100%
Iodine (as hydrolyzed protein complex)	150 mcg	100%
Magnesium (as magnesium oxide)	500 mg	125%
Zinc (as amino acid chelate)	50 mg	333%
Selenium (as hydrolyzed protein complex)	200 mcg	286%
Copper (as amino acid chelate)	2 mg	100%
Manganese (as amino acid chelate)	10 mg	500%
Chromium (as hydrolyzed protein complex)	200 mcg	167%
p-Aminobenzioc Acid (PABA)	25 mg	*
Betaine HCl	100 mg	*
Pancreatin 4X	75 mg	*
Inositol	36 mg	*
Hesperidin	35 mg	*
Rutin	25 mg	*
Boron (hydrolzed protein complex)	3 mg	*

* Daily Value (DV) not established.
Other ingredients: Micosolle®, a silica-based excipient containing a non-ionic surfactant, cellulose and modified cellulose, silica, stearic acid, pharmaceutical glaze, magnesium stearate, natural flavor and annatto as natural source of color.

OPTIVITE PMT (OPTIMOX)

INGREDIENT	AMOUNT PER 6 TABLETS	%DV
Vitamin A (as retinyl palmitate and 60% as beta-carotene)	12500 IU	250%
Vitamin C	1500 mg	2500%
Vitamin D (as cholecalciferol)	100 IU	25%
Vitamin E (as d-alpha tocopheryl succinate)	100 IU	333%
Thiamin (as thiamine mononitrate)	25 mg	1666%
Riboflavin	25 mg	1471%
Niacin (as niacinamide)	50 mg	250%
Vitamin B6 (as pyridoxine HCl)	300 mg	15000%
Folic Acid	200 mcg	50%
Vitamin B12 (as hydroxocobalamin)	60 mcg	1000%
Biotin	60 mcg	20%
Pantothenic Acid (as calcium pantothenate)	25 mg	250%
Iron (as amino acid chelate)	15 mg	83%
Iodine (as hydrolyzed protein complex)	75 mcg	50%
Magnesium (as magnesium oxide)	250 mg	63%
Zinc (as amino acid chelate)	25 mg	167%
Selenium (as hydrolyzed protein complex)	100 mcg	143%
Manganese (as amino acid chelate)	10 mg	500%
Chromium (as hydrolyzed protein complex)	100 mcg	83%
Potassium (as hydrolyzed protein complex)	48 mg	1%
Choline (from choline bitartrate)	313 mg	*
Citrus Bioflavonoids	250 mg	*
Betaine HCl	100 mg	*
Pancreatin 4X	75 mg	*
Inositol	36 mg	*
p-Aminobenzioc Acid (PABA)	25 mg	*
Rutin	25 mg	*

* Daily Value (DV) not established.
Other ingredients: Stearic acid, carnauba wax, hydroxypropyl methlcellulose, silica, magnesium stearate, pharmaceutical glaze, titanium dioxide, and natural flavors.

PROCYCLE PMS PROPRIETARY FORMULA BY AMERICAN PRO-LIFE ENTERPRISE

INGREDIENT	AMOUNT PER 4 TABLETS	%DV
Vitamin A (40% Palmitate and 60% beta-carotene)	12500 IU	250%
Vitamin C (ascorbic acid)	1500 mg	2500%
Vitamin D3 (cholecalciferol)	200 IU	100%
Vitamin E (natural d-alpha tocopherol succinate)	200 IU	666%
Vitamin B1 (thiamin HCl)	25 mg	1666%
Vitamin B2 (riboflavin)	25 mg	1470%
Niacinamide	25 mg	125%
Vitamin B6 (as pyridoxine HCl)	300 mg	15000%
Folic Acid	800 mcg	200%
Vitamin B12 (as hydroxocobalamin)	62.5 mcg	1041%
Biotin	62.5 mcg	20%
Pantothenic Acid (as calcium pantothenate)	25 mg	250%
Iodine (as hydrolyzed protein complex)	75 mcg	50%
Magnesium (as magnesium oxide)	300 mg	75%
Zinc (as amino acid chelate)	25 mg	167%
Selenium (as hydrolyzed protein complex)	200 mcg	285%
Manganese (as amino acid chelate)	10 mg	500%
Chromium (as hydrolyzed protein complex)	200 mcg	166%
Potassium (as hydrolyzed protein complex)	48 mg	1%
Propietary Blend Choline (bitartrate), Citrus Bioflavonoids, Betaine HCl, Pancreatin 4X (provides protease, amylase and lipase), PABA (Para-Aminobenzoic Acid), Rutin and Inositol	830.8 mg	*

* Daily Value (DV) not established.
Other ingredients: Special Plant Cellulose, Vegetable Stearates, Natural Silica, Natural Color Coat, and Magnesium Stearate.

FERTILITY BLEND FOR WOMEN (DAILY WELLNESS)

INGREDIENT	AMOUNT PER 3 CAPSULES	%DV
Vitamin E (as d-alpha tocopheryl succinate)	150 IU	500%
Vitamin B6 (as pyridoxine hydrochloride)	6 mg	300%
Vitamin B12 (as cyanocobalamin)	400 mcg	100%
Folate (as folic acid)	400 mcg	100%
Iron (as gluconate)	9 mg	50%
Magnesium (as oxide)	400 mg	100%
Zinc (as gluconate)	15 mg	100%
Selenium (as soduim selenate)	70 mcg	100%
Proprietary Blend	1080 mg	*
L-arginine, Green Tea (Camelia sinensis)-standardized leaf extract, Chasteberry (Vitex agnus-castus)-standardized berry extract		

* Percent Daily Values (%DV) are based on a 2000-calorie diet.
** Daily Value (DV) not established.
Other ingredients: Hypromellose, rice flour, magnesium stearate, silicon dioxide

PROFESSIONAL PRE-NATAL FORMULA (LIFETIME)

INGREDIENT	AMOUNT PER 6 TABLETS	%DV
Vitamin A (as Beta-Carotene)	5000 IU	100%
Vitamin A (as Palmitate)	5000 IU	100%
Vitamin C (as Ascorbic Acid)	1000 mg	1667%
Vitamin D-3	400 IU	100%
Vitamin E (as D-Alpha Tocopherol)	400 IU	1333%
Vitamin B1 (as Thiamin Mononitrate)	75 mg	5000%
Vitamin B2 (as Riboflavin)	75 mg	4412%
Niacinamide	100 mg	500%
Vitamin B6 (as Pyridoxine HCl)	300 mg	15000%
Folic Acid	800 mcg	200%
Vitamin B12 (as Cyanocobalamin)	75 mcg	1250%
Biotin (as D-Biotin)	300 mcg	100%
Pantothenic Acid (D-Calcium Pantothenate)	27 mg	750%
Calcium (as Amino Acid Chelate), Citrate & Carbonate	800 mg	80%
Iodine (kelp)	150 mcg	100%
Magnesium (as Amino Acid Chelate, oxide)	500 mg	125%
Zinc (as Amino Acid Chelate)	25 mg	167%
Selenium (as Amino Acid Chelate)	100 mcg	143%
Copper (as Amino Acid Chelate)	2 mg	100%
Manganese (as Amino Acid Chelate)	10 mg	500%
Chromium (as Amino Acid Chelate)	100 mcg	83%
Molybdenum (as Amino Acid Chelate)	75 mg	100%
Choline Bitartrate	75 mg	*
Inositol	75 mg	*
Lemon Bioflavinoids	300 mg	*

APPENDIX B:
FOCUS ON INFERTILITY

I will say to the north: Give them up! and to the south: Hold not back! Bring back my sons from afar, and my daughters from the ends of the earth. — Isaiah 43:6

The Couple to Couple League offers a systematic self-help approach to infertility that may help you to achieve pregnancy. Even if it does not help you directly, it will c ertainly tip the balance in favor of pregnancy as you seek medical care.

For six to nine months, implement all of the self care options outlined below as a couple: charting and timing of intercourse, improved diet and nutritional supplementation for both spouses, and self help targeted to the particular situation that seems to fit — weight gain if you are underweight, weight loss if you are overweight, and so forth. If in those six to nine months you do not become pregnant, continue the self-help strategies, but seek ethical medical intervention from a physician who is supportive of your moral values and is knowledgeable about or at least open to nutrition and nutritional supplements.

A. FOR 6–9 MONTHS, BOTH SPOUSES SHOULD IMPLEMENT ALL OF THE SELF-HELP OPTIONS THAT SEEM TO APPLY.

1. Take the CCL course, learn Natural Family Planning, and chart your cycles.
2. Time marital relations to the most fertile days of the cycle.

   a. Abstain for a few days before ovulation is expected.

   b. Have relations in an every-other-day pattern during the fertile time.

   c. Remain lying down for a short time after relations.

   d. If the mucus pattern is poor, the wife can use an over-the-counter product called Robitussin to improve her mucus secretion.

3. Make positive lifestyle changes.

   a. The husband should switch to wearing boxer shorts if his fertility status is unknown, or if he lives or works in a hot environment.

   b. Both spouses should quit smoking and avoid second-hand smoke.

   c. Alcoholic beverages should be used only in moderation.

   d. At least the wife should limit caffeine to the equivalent of two cups of coffee daily.

   e. The wife should try to lose or gain weight as needed.

   f. For men, weight is not so critical, unless significant overweight or obesity is involved.

   g. Get enough sleep, which along with better nutrition is a key to good health.

A dark bedroom improves sleep and may improve the woman's reproductive hormones.

4. Both spouses should improve their diet as explained in Chapter 1.

5. Both spouses should take basic supplements as explained in Chapter 3.

   a. For men: The vitamin Androvite for Men and flax oil and/or fish oil "covers all the bases."

   b. For women, use a good multivitamin/multimineral, flax oil and/or fish oil, and other supplements as indicated by your chart and symptoms.

6. Use the NFP chart and other symptoms as detailed in Part 2 to make an educated guess as to what might be contributing to your infertility. Your CCL instructor may be able to help you.

7. Men, consider Chapter 15 to improve your fertility if there is any doubt.

If you get pregnant within those six to nine months of self help — wonderful! You won't be able to say exactly what might have helped, but you won't care! Your self care will have been the best preparation for a healthy pregnancy, so continue the good nutrition and vitamins, minerals, and flax oil or fish oil, with the approval of your health care professional.

B. IF YOU ARE UNSUCCESSFUL IN THOSE SIX TO NINE MONTHS, CONTINUE YOUR SELF-HELP STRATEGIES, BUT ALSO LOOK FOR ETHICAL, PRUDENT MEDICAL INTERVENTION.

1. Do not wait longer than twelve months to do so.

2. Consult a fertility specialist rather than a family doctor or an obstetrician/gynecologist. A specialist who works with infertile couples on a daily basis is better able to offer you specific options based on your particular situation.

   a. Choose a specialist who respects your moral beliefs.

   b. Get a complete physical and hormonal evaluation.

   c. Make sure the doctor can understand chart problems.

   d. If at all possible, employ a doctor who uses a holistic approach that includes attention to nutrition, body weight, and lifestyle factors.

3. Proceed in a conservative, stair-step fashion.

   a. Many doctors will start with a trial of Clomid or metformin before extensive testing. This can be a prudent starting point.

   b. If you have had children or have miscarried previously, make sure there is a good reason if the doctor suggests semen evaluation or a test to see if your tubes are open. Request ethical semen collection, if necessary.

c. Be sure that ultrasounds and hormone tests are done at times consistent with what your NFP chart shows rather than with arbitrary cycle days.

If you get pregnant with such care, wonderful! Who knows how much of a difference all your self help contributed!

C. IF YOU ARE STILL UNSUCCESSFUL, MAKE A DECISION AS TO HOW LONG YOU WILL CONTINUE, HOW MUCH MONEY YOU WILL SPEND ON INFERTILITY CARE, AND HOW MUCH ETHICAL INTERVENTION YOU WILL UNDERTAKE.

1. Consider your age, your finances, your own feelings about having another child, and whether or not it would still be possible or likely for you to conceive without medical care.

2. If you are Catholic, recognize that not all expensive and high-tech fertility care is immoral or forbidden by the Church. Make sure you know what is and what is not approved.

D. IF YOUR INFERTILITY PERSISTS AND YOU CONTINUE TO LONG FOR A CHILD, FOLLOW YOUR HEART AND CONSIDER ADOPTING A CHILD OR CHILDREN.

1. Infertility with longing for a child may be a call from God to place a child needing a home into your family.

2. Adopting a child is not identical to giving birth, but it has a wonder and charm all its own that many people do not appreciate until they do adopt a child.

3. If it is a baby that is your heart's desire, you are most likely not too old to adopt a child from a country where adoptive parents are in short supply.

E. IN ANY CASE, PRAY ALWAYS FOR YOUR FAMILY AND FOR THE GRACE OF GOD TO MAKE PRUDENT DECISIONS AND TO LIVE WITH THOSE DECISIONS.

QUESTIONS AND ANSWERS

Q: What is Robitussin? How do I use it?

Robitussin is actually a cough medicine that makes nasal mucus more fluid. It also makes cervical mucus more fluid. Use the plain kind which contains the ingredient "guaifenesin" only. Any other variations of Robitussin, which contain other ingredients, may dry up mucus. Use plain Robitussin according to labeled directions on days of marital relations. While this recommendation may seem odd, it has helped many couples to conceive.

Q: My husband needs a semen analysis and we are trying to do this ethically. Where can we obtain a perforated condom?

A special type of condom is available from Apex Medical Technologies, Inc. The condom is thin, non-spermicidal and non-latex, and is only handled by the couple at home, who perforate it before having normal relations. Instructions are included for collecting the sample. (See "Resources.")

Q: When should couples who have already had children seek fertility care?

Answering the question of when to seek fertility care is not so hard for a couple in their fertile years who have never had children. Once twelve months of regular intercourse have passed without conceiving, most couples strongly suspect that something is wrong. Their friends, family, and doctor will assure them that that is not the ordinary way things happen. (If you are over 35, consider seeking fertility care after six months of infertility.)

It is for couples who have already had children that the question is harder to answer. The birth of a previous child or children reassures both of them that they are fertile, that having had a baby before is evidence that they can do it again. Yet all too often I meet couples in their fertile years who truly desire more children, but have not sought out fertility help after three, four, or five or more years of infertility. Do not wait more than twelve months.

Q: I already have [three, four, five, six] children; how can I call this infertility?

Are you in your fertile years? The limit of human female fertility is about age 48; on average fertility declines sharply after ages 42-45. Have you tried without success to conceive for at least six months to a year? Have you been able to rule out reversible causes such as underweight? If you answer yes to the above three questions, your situation is called secondary infertility, which means difficulty in conceiving after having had children. The number of children you have already had is not part of the definition.

Q: I already have [three, four, five, six] children; will the doctor laugh me out of the office if I go there for infertility?

An NFP user with six children went through menopause at age 41. She was given the diagnosis in the office of a fertility specialist. She phoned me to ask about nutritional approaches. True menopause, with no periods and constant high levels of FSH and LH, is irreversible, both nutritionally and medically. But I asked her a question: What did the doctor think of you, with six children, including preschoolers, seeking infertility treatment? Her answer was striking: The doctor had lived in Salt Lake City, Utah, where there is a high proportion of residents who are practicing Mormons, a faith which highly respects large families. He said that it was not uncommon for a Mormon woman to come to him in her early forties for fertility treatment, even though she might already have seven or eight children! So he was quite compassionate. By the way, this family dealt with this diagnosis in a wonderful way — they adopted a baby with special needs.

Q: Should I think that maybe God does not want us to have another child?

May I share my Catholic beliefs with you? God is the Lord of LIFE, and a soul for him in eternity procreated by a husband and wife is in keeping with His will! "Be fruitful and multiply" is a quote from Him.

All too often it seems to me that couples experiencing secondary infertility wonder if God is withholding children from them. I think the explanation is this: In most cases secondary infertility is hormonal in nature; it cannot be visualized like, for example, a fibroid tumor which is blocking the tubes. I do not imagine a woman who finds that she has a fibroid tumor that is causing her infertility would say that the fibroid tumor is evidence that "God does not want us to have another child." No, she most likely will have the surgery to remove the tumor. Hormonal imbalances and other less obvious factors may be more difficult to diagnose, but just because they cannot be seen does not mean that it is God preventing conception.

Let me use an analogy. If a young woman changes physically so that she notices very low basal temperatures, hair loss, coldness, fatigue, weight gain, and sluggish reflexes, yet nothing hurts and she still can tend to her home duties, should she conclude that God desires her to be a tired, low energy person? Of course not. If she is prudent she will go to considerable trouble to find the source of her problem. If it turns out to be a thyroid dysfunction, should she not be encouraged to take the thyroid hormone that can correct her problems and restore her good health?

Q: What if my family doctor says just to wait?

Again, CCL advises six to nine months of charting, timing, weight gain or loss, and the vitamins and minerals which make the greatest difference to fertility. I am distressed to find that couples will wait longer than a year to seek help, having done all the self care without success. If the wife is in her prime fertile years—say, up to age 35—perhaps only time is lost. But if the wife is older than that, delay while waiting for another pregnancy could mean the difference between giving birth to more children or not.

Q: Is it necessary to treat a physical disorder that doesn't hurt?

No, it is not, as long as the disorder is not life-threatening. Infertility is not life-threatening, and one could argue that it does not hurt like arthritis or a bad back. But it hurts one's heart in a way that those who have not suffered from it can hardly appreciate.

I JUST WANT TO DO THINGS NATURALLY.

The Catholic Church admonishes that when it comes to having children, we must do things naturally. That is, we may only conceive children by intercourse between husband and wife. As is obvious from this book, I am a strong advocate of natural self-help ways of improving fertility. Better diet, weight gain or loss, vitamin and mineral supplements, and timing of intercourse are all ways of improving the chances. However, if these measures do not work in six to nine months, CCL is wise to suggest that you seek ethical medical assistance for diagnosis and treatment.

Let me repeat my previous analogy: If you have symptoms of low thyroid function, it is wise to look at your intake of iodine, essential fatty acids, and other vitamins and minerals. But, what if attention to good nutrition makes no difference? Wouldn't a prudent person seek medical help for proper diagnosis? Would he or she not take thyroid hormone as a medication in an attempt to correct overall health?

FERTILITY TREATMENT TAKES INJECTIONS, ULTRASOUNDS, AND CONSTANT DOCTOR VISITS. IT'S JUST TOO HIGH-TECH AND EXPENSIVE.

May I continue the analogy with thyroid function one more time? If a woman is diagnosed with low thyroid function, after a period of testing and adjustment, she can take a pill every day that can correct her hormonal problems. Why? Thyroid hormone is naturally secreted in a constant fashion, so one day's dose is the same as the next. Thyroid hormone, a small molecule derived from an amino acid, is not destroyed by the stomach or intestinal secretions, and it can be readily absorbed into the blood. Yes, it does take diagnosis and adjustment, but in theory and in practice, replacing thyroid hormone is relatively easy. Either synthetic thyroid hormone or hormones from slaughterhouse animals can be used, and the expense is modest.

In some cases, fertility treatment may just require oral supplements of thyroid medication, or the oral drugs Clomid or metformin. But there are reasons that some ethical fertility treatments involve injections and ultrasounds as well as significant expense. The fertility hormones FSH and LH are secreted in a manner that varies markedly throughout the cycle. Because they are protein hormones, they must be injected; otherwise the digestive system will destroy them. Progesterone may need to be injected in some cases, though other routes can also be used. In order to inject the right amount of hormone at the right time, ultrasounds of the developing follicles are essential.

Furthermore, if FSH and LH are required, they must come from human beings. It is very expensive to purify these hormones from huge quantities of urine from postmenopausal women. The changing pattern of hormone secretion and the nature of the hormones certainly makes hormone therapy for infertility more complicated than replacement of thyroid hormone, as in the example above.

Q: **So would you recommend some of those high-tech fertility procedures?**

Let me restate CCL's recommendation for infertility: For six to twelve months, try all of the self-help options in this book that are generally useful or are specific to your situation. If after that time you are still not pregnant, continue the self care, but seek ethical medical care from a physician who is respectful of your moral beliefs and at least open to the role of nutrition.

Yes, this is a book that emphasizes nutrition for fertility. But ethical medical treatments are not incompatible with nutritional self care, and the two together may make the difference.

I wish you all the children that your hearts desire.

APPENDIX C:
NATURALLY IMPROVING WOMANLY DESIRE

Note: This originally appeared as an article in Family Foundations *magazine, and is similar in content to the section on "Low Desire" in Chapter 14.*

Here's a situation that comes up fairly often. A wife, otherwise happily married, finds that her desire for marital intimacy occurs only during the fertile time, when she and her husband are abstaining in order to avoid a pregnancy. When she enters the infertile phase (Phase III), her desire seems to fade. It is a dismaying situation for both the husband and the wife. It provides all too much opportunity for misunderstanding, as the husband may feel that his physical attention is unwelcome, and the wife may conclude that he is insensitive to her moods. Is there a "quick fix" for such a problem? If not, is there a way to progressively improve it?

It is true that we humans we vary in our appetites, our preferences, and certainly in sexual desire. That said, though, women are normally sexually responsive during all phases of their cycles. Studies show that desire tends to peak around the time of ovulation and then again in the premenstrual time. Womanly desire occurring only during the preovulatory time is a mild form of low sexual desire. But husband and wife can work together to improve her **libido**, as it is called, for the overall satisfaction of their marriage.

To begin, let's look at some "quick fixes"—strategies that can help the couple right now, as they enter and continue in Phase III. These ideas are also be practical for couples in which the woman is not cycling and not abstaining. For example, a woman may be breastfeeding without abstinence, or in the permanent infertility of the postmenopausal years, or experiencing long term infertility with or without cycles. Once we tackle the short term, we'll look at underlying causes and self care for them.

QUICK FIXES

1) First and foremost, get enough sleep! A good night's sleep every night is the goal, but when small children or other situations make enough sleep difficult, look to that special day itself. Can you sleep in? Or fit in a nap in the morning, after lunch, or after dinner? Is "screen time" interfering with sleep time? Is excess exercise leaving you exhausted? Can time be made for relations in the morning, or at some other time when both of you are rested? Take one day at a time, planning for the expected time of infertility.

2) Reduce stress. Sleep itself is a terrific way to decrease your stress hormones. So is prayer, which can be done with or apart from your spouse. When we pray, we also give thanks to God, which helps dispel anger and frustration at the little things in life. And those little annoyances can seem big when womanly desire is low! An "attitude of gratitude" comes with praying. I love the prayer of St. Francis, which helps us to live in the moment: "Lord, give me the courage to change the things I can, the ability to accept the things I cannot change, and the wisdom to know the difference."

Related to stress, consider if you **have confidence in the effectiveness of NFP.** Fear of pregnancy can inhibit desire. If you would like to double check this month's chart, your Teaching Couple or CCL Central can verify you that yes, your signs show you to be in Phase III, a highly infertile time. Resolve to keep better charts or take a refresher course if needed for future confidence.

3) A sense of humor is a great ally for the ups and downs of marriage. C.S. Lewis wrote in his classic book, *The Fours Loves*, that "Venus," as he termed sexual desire, is nothing if not fickle. If you are dealing with low sexual desire, see if you identify with his spot-on perspective, published in 1971:

[Venus] herself is a mocking, mischievous spirit, far more elf than deity, and makes game of us. When all external circumstances are fittest for her service she will leave one or both the lovers totally indisposed for it. When every overt act is impossible and even glances cannot be exchanged–in trains, in shops, and at interminable parties–she will assail them with all her force. An hour later, when time and place agree, she will have mysteriously withdrawn, perhaps from only one of them. But sensible lovers laugh. It is all part of the game..."[1]

As you can see, it's not just NFP users who deal with disappearing and reappearing desire!

4) Employ "for the moment" strategies: All of five senses are involved with womanly (and male) desire. For example, dark chocolate has the reputation as the food of lovers. It pleases the taste buds, but it also contains caffeine-like compounds that help overcome the original enemy, fatigue. Likewise, the sense of smell is related to desire. Aromatherapy, or the use of essential oils such as cedarwood oil, sandalwood oil, jasmine oil, and many others, may be worth trying during those special times. If you are interested in more information on this topic, you can safely Google the word "aromatherapy" without accidentally accessing immoral websites.

Some women are tempted to view sexy movies in an attempt to increase their libido. Please, don't be seduced by such images of other people. Instead, a wonderful way of using the sense of vision for sexual desire is to spend a little time looking at photos of your wedding, of family outings, or of other fun and meaningful family events that rekindle the memories of why you are so much in love with your husband. Talking and cuddling outside the bedroom about your past and future together combines the senses of hearing and touch. Deep communication resolves petty annoyances and strengthens your bond. For most woman, the emotional simply cannot be separated from the physical.

UNDERLYING CAUSES OF LOW SEXUAL DESIRE

Perhaps you have tried all of the above, and you have concluded that there is a physical issue that has reduced your desire. You may be right, and your chart and your own self-awareness can help you get to the root of your loss of desire.

1. Low thyroid function is a common cause of low desire in women. Very low temperatures, with preovulatory temperatures in the range of 97.3 and below, are a good indicator of low thyroid function. Other signs are weak changes in mucus as the cycle proceeds, both before and after ovulation. Short luteal phase, discussed below, is very common when basal temperatures are low. Self-care in many cases can make a difference. Improve your diet generally. Watch out for sugary and starchy foods that may cause yeast overgrowth, as described in Chapter 10. Take a comprehensive multivitamin/multimineral. Add flax oil or fish oil to provide the fatty acids that nourish all glands.

If self care does not enable you to have better cycles, better charts, or better libido, it may be worth the time and expense to consult with a compassionate physician who is an expert in thyroid function.

2. Short luteal phase may be related to low desire. If your chart shows a poor temperature shift, and Phase III is considerably shorter than the charts shown in *The Art of Natural Family Planning*, it may be that your progesterone, which rises to its highest level after ovulation, is lower than ideal. Normal levels of progesterone contribute to better overall cycles as well as to improved desire, at least in some women. Chapter 8 has detailed, referenced information on raising progesterone. Optivite PMT and a similar supplement, ProCycle PMS, contain vitamin and mineral intended to raise progesterone. Vitamin B6 and vitamin C are particularly useful for this, and along with other nutrients, are found in appropriate amounts in both of these products.

3. Adrenal hormones can help or hinder sexual desire. The adrenal glands, which sit atop each kidney, produce steroid hormones that perform various functions in the body. The stress hormone cortisol is the "bad" hormone which rises in response to long term stress. In large amounts, it interferes with estrogen, progesterone, and testosterone, and can disrupt the cycle and decrease desire. Getting enough sleep and maintaining steady blood glucose levels are the two best ways to reduce cortisol. In both sexes, the adrenal glands also produce testosterone. Far more is produced by the testes in men, but in women, the adrenals are the usual source of testosterone, which boosts libido. Reducing stress is helpful to overall reproductive function, but even if stress is an unavoidable part of your life, vitamin and mineral supplements can normalize the adrenals' hormones. These active glands depend on vitamin C, several B vitamins, many minerals, and fatty acids for optimum function. My favorite supplement for adrenal health is Androvite for Men, which is made to support testicular health. The adrenal glands are much like the testes in their nutritional needs, though women who take Androvite do not need a full dose.

4. Overweight or obesity can affect hormones and desire. Body fat is a source of estrogen, which if excess competes with progesterone's functions. Body fat also turns testosterone from the adrenal glands into estrogen. Losing excess body fat can improve both progesterone and testosterone levels, which in turn improves desire. Weight loss of course is easier said than done, but you do not need to achieve your ideal weight to benefit. The right diet for you is any sensible, gradual one that you prefer. I do believe that a support group for weight loss is a great help, no matter if you choose low calories, low carbohydrates or low fat.

5. Depression decreases sexual desire. Good nutrition, enough sleep, the right amount of outdoor exercise, stress reduction, and an active prayer life all contribute to healthy moods. If you or your spouse feel that your moods are often dark and that normal activities seem too heavy to handle, look to good medical care. At the same time, begin or keep up good health habits. Do realize, though, that women can experience low libido without being depressed.

OTHER SITUATIONS THAT MAY AFFECT WOMANLY DESIRE

BREASTFEEDING. The most profound natural change in hormones in the human species occurs after birth, as the placenta, which had been producing large amounts of estrogen and progesterone, is passed after the baby is born. These hormones may remain low for many months as a woman breastfeeds. It is entirely normal that her desire may be lower than usual. Ideal nutrition, strategies to overcome lack of sleep, and the "quick fixes" listed above may be helpful. Low thyroid function is common after childbirth and while nursing, but it usually resolves on its own. Desire can return long before fertility returns, as the body adjusts to the change in hormonal status and adrenal hormones, including testosterone, are produced.

PRE- AND POST MENOPAUSAL YEARS. I have always been amazed that for years and years books and magazine articles assure women that "after menopause, desire may even increase as the fear of pregnancy disappears." This trite explanation of womanly desire flies in the face of modern practice, in which all too many women have undergone tubal ligations years earlier, and in which a growing number of women would actually like to have children as they enter their mid-forties. Yet there is a grain of truth: As the levels of the steroid hormones estrogen and progesterone drop, testosterone from the adrenal glands is "unmasked"; that is, its function is no longer overshadowed by estrogen and progesterone. Testosterone stimulates sexual desire in women as well as men, so that a rise in desire during the premenopausal time or after menopause is common. The best approach to maintaining desire during this time of life and afterward is good nutrition aimed at supporting the adrenal glands. Womanly desire continues long after menopause.

END NOTES

CHAPTER 1

1 Vanputte, C, Regan, J, and Russo, A. *Seeley's Anatomy and Physiology*, 11th ed. (New York: McGraw-Hill, 2017, p. 929). The essential amino acids are histidine, isoleucine, leucine, lysine, methionine, phenylalanine, threonine, tryptophan, and valine.

2 Chavarro, J., Willett, W., and Skerrett, P. *The Fertility Diet* (New York: McGraw-Hill, 2008, p. 81). If a "serving" of a food contains less than 0.5 grams of *trans* fat, it may be labeled "0 *trans* fats." Essentially no amount of *trans* fat is healthy, but 2.0 grams per day is considered acceptable by the U.S. Food and Drug Administration. This labeling policy makes it necessary to check for the presence of the terms "partially hydrogenated" or "fully hydrogenated" whether or not a product advertises "0 *trans* fat" per serving.

3 Missmer, S., Chavarro, J., Malspeis, S., et al. "A prospective study of dietary fat consumption and endometrioisis risk" (Reproductive Epidemiology 2010, 25: 1528-1535).

4 Chavarro, J., Rich-Edwards, J., Rosner, B., et al. "Dietary fatty acids and the risk of ovulatory infertility" (*Am. J. Clin. Nutr.* 2007, 85:231-237).

5 Chavarro, J., Rich-Edwards, J., Rosner, B., et al. "A prospective study of dairy foods intake and anovulatory infertility" (*Human Reprod.* 2007, 22:1340-1347).

6 Nettleton, J., et al "Diet soda intake and risk of incident metabolic syndrome and type 2 diabetes in the Multi-Ethnic Study of Atherosclerosis (MESA)" (*Diabetes Care* 2009, 32:688-694).

7 Suez, J., Korem, T., Zeezi, D., et al. "Artificial sweeteners induce glucose intolerance by altering the gut microbiota" (*Nature* 2014, 514:181-186).

8 Chavarro, J., Willett, W., and Skerrett, P. (2008, p.147).

9 Dhingra, R., Sullivan, L., Jacques, P., et al. "Soft drink consumption and the risk of developing cardiometabolic risk factors and the metabolic syndrome in middle-aged adults in the community" (*Circulation* 2007, 116:480-488).

10 Gold, E., Bair, Y., Block, G., et al. "Diet and lifestyle factors associated with pre-menstrual symptoms in a racially diverse community sample: Study of women's health across the nation (SWAN)" (*J. Women's Health* 2007,16:641-656); Rossignol, A., and Bonnlander, H. "Caffeine-containing beverages, total fluid consumption, and premenstrual syndrome" (*Am. J. Public Health* 1990, 80:1106-1109).

11 Derbyshire, E. "Dietary factors and fertility in women of childbearing age" (*Nutrition and Food Science* 2007, 37:100-104).

12 Weng, X., Odouli, R., and Li, D. "Maternal caffeine consumption during pregnancy and the risk of miscarriage: A prospective cohort study" (*J. Obst. Gynecol.*, January 2008, pp. 1e1-1e8).

CHAPTER 2

1 The dairy goat breed that we have been happiest with is the Saanan breed. Recognizable by their all-white color and upright ears, they are gentle, quiet, heavy-milking goats that have been bred commercially. We have also enjoyed the "earless" LaMancha goats, which are sturdy, quiet, and good milkers. We have kept the long-eared Nubian breed as well. Nubians are gentle, but, according to their detractors, a bit noisy. They produce milk with 6-8% butterfat, which is best for cheese-making. While many folks have started raising dwarf milk goats, please remember that if you are interested in milk and meat, you will do far better to choose the standard size. Standard breed adults weight about 120-160 pounds, which is very manageable, even in a family with small children.

CHAPTER 3

1 Ulven, S., Kirkhus, B., Lamglait, A., et al. "Metabolic effects of krill oil are essentially similar to those of fish oil but at lower dose of EPA and DHA, in healthy volunteers" (*Lipids* 2011, 46:37-46) The EPA and DHA of krill oil are complexed in a phospholipid form, so that two fatty acids are part of a molecule with a water-soluble end (the phospholipid head). In fish oil, three EPA and/or DHA molecules or other fatty acids are complexed to form triglycerides, making the entire molecule lipid soluble. It is easier for the body to assimilate the phospholipid form.

2 Saldeen, P., and Saldeen, T. "Women and omega-3 fatty acids" (*Obstet. Gynecol. Survey* 2004, 59:722-733).

3 Ibid.

4 Mora-Esteves, C., and Shin, D. "Nutrient supplementation: Improving male fertility fourfold" (*Seminars in Reproductive Medicine* 2013, 31:293-300); Agarwal, A.,

Aponte-Mellado, A., Premkumar, B., et al. "The effects of oxidative stress on female reproduction: a review" (*Reprod. Biol. Endocrinol.* 2012, 10:49)

5 Conhaire, F., El Garem, Y., Mahmoud, A., et al. "Combined conventional/antioxidant 'Astaxanthin' treatment for male infertility: a double-blind, randomized trial" (*Asian J. Andrology* 2005, 7:257-262)

6 Stine, M., Kirkhus, B., Lamglait, A., et al. "Metabolic effects of krill oil are essentially similar to those of fish oil but at lower dose of EPA and DHA, in healthy volunteers" (*Lipids* 2011, 46:36-46)

7 "Meet Dr. Chavarro" by Megan Miller. *Family Foundations*, March/April 2011, pp.22-23.

8 Henmi, H., Endo, T., Kitajima, Y., et al. "Effect of ascorbic acid supplementation on serum progesterone levels in patients with a luteal phase defect" (*Fertil. Steril.* 2003, 80: 459-461).

9 Minguez-Larcon, L., Mendiola, J., Lopez-Espin, J., et al. "Dietary intake of antioxidant nutrients is associated with semen quality in young university students" (*Human Reprod.* 2012, 37:2807-2814).

10 See Appendix A, "Labeled Contents of Recommended Supplements." Guy Abraham, M.D., formulated both Optivite PMT and Androvite for Men.

11 Crook, W., Dean, C., and Crook, E. *The Yeast Connection and Women's Health* (Jackson, TN: Professional Books, 2005, p. 240).

12 "Forward Plus Daily Regimen" www.drwhitaker.com/multivamins-2/forward-plus-daily-regimen/ (April,2015).

13 Murray, Michael T., N.D. *Stress, Anxiety, and Insomnia: What the Drug Companies Won't Tell You and Your Doctor Doesn't Know* (Mind Publishing 2012, pp. 55-56).

14 Lee, J., with Hopkins, V. *What Your Doctor May Not Tell You About Menopause* (New York: Warner Books, 2004, pp. 418-424).

15 Raffelock, D., Rountree, R., and Hopkins, V. *A Natural Guide to Pregnancy and Postpartum Health* (New York: Avery, 2002, pp. 129-149).

16 Teitelbaum, J. and Feidler, C. *Beat Sugar Addiction Now! The Cutting-Edge Program That Cures Your Type of Sugar Addiction and Puts You on the Road to Feeling Great—and Losing Weight!* (Fair Winds Press, 2010, pp.).

17 Smith, M., M.D., with Lovelady, S. *The Supplement Pyramid* (Basic Health Publications, 2014, pp. 53-54)

18 The gene involved codes for the enzyme methylenetetrahydrofolate reductase (abbreviated the MTHFR gene—think Monday-THursday-FRiday to remember it).

19 Seibel, M. "The role of nutrition and nutritional supplements in women's health" (*Fertil. Steril* 1999, 72:579-591).

CHAPTER 4

1 Soares, C. "Characteristics of sleep disorders in women" (*Psychiatric Times* 2013, 30:2).

2 Davis, A., *Let's Get Well* (New York: Harcourt Brace Jovanovich, Inc., 1972, pp. 22-31).

3 Abraham, G., personal communication to M. Shannon (April 10, 1991).

4 Glynn, L., Davis, E., and Sandman, C. "New insights into the role of perinatal HPA-axis dysregulation in postpartum depression" (*Neuropeptides* 2013, 47:363-370).

5 Ibid.

6 Levant, B. "N-3 (omega-3) fatty acids in postpartum depression: implications for prevention and treatment" (*Depression Research and Treatment* 2011, 2011:Art. ID 467349).

CHAPTER 5

1 Patel,. S., Malhotra, A., White, D., et al. "Association between reduced sleep and weight gain in women" (*Am. J. Epidemiology* 2007, 164: 947-954).

2 Roberts, H., *Aspartame (NutraSweet): Is It Safe?* (Philadelphia: The Charles Press, 1990, pp. 168-172).

3 Gittleman, A. *Get the Sugar Out!* 2nd ed. (New York: Three Rivers Press, 2008, p. 69).

4 Hibbeln, J., Davis, J., Steer, C., et al. "Maternal seafood consumption in pregnancy and neurodevelopment outcomes in childhood (ALSPAC study: an observational cohort study)" (*The Lancet* 2007, 369:578-585).

5 Davis, A. *Let's Cook It Right* (New York: Signet Books, 1970, p. 15).

6 Whitaker, Julian, M.D. "Why Children Should Take Supplements" (*Health and Healing* 2001 11(9), 1-3).

INTRO TO PART 2

1 Fuchs, N., Hakim, M., and Abraham, G. "The effect of a nutritional supplement, Optivite for Women, on premenstrual tension syndromes: I. Effect on blood chemistry and serum steroid levels during the midluteal phase" (*J. Appl. Nutr.* 1985, 37:1-11).

2 Henmi, H., Endo, T., Kitajima, Y., et al. "Effect of ascorbic acid supplementation on serum progesterone levels in patients with a luteal phase defect" (*Fertil. Steril.* 2003, 80: 459-461).

3 Gaskins, A., Mumford, S., Chavarro, J., et al. "The impact of dietary folate intake on reproductive function in premenopausal women: A prospective cohort study" (*PLoS ONE* 2012, 7:79: e46276).

4 Hassold T., and Hunt, P. "Maternal age and chromosomally abnormal pregnancies: What we know and what we wish we knew" (*Curr. Open. Pediatr.* 2009, 21:703-708).

5 Allen, G., Freeman, S., Druschel, C., et al. "Maternal age and risk for trisomy 21 assessed by the origin of chromosome nondisjunction: a report from the Atlanta and National Down Syndrome Projects" (*Human Genetics* 2009, 125:41-52). At least in trisomy 21, it has been shown that the genetic error may also occur during meiosis II. However, that error is thought to be a consequence of an error in meiosis I: "Thus, as is true for most other autosomal chromosomes....the majority of chromosome 21 maternal meiotic errors may begin during meiosis I" (p. 42).

6 Sugiura-Ogasawara, M., Ozaki, Y., Katano, K., et al. "Abnormal embryonic karyotype is the most frequent cause of recurrent miscarriage" (*Human Reprod.* 2012, 27:2297-2303).

7 Allen, Freeman, Druschel et al. (2009).

8 Bentov, Y., Esfandiari, N., Burstein, E., et al. "The use of mitochondrial nutrients to improve the outcome of infertility treatment in older patients" (*Fertil. Steril.* 2010, 93: 272-275); Bentov, Y., Casper, R. "The aging oocyte—can mitochondrial function be improved?" (*Fertil. Steril.* 2013, 99:18-22).

9 Agarwal, A., Aponte-Mellado, A., Premkumar, B., et al. "The effects of oxidative stress on female reproduction: a review" (*Reprod. Biol. Endocrinol.* 2012, 10:49).
10 Santangelo, C., Vari, R., Scazzocchio, B., et al." Review Article: Management of reproduction and pregnancy comlications in maternal obesity: Which role for dietary phenols?" (*International Union of Biochemistry and Molecular Biology*, 2014, 40:79-102).

11 Mora-Esteves, C., and Shin, D. "Nutrient supplementation: Improving male fertility four-fold" (*Semin. Reprod. Med.* 2013, 31:293-300).

CHAPTER 6

1 Beck, S., and Abraham, G. *Optivite PMT and Gynovite Plus Total Dietary Programs for Premenstrual Syndrome and Menopause with Answers to the Most Commonly Asked Questions* (Torrance, CA: Optimox Corp., 1992, p. 26).

2 If you are bothered by acne, see the question and answer that covers this topic in Chapter 16.

3 Abraham, G. "Nutritional factors in the etiology of the premenstrual tension syndromes" (*J. Reprod. Med.* 1983, 28:446-464).

4 Abraham, G., and Rumley, R. "Role of nutrition in managing the premenstrual tension syndromes" (*J. Reprod. Med.* 1987, 32:405-422).

5 Goei, G., Ralston, J., and Abraham, G. "Dietary patterns of patients with premenstrual tension" (*J. Appl. Nutr.* 1982, 34:9-17).

6 Abraham, G. (1983).

7 Goei, G., Ralston, J., and Abraham, G. (1982).

8 Abraham, G., and Rumley, R. (1987).

9 Delitala, G., Masala, A., Alagna, S., et al. "Effect of pyridoxine on human hypophyseal trophic hormone release: A possible stimulation of hypothalamic dopaminergic pathway" (*J. Clin. Endocrinol. Metab.* 1976, 42:603ff); Abraham, G. "Nutrition and the premenstrual tension syndromes" (*J. Appl. Nutr.* 1984, 36:103-124).

10 Abraham, G., and Rumley, R. (1987).

11 Hargrove, J., and Abraham, G. "Effect of vitamin B6 on infertility in women with the premenstrual tension syndrome" (*Infertility* 1979, 2:315ff).

12 Abraham, G., and Hargrove, J., "Effect of vitamin B6 on premenstrual symptomatology in women with premenstrual tension syndromes: A double blind crossover study" (*Infertility* 1980, 3:155ff); Williams, M., Harris, R., and Dean, B., "Controlled trial of pyridoxine in the premenstrual syndrome" (*J. Int. Med. Res.* 1985,13:174ff); Wyatt, K., Dimmock, P., Jones, P., et al. "Efficacy of vitamin B6 in the treatment of premenstrual syndrome: systematic review" (*Br. Med. J.* 1999, 318:1375-1381); Canning, S., Waterman, M., and Dye, L. "Dietary supplements and herbal remedies for premenstrual syndrome (PMS): A systematic research review of the evidence for their efficacy" (*J. Reprod. and Infant Psychol.* 2007, 24:363-378); Kashanian, M., Mazinani, R., and Jalalmanesh, S. "Pyridoxine (vitamin B6) therapy for premenstrual syndrome" (*Int. J. Obstet. Gynecol.* 2007, 96:43-44).

13 Henmi, H., Endo, T., Kitajima, Y., et al. "Effect of ascorbic acid supplementation on serum progesterone levels in patients with a luteal phase defect" (*Fertil. Steril.* 2003, 80: 459-461).

14 Fuchs, N., Hakim, M., and Abraham, G. "The effect of a nutritional supplement, Optivite for Women, on premenstrual tension syndromes: I. Effect on blood chemistry and serum steroid levels during the midluteal phase" (*J. Appl. Nutr.* 1985, 37:1-11).

15 Abraham, G., and Rumley, R. (1987).

16 Abraham, G. (1983).

17 Abraham, G., and Lubran, M. "Serum and red cell magnesium levels in patients with premenstrual tension" (*Am. J. Clin. Nutr.* 1981, 34:2364-2366).

18 Goei, G., Ralston, J., and Abraham, G. (1982).

19 Bendich, A. "The potential for dietary supplements to reduce premenstrual syndrome (PMS) symptoms" (*J. Amer. Coll. Nutr.* 2000, 19:3-12); Girman, A., Lee, R., and Kligler, B. "An integrative medicine approach to premenstrual syndrome"(*Clin. J. Women's Health* 2002, 2:116-127); Quaranta, S., Buscaglia, M., Meroni, M., et al. "Pilot study of the efficacy and safety of a modified-release magnesium 250 mg tablet (Sincromag®) for the treatment of premenstrual syndrome" (*Clin. Drug. Invest.* 2007, 27:51-58).

20 Abraham, G., and Rumley, R. (1987).

21 Abraham, G. (1983).

22 Goei, G., Ralston, J., and Abraham, G. (1982).

23 Abraham, G. (1983).

24 Abraham, G., and Rumley, R. (1987).

25 Abraham, G. (1984).

26 Abraham, G., and Taylor, R. "Premenstrual Tension Syndromes" in *Current Therapy in Obstetrics and Gynecology*, edited by E. Quilligan, M.D., and F. Zuspan, M.D. (Philadelphia: W.B. Saunders Co., 1990, pp. 100-105).

27 "The monounsaturates and polyunsaturates should come predominantly from vegetables oils in order to emphasize oleic, cis-linoleic, and alpha-linolenic acid. Good sources of these unsaturated fatty acids are, respectively, olive, safflower, and flaxseed oil. The ingestion of animal fats and hydrogenated vegetables should be curtailed in order to minimize the intake of arachidonic acid, saturated fatty acids, and trans-unsaturated fatty acids." Abraham, G., and Taylor, R. (1990).

28 Abraham, G. (1983); Beck, S., and Abraham, G. (1992, p. 3).

29 Abraham, G., and Taylor, R. (1990).

30 Rossignol, A., and Bonnlander, H. "Caffeine-containing beverages, total fluid consumption, and premenstrual syndrome" (*Am. J. Public Health* 80:1106-1110, 1990).

31 Beck, S., and Abraham, G. (1992, p. 27).

32 Teitelbaum, T., M.D. *Beat Sugar Addiction Now!* (Beverly, MS: Fairwinds Press 2010, p.118).

33 Roberts, H., *Aspartame (NutraSweet): Is It Safe?* (Philadelphia: The Charles Press, 1990, pp. 168-172).

34 Goei, G., and Abraham, G. "Effect of a nutritional supplement, Optivite, on symptoms of premenstrual tension" (*J. Reprod. Med.* 1983, 28:527-531).

35 Abraham and Rumley (1987); Chakmakjian, Z., Higgins, C., and Abraham, G. "The effect of a nutritional supplement, Optivite for Women, on premenstrual tension syndromes: II. Effect on symptomatology, using a double-blind crossover design" (*J. Appl. Nutr.* 1985, 37:12ff); Stewart, A., "Clinical and biochemical effects of nutritional supplementation on the premenstrual syndrome" (*J. Reprod. Med.* 1987, 32:435-441); London, R., Bradley, L., and Chiamori, N. "Effect of a nutritional supplement on premenstrual symptomatology in women with premenstrual syndrome: A double blind longitudinal study" (*J. Am. Coll. Nutr.* 1991, 10:494-499).

36 Kashanian, Mazinani, and Jalamanesh (2007).

37 Hemni, H., Endo, T., Kitajima, Y., et al. (2003).

38 Fuchs, N., Hakim, M., and Abraham, G. (1985).

39 Optimox Corp. (www.Optimox.com, March 24, 2009).

40 Abraham, G., and Rumley, R. (1987).

41 Beck, S., and Abraham, G. (1992, p. 18).

42 Wakeman, M, "An open-label pilot study to assess the effectiveness of krill oil with added vitamins and phytonutrients in the relief of symptoms of PMS" (*Nutrition and Dietary Supplements* 2013, 5:17-25).

43 Schellenberg, R. "Treatment for the premenstrual syndrome with *Vitex agnus* *castus* fruit extract: prospective, randomized, placebo controlled study" (*Br. Med. J.* 2001, 322:134-137).

44 Girman, A., Lee, R., and Kligler, B. (2002).

45 Wutteke, W. "Dopaminergic action of extracts of *Vitex agnus castus*" (*Forschende Komplementarmedizen* 1996, 6:329-330).

46 Westphal, L., Polan, M., and Trant, A. "Double-blind, placebo-controlled study of FertilityBlend: a nutritional supplement for improving fertility in women" (*Clin. Exp. Obst. & Gyn.* 2006, xxxiii:205-208).

47 Thys-Jacobs, S., McMahon, D., and Bilezikian, J. "Cyclical changes in calcium metabolism across the menstrual cycle in women with premenstrual dysphoric disorder" (*J. Clin. Endocrinol. Metab.* 2007, 92:2952-2959).

48 Bertone-Johnson, E., Hankinson, S., Benich, A., et al. "Calcium and vitamin D intake and risk of incident premenstrual syndrome" (*Arch. Intern. Med.* 2005, 165:124601252).

49 Bertone-Johnson, E., Chocano-Bedoya, P., Zagarins, S., et al. "Dietary vitamin D intake, 25-dydroxyvitamin D3 levels and premenstrual syndrome in a college-age population" (*Journal of Steroid Biochemistry and Molecular Biology* 2010, 121:434-437).

50 Thys-Jacobs, S., Starky, P., Bernstein, D., et al. "Micronutrients and the premenstrual syndrome: the case for calcium" (*J. Am. Coll. Nutr.* 2000, 19:220-227); Sutariya, S., Talsania, N., Shah, C., et al. "An interventional study (calcium supplementation & health education) on premenstrual syndrome—effect on premenstrual and menstrual symptoms" (*National Journal of Community Medicine* 2011, 2:100-104).

51 Bertone-Johnson, E., Hankinson, S., Bendich, A., et al. (2005).

52 2007-08 "PMS: How Far Have We Really Come?" (*Women's Health America Online Newsletter* (www.womenshealth.com, August, 2007).

53 Barron, M. "Light exposure, melatonin secretion, and menstrual cycle parameters: an integrative review" (*Biol. Res. Nursing* 2007, 9:49-69).

54 Bertone-Johnson, E., Hankinson, S., Bendich, A., et al. (2005).

55 Soares, C. "Characteristics of sleep disturbances in women" (*Psychiatric Times* 2013, 30(7):1-3); Karamen, H., Tanriverdi, G., and Degirmenci, Y. "Subjective sleep quality in premenstrual syndrome" (*Gynecological Endocrinology* 2012, 28:661-664).

56 Beck, S., and Abraham, G. (1992).

57 Shrim, A. Boskovic, C., Maltepe, Y., et al. "Pregnancy outcome following use of large doses of vitamin B6 in the first trimester" (*J. Obstet. Gynecol.* 2006, 26:749-751).

CHAPTER 7

1 Livdans, A., Harvey, P., and Larkin-Thier, S. "Menorrhagia: A synopsis of management focusing on herbal and nutritional supplements, and chiropractic" (*J. Can. Chiropr. Assoc* 2007, 51:235-246).

2 Livdans, A., Harvey, P., and Larkin-Thier, S. (2007).

3 Rothman, K., and Moore, L. "Teratogenicity of high vitamin A intake" (*NEJM* 1995, 333:1369-1373). Beta-carotene, which is not pre-formed vitamin A, can be taken in amounts far higher than the guideline given here.

4 Livdans, A., Harvey, P., and Larkin-Thier, S. (2007).

5 Hudson, T. "Using nutrition to relieve primary dysmenorrhea" (*Alt. & Comp. Therapies*, June 2007, pp. 125-128).

6 Soares, C. "Characteristics of sleep disorders in women" (*Psychiatric Times*, 2013, 30:p.2-2).

7 Haidari, F., Akrami, A., Sarhadi, M., et al. "Prevalence and severity of primary dysmenorrhea and its relation to anthropometric parameters" (*J. of Faculty of Nursing and Midwifery*, Tehran University of Medical Sciences 2011, 17:85).

8 Proctor, M., and Farquhar, C. "Diagnosis and management of dysmenorrhea" (*Br. Med. J.* 2006, 332:1134-1138).

9 Visvanathan, N., and Wyshak, g. "Tubal ligation, menstrual changes, and menopausal symptoms" (*J. Women's Health and Gender-Based Medicine* 2000, 9:521-527); Kutlar, I., Ozkur, A., Balat, O., et al. "Effects of three different sterilization methods on utero-ovarian Doppler blood flow and serum levels of ovarian hormones" (*Euro. J. Obstet. Gynecol. and Reprod. Biol.* 2005, 122:112-117).

10 Livdans, A., Harvey, P., and Larkin-Thier, S. (2007).

11 Derman, O., Kanbur, N., Tokur, T., et al. "Premenstrual syndrome and associated symptoms in adolescent girls" (*Euro. J. Obstet. Gynecol. and Reprod. Biol.* 2004, 116:201-206).

12 Puder, J. , Blum, C., Mueller, B., et al. "Menstrual cycle symptoms are associated with changes in low-grade inflammation" (*Euro. J. Clin. Invest.* 2006, 36:58-64).

13 Horrobin, D. "The role of essential fatty acids and prostaglandins in the premenstrual syndrome" (*J. Reprod. Med.* 1983, 28:465-468).

14 Abdul-Razzak, K., Ayoub, M., Abu-Taleb, A., et al. "The influence of dietary intake of dairy products on dysmenorrhea" (*J. Obstet Gynaecol. Res.* 2010, 36:377).

15 Proctor, M., and Farquhar, C. (2006).

16 Hanson, S., and Knudsen, U. "Endometriosis, dysmenorrhoea and diet" (*Euro. J. Obstet. Gynecol. and Reprod. Biol* 2013, 169:162-171).

17 Rahbar, N., Asgharzadeh, N., and Ghorbani, R. "Effect of omega-3 fatty acids on intensity of primary dysmenorrhea" (*International J. of Gynecol. and Obstet.* 2012, 117: 45-47).

18 Harel, Z., Biro, F., Kottenhahn, R., et al. "Supplementation with omega-3 poly-unsaturated fatty acids in the management of dysmenorrhea in adolescents" (*Am. J. Obstet. Gynecol.* 1996, 174:1335-1338).

19 Deutch, B., Jorgensen, E., and Hansen, J. "Menstrual discomfort in Danish women reduced by dietary supplements of omega-3 PUFA and B12" (*Nutr. Res.* 2000, 20: 621-631).

20 Saldeen, P. and Saldeen, T. "Women and Omega-3 fatty acids" (*Obstet. Gynecol. Survey* 2004, 59:722-730).

21 Ziaei, S., Faghihzadeh, S., Sohrabvand, F., et al. "A randomised placebo-controlled trial to determine the effect of vitamin E in treatment of primary dysmenorrhea" (*Br. J. Obstet. Gynecol.* 2001, 108:1181-1183); Dennehy, C. "The use of herbs and dietary supplements in gynecology: an evidenced-based review" (*J. Midwifery & Women's Health* 2006, 51:402-409).

22 Dennehy, C. (2006); Proctor, M., and Farquhar, C. (2006).

23 Abdul-Razzak, K., Ayoub, M., Abu-Taleb, A., et al. (2010).

24 Abdul-Razzak, K., Obeidat, B., Al-Farras, M., et al. "Vitamin D and PTH status among adolescent and young females with severe dysmenorrhea" (*J. Pediatr. Adolesc. Gynecol.* 2014, 27:78-82).

25 Lasco, A., Catalano, A., and Benvenga, S. "Improvement of primary dysmenor-rhea caused by a single oral dose of vitamin D: results of a ramdomized, double-blind, placebo-controlled study" (*Arch. Intern. Med.* 2012, 172:366-367).

26 Witz, C., and Burn, W. "Endometriosis and infertility: Is there a cause and effect relationship?" (*Gyn. And Obstet. Invest.* 2002, 5(suppl:)2-11).

27 Osteen, K., Bruner-Tran, K., and Eisenberg, E. "Reduced progesterone action during endometrial maturation: a potential risk factor for the development of endome-triosis" (*Fert. Steril.* 2005, 83:529-537); Bulun, S., Cheng, Y., Yin, P., et al. "Progesterone resistance in endometriosis: link to failure to metabolize estradiol" (*Molec. and Cell. Endocrinol* 2006, 248:94-103).

28 Sekhon, L., Gupta, S., Kim, Y. et al. "Female fertility and antioxidants" (*Current Women's Health Reviews*, 2010, 6:84-94); Augoulea, A., Mastorakos, G., Lambrinoudaki, I., et al. "The role of oxidative-stress in the endometriosis-related infertility" *Gynecological Endocrinol.* 2009, 25:75-81); Prieto, L., Quesada, J., Cambero, O., et al. "Analysis of follicular fluid and serum markers of oxidative stress in women with infertility related to endometriosis" (*Fertil. Steril.* 2012, 98:126-130).

29 Hilgers, Thomas W. "Endometriosis and Its Effects on Fertility" in *The NaPro Technology Revolution: Unleashing the Power in a Woman's Cycle* (New York: Beaufort Books, 2010, pp.282-283).

30 Cunha-Filio, J., Gross, J., Lemos, N., et al. "Hyperprolactinemia and luteal insufficiency in infertile patients with mild and minimal endometriosis" (*Horm. Metab. Res.* 2001, 33:216-220).

31 Hargrove, J., and Abraham, A. "The ubiquitousness of premenstrual tension in gynecologic practice" (*J. Reprod Med.* 1983, 28:435-437).

32 Hargrove, J., and Abraham, A. "Abnormal luteal function in women with endometriosis" (*Fertil. Steril.* 1983, 34:302).

33 Hilgers, Thomas W. (2010).

34 Missmer, S., Chavarro, J., Malspeis, S., et al. "A prospectivie study of dietary fat consumption and endometrioisis risk" (*Reproductive Epidemiology* 2010, 25:1528-1535).

35 Hanson and Knudsen (2013).

36 Harris, H., Chavarro, J., Malspeis, S., et al. "Dairy-food, calcium, magnesium, and vitamin D intake and endometriosis: A perspective cohort study" (*Am. J. Epidemiology* 2013, 177:420-430).

37 Prieto, L., Quesada, J., Cambero, O., et al. "Analysis of follicular fluid and serum markers of oxidative stress in women with infertility related to endometriosis" (*Fertil. Steril.* 2012, 98:126-130); Sekhon, L., Gupta, S, et al. "Female fertility and antioxidants" (*Current Women's Health Reviews* 2010, 6:84-95); Augoulea, A., Mastorakos, G., Lambrinoudaki, I., et al. "The role of the oxidative-stress in the endometriosis-related infertility" (*Gynecological Endocrinology* 2009, 25:75-81).

38 Sesta, F., Pietropolli, A., Capozzola, T., et al. "Hormonal suppression treatment of dietary therapy versus placebo in the control of painful symptoms after conservative surgery for endometriosis stage III-IV. A randomized comparative trial" (*Fertil. Steril.* 2007, 88:1541-1547).

39 Lark, S. "End the Pain of Endometriosis" (*Women's Wellness Today,* June, 2008, pp. 6-7).

40 Kohama, T., Herai, K., and Inoue, M. "Effect of French maritime pine bark extract on endometriosis as compared with leuprorelin acetate" (*J. Reprod. Med.* 2007, 52: 703-708).

41 Schwertner, A., Conceicao dos Santos, C., Costa, G., et al. "Efficacy of melatonin in the treatment of endometriosis: A phase II, randomized, double blind, placebo-controlled trial (*Pain* 2013, 154:874-881).

42 Crook, W., Dean, C., and Crook, E. *The Yeast Connection and Women's Health* (Jackson, TN: Professional Books, 2005, p.74).

CHAPTER 8

1 Gibbs, J., Williams, N., Mallinson, R., et al. "Effect of high dietary restraint on energy availability and menstrual status" (*Med. Sci. Sports Exerc.* 2013, 45:1790-1797).

2 Bruchalski, J. (Personal communication to M. Shannon, October 6, 2008). John Bruchalski, M.D., is an NFP-only obstetrician/gyneoclogist at the Tepeyac OB/GYN in Fairfax, VA.

3 Roberts, C., and Murphy, A. "Endocrinopathies associated with recurrent pregnancy loss" (*Sem. in Reprod. Med.* 2000, 18:357-362).

4 Hilgers, T., M.D. *The NaproTechnology Revolution: Unleashing the Power in a Woman's Cycle* (New York:Beaufort Books, 2010, p. 161).

5 Roberts, C., and Murphy, A. (2000).

6 Check, J. "Ovulation defects despite regular menses: Part III" (*Clin. Exp. Obst. & Gyn.* 2007, XXXIV: 133-136).

7 McIntosh, E. "Treatment of women with the galactorrhea-amenorrhea syndrome with pyridoxine (vitamin B6)" (*J. Clin. Endocrinol Metab.* 1976, 1192ff).

8 Hargrove, J., and Abraham, G. "Effect of vitamin B6 on infertility in women with the premenstrual tension syndrome" (*Infertility* 1979, 2:315-317).

9 Henmi, H., Endo, T., Kitajima, Y., et al. "Effect of ascorbic acid supplementation on serum progesterone levels in patients with a luteal phase defect" (*Fertil. Steril.* 2003, 80:459-461).

10 Abraham, G. "Nutritional factors in the etiology of the premenstrual tension syndromes" (*J. Reprod. Med.* 1983, 28:446-464).

11 Fuchs, N., Hakim, M., and Abraham, G. "The effect of a nutritional supplement,

Optivite for Women, on premenstrual tension syndromes: I. Effect on blood chemistry and serum steroid levels during the midluteal phase" (*J. Appl. Nutr.* 1985, 37:1-11).

12 Kasse-Annese, B., and Danzer, H. *The Complete Guide to the Treatment of Premenstrual Problems* (Santa Monica, CA: Patterns Publishing, 1984, p. 65).

13 *Family Foundations* (Couple to Couple League, July/August 2014, pp. 36-37).

14 Westphal, L., Polan, M., and Trant, A. "Double-blind, placebo-controlled study of FertilityBlend: a nutritional supplement for improving fertility in women" (*Clin. Exp. Obst. & Gyn.* 2006, xxxiii:205-208).

15 Westphal, L., Polan, M., and Trant, A. (2006).

16 Milewicz, A., Gejdel, E., Sworen, H., et al. "Vitex agnus castus-extrakt zur behandlung von regeltempoanomalien infolge latenter hyperprolaktinamie" (*Arzneimettel-Forschung* 1993, 43:752-756; reviewed in Fugh-Berman, A., and Kronenberg, F. "Complementary and alternative medicine (CAM) in reproductive-age women: a review of randomized controlled studies" (*Reproductive Toxicology* 2003, 17:137-152).

17 Goswami, B., Patel, S., Chatterjee, M., et al. "Correlation of prolactin and thyroid hormone concentration with menstrual patterns in infertile women" (*J. Reprod. Infertil.* 2009, 10:207-212).

18 Goswami, B., Patel, S., Chatterjee, M., et al. (2009).

19 Poppe, K., Velkeniers, B., and Glinoert, D. "Thyroid disease and female reproduction" (*Clin. Endocrinol.* 2007, 66:309-321).

20 Shomon, M. *The Thyroid Hormone Breakthrough: Overcoming Sexual and Hormonal Problems at Every Age* (New York: Collins, an imprint of HarperCollins, 2006, pp. 33-34, 37).

21 Lark, S. "Solutions for a Healthy Thyroid" (*Women's Wellness Today* 2007, 14:1-5).

22 Shomon, M. (2006, pp. 82-86).

23 Shomon, M. (2006, p. 80).

24 Balch, P. *Prescription for Nutritional Healing*, 5th ed. (New York: Avery Press, 2010, p. 518).

25 Melotte-Athmer, A. "Iodine needed for proper thyroid function" (*CCL News* 1986, 12(5):3).

26 Norris, K. "Case study—The management of hypothyroidism" (*ACNEM Journal* 2015, 34[(1]).

27 Ashok, K., Sarma, D., and Saikia, U. "Selenium and the thyroid: A close-knit connection" (*Indian J. Endocrinol. Metab.* 2012, 16[Supl. 2: S354-S355]).

28 Nacamulli, D., Mian, C., Petriccca, D., et al. "Influence of physiological dietary selenium supplementation on the natural course of autoimmune thyroiditis" (*Clin. Endocrinol.* 2010, 73:535-539).

29 Norris (2015).

30 Androvite for Men, while formulated to improve male reproductive function, is safe for women, even during pregnancy, as long as they have their doctor's approval.

31 Duntas, L. "The role of iodine and selenium in autoimmune thyroiditis" (*Horm. Metab. Res.* 2015, 47:721-726).

32 Bhuyan, A., Sarma, D., and Saikia, U. "Selenium and the thyroid: A close-knit connection" (*Indian J. Endocrinol. Metab.* 2012, 16:S354-S355).

33 De Souza, M., Van Heest, J., Demers, L., et al. (2003).

34 Frisch, R. *Female Fertility and the Body Fat Connection* (Chicago: University of Chicago Press, 2002, p. 99).

35 Franklyn, J. "Subclinical thyroid disorders–Consequences and implications for treatment" (*Annales d'Endocrinologie* 2007, 68:229-230).

36 Barnes, B., and Galton, L. *Hypothyroidism: The Unsuspected Illness* (New York: Harper and Row, 1976, p. 136).

37 Puglio, P. "Hypothyroidism: The relationship to menstrual disorders." (*Women's Health Connections,* Complementary Issue II). Available through the Barnes Foundation, P.O Box 110098, Trumbull, CT 06611. Telephone 203-261-2101; or www.brod-abarnes.org.

38 Barnes, B., and Galton, L. (1976, p. 46).

39 Sharma, N., and Sharma, A. "Thyroid profile in menstrual disorders" (*JK Science* 2012, 14:14-17).

40 Franklyn, J. (2007).

41 Frisch, R. (2002, pp. 75-78).

42 Frisch, R. (2002, p. 17).

43 Frisch, R. (2002, pp. 85-88).

44 Frisch, R. (2002, p. 141).

45 Manore, M. "Nutritional recommendations and athlete menstrual dysfunction" (*Int. Sports Med J.* 2004, 5:45-55).

46 De Souza, M., Toombs, R., Scheid, J., et al. "High prevalence of subtle and severe menstrual disturbances in exercising women: Confirmation using daily hormone measures" (*Human Reprod.* 2010, 25:491-503).

47 Manore, M., Kam, L., and Loucks, A. "The female athlete triad: Components, nutrition issues, and health consequences" (*J. Sports Science* 2007, 25 S1):S61-S71).

48 Manore, Kam, and Loucks, 2007.

49 Manore, Kam, Loucks, 2007.

CHAPTER 9

1 Rotterdam ESHRE/ASRM-Sponsored Consensus Workshop Group. "Revised 2003 consensus on diagnostic criteria and long-term health risks related to polycystic ovary syndrome" (*Fertil. Steril.* 2004, 81:19-25).

2 Norman, R., Dewailly, D., Legro, R., et al. "Polycystic ovary syndrome" (*The Lancet* 2007, 370:685-697).

3 Norman, R., Dewailly, D., Legro, R., et al. (2007).

4 Velija-Asimi, Z., Ascic-Buturovic, B., and Pesto, S. "The role of subclinical hypothyroidism in polycystic ovary syndrome" (*Medicinski Zurnal* 2009, 15:34-35).

5 Singla, R., Gupta, Y., Khemani, M., et al. "Thyroid disorders and polycystic ovary syndrome: An emerging relationship" (*Indian Journal of Endocrinology and Metabolism* 2015, 19:25ff).

6 Sinha, U., Sinharay, K., Longkumer, T., et al. "Thyroid disorders in polycystic ovarian subjects: A tertiary hospital based cross-sectional study from Eastern India" (*Indian Journal of Endocrinology and Metabolism* 2013, 17:304ff).

7 Singla, R., Gupta, Y., Khemani, M., et al. (2013).

8 Norman, R., Dewailly, D., Legro, R., et al. (2007).

9 Moran, L., Pasquali, R., Teede, H., et al. "Treatment of obesity in polycystic ovary syndrome: A position statement of the Androgen Excess and Polycystic Ovary Syndrome Society" (*Fertil. Steril.* 2009, 92:1966-1982).

10 Franks, S., Robinson, S., and Willis, D. "Nutrition, insulin, and polycystic ovary syndrome" (*Reviews of Reproduction* 1996, 1:47-53).

11 Franks, S., Robinson, S., and Willis, D. (1996).

12 Kasin-Karakas, S., Cunningham, W., and Tsodikov, A. "Relation of nutrients and hormones in polycystic ovary syndrome" (*Am. J. Clin.* 2007, 85:688-694).

13 Liepa, G., Sengapta, A., and Karsies, D. "Polycystic ovary syndrome (PCOS) and other androgen excess-related conditions: Can changes in dietary intake make a difference?" (*Nutrition in Clin. Prac.* 2008, 23:63–71).

14 Sorensen, L., Soe, M., Halkier, H., et al. "Effects of increased dietary protein-to-carbohydrate rations in women with polycystic ovary syndrome" (*Am. J. Cin Nutr.*, 2012, 95:39-48).

15 Moran, L., Ko, H., Misso, M., et al. "Dietary composition in the treatment of polycystic ovary syndrome: A systematic review to inform evidence-based guidelines" (*Journal of the Academy of Nutrition and Dietetics* 2013, 113:520-545).

16 Chavarro, J., Willett, W., and Skerrett, P. *The Fertility Diet* (New York: McGraw-Hill 2008, p. 183).

17 Chavarro, J., Rich-Edwards, J., Sosner, B., et al. "Dietary fatty acid intake and the risk of ovulatory infertility" (*Am. J. Clin. Nutr.* 2007, 85:231-237).

18 Chavarro, J. Personal communication to M. Shannon (Mar. 17, 2008). "In the overwhelming majority of cases the underlying condition affecting ovulation was PCOS although there were other conditions that we considered as accurate reports of 'ovulatory infertility' such as anovulation due to hyperprolactinemia, hypothyroidism, hypopituitarism and premature ovarian failure."

19 Chavarro, J., Willett, W., and Skerrett, P. (2008, pp. 147, 184).

20 Gittleman, A. *Get the Sugar Out!*, 2nd ed. (New York: Three Rivers Press, 2008, pp. 14-16).

21 Chavarro, J., Rich-Edwards, J., Rosner, B., and Willett, W. "A prospective study of dairy foods intake and anovulatory infertility" (*Human Reprod.* 2007, 22:1340-1347).

22 Dhingra, R., Sullivan, L., Jacques, P., et al. "Soft drink consumption and the risk of developing cardiometabolic risk factors and the metabolic syndrome in middle-aged adults in the community" (*Circulation* 2007, 116:480-488).

23 Nettleton, J., Lutsey, P., Wang, Y., et al. "Diet soda intake and risk of incident metabolic syndrome and type 2 diabetes in the multi-ethnic study of atherosclerosis (MESA)" (2009, *Diabetes Care* 32:688-694).

24 Roberts, H., *Aspartame (NutraSweet): Is It Safe?* (Philadelphia: The Charles Press, 1990, pp. 147-150).

25 Roberts (1990, pp. 194-195).

26 Suez, J., Korem, T., Zeevi, D., et al. "Artificial sweeteners induce glucose intolerance by altering the gut microbiota" (*Nature* 2014, 514:181ff).

27 Chavarro, J., Rich-Edwards, J., Rosner, B., et al. "Use of multivitamins, intake of B vitamins, and risk of ovulatory infertility" (*Fertil. Steril.* 2008, 89:668-676).

28 Guzelmeric, K., Alkan, N., Pirimoglu, M., et al. "Chronic inflammation and elevated homocysteine levels are associated with increased body mass index in women with polycystic ovary syndrome" (*Gynecol. Endocrinol.* 2007, 23:505-510).

29 Kilicdag, E., Bagis, T., Tarim, E., et al. "Administration of B-group vitamins reduces circulating homocysteine in polycystic ovarian syndrome patients treated with metformin: a randomized trial" *Human Reprod.* 2005, 20:1521-1528) [The amounts studied were 500 mg vitamin B1, 500 mg B6, and 2,000 mcg B12 daily, or folic acid (348 mcg daily)].

30 Schachter, M., Raziel, A., Strassburger, D., et al. "Prospective, randomized trial of metformin and vitamins for the reduction of plasma homocysteine in insulin-resistant polycystic ovary syndrome" (*Fertil. Steril.* 2007, 88:227-230).

31 Constantino, D., Minozzi, G., Minozzi, F., et al. "Metabolic and hormonal effects of myo-inositol on women with polycystic ovary syndrome: a double-blind trial" (*Eur. Rev. Med. Pharmacol.* Sci. 2009, 13:105-110).

32 Pizzo, A., Lagana, A., and Barbaro, L. "Comparisin between effects of myo-inositol and D.chiro-inositol on ovarian function and metabolic facors in women with PCOS" (*Gynecol. Endocrinol.* 2014, 30:205-208).

33 Genazzani, A., Lanzoni, C., Ricchieri, F., et al. "Myoinositol administration positively affects hyperinsulinemia and hormonal parameters in overweight patients with polycystic ovary syndrome" (*Gynecol. Endocrinol.* 2008, 24:139-144).

34 D'Anna, R., DiBenedetto, V., Rizzo, P., et al. "Myo-inositol may prevent gestational diabetes in PCOS women" (*Gynecol. Endocrinol.* 2012, 28:440-442).

35 Hahn, S., Haselhorst, U., Tan, S., et al. "Low serum 2,5-hydroxyvitamin D concentrations are associated with insulin resistance and obesity in women with polycystic ovary syndrome" (*Exp. Clin. Endocrinol. Diabetes* 2006, 114:557-583).

36 Moran, L., Teede, H., and Vincent, A. "Vitamin D is independently associated with depression in overweight women with and without PCOS" (*Gynecol. Endocrinol.* 2015, 31:179-182).

37 Jamilian, M., and Asemi, Z. "Chromium supplementation and the effects on metabolic staus in women with polycystice ovary syndrome: A randomized, double-blind, placebo-controlled trial" (*Ann. Nutr. Metabl.* 2015, 67:42-47); Personal communication to M. Shannon (October 12, 1996) Julian Whitaker, M.D. stated that 400 mcg of chromium is safe during pregnancy.

38 Whitaker, J. "Weight Loss is Not Just About Fat" (*Health and Healing* 1997, 7:5-8).

39 Kasim-Karakas, S., Almario, R., Gregory, L., et al. "Metabolic and endocrine effects of a PUFA rich diet in PCOS (*J. Clin. Endocrinol. Metab.* 2004, 89:615–620).

40 Mohammadi, E., Rafraf, M. Farzadi, L., et al. "Effects of omega-3 acids supplementation on serum adiponectin levels and some metabolic risk factors in women with polycystic ovary syndrome" (*Asia Pac. J. Clin.* 2012, 21:511-518). EPA is the abbreviation for eicosapentaenoic acid; DHA is the abbreviation for docosahexanoic acid.

41 Nadjarzadeh, A., Dehghani-Firouzabadi, R., Daneshbodi, H., et al. "Effect of omega-3 supplementation of visfatin, adiponectin, and anthropometric indices in women with polycystic ovarian syndrome" (*J. Reprod. Infertil.* 2015, 16:212-220).

42 Saldeen, P., and Saldeen, T. "Women and omega-3 fatty acids" [CME Review Article] (*Obstet. Gynecol. Survey* 2004, 59:722-730).

43 Suez, J., Korem, T., Zeevi, D., et al. (2014).

44 Tremellen, K., and Pearce, P. "Dysbiosois of gut microbiota (DOGMA)—A novel theory for the development of polycystic ovarian syndrome" (*Medical Hypot*hesis 2012, 79:104-112).

45 Dean, C. "Understanding the Weight Connection" in Crook, W., Dean, C., and Crook, E. *The Yeast Connection and Women's Health* (Jackson, TN: Professional Books, 2005, pp.245-252).

46 Moran, L., et al. "Exercise and lifestyle modification in PCOS [Symposium: Effects of lifestyle modification in PCOS]" (*Reprod. BioMedicine Online* 2002, pp. 573-578).

47 Randeva, H., Lewandowski, K., Drzewoski, J., et al. "Exercise decreases plasma total homocysteine in overweight young women with polycystic ovary syndrome" (*J. Clin. Endocrinol. Metab.* 2002, 87:4496-4501).

48 "Nutrition Information Leads to Much-Desired Pregnancy," Letter to the Editor (*Family Foundations*, Sept.-Oct. 2001, p. 25).

49 Shomon, M. *The Thyroid Hormone Breakthrough: Overcoming Sexual and Hormonal Problems at Every Age* (New York: Collins, an imprint of HarperCollins, 2006, pp. 33, 37).

50 Lee, J., and Hopkins, V. *Dr. John Lee's Hormone Balance Made Simple* (New York: Warner Wellness, 2006, pp. 102-103).

51 Moran, L., Teede, H., and Vincent, A. (2015).

CHAPTER 10

1 Shapira, I., Sultan, K, Lee, A., et al. "Evolving concepts: How diet and the intestinal microbiome act as modulators of breast malignancy" (*ISRN Oncology* 2013: Article ID 693920); Isolauri, E., Rautava, S., Collado, M., et al. "Role of probiotics in reducing the risk of gestational diabetes"(*Diabetes, Obesity, and Metabolism* 2015, 17:713-719).

2 Crook, W., M.D, Dean, C., M.D., and Crook, E. *The Yeast Connection and Women's Health* (Jackson TN: Professional Books (2005), p. 3-4).

3 Galland, L. "Foreword" in *The Yeast Connection and Women's Health*, by William G. Crook, M.D., with Carolyn Dean, M.D. (Jackson, TN: Professional Books, 2005, pp. xi-xiv).

4 Crook, W. *The Yeast Connection and Women's Health* (Jackson, TN: Professional Books, 2005, pp. 12-13).

5 Smith, K. "Purging out the yeast: An informal study of yeast overgrowth" (An unpublished document provided by K. Smith to M. Shannon, June, 2004).

6 Suez, J., Korem, T., Zeevi, D., et al. "Artificial sweeteners induce glucose intolerance by altering the gut microbiota" (*Nature* 2014, 514:181ff).

7 Lark, S. "The Countless Pros of Probiotics" (*Women's Wellness Today*, March, 2008, pp.1-5).

8 Shapira, I., Sultan, K, Lee, A., et al., 2015.

9 Crook and Dean, 240.

10 Crook and Dean, 223-224.

11 Teitelbaum, J., M.D. *Beat Sugar Addiction Now!* (Beverly, MA, Fair Winds Press, 2015, p. 99).

12 Schwarzbein, D. *The Schwarzbein Principle II: The Transition* (Deerfield Beach, FL: Health Communications 2002, p. 378).

13 Berenson, A., and Rahman, M. "Effect of hormonal contraceptives on vitamin B12 level and the association of the latter with bone mineral density" (*Contraception* 2012, 86:481-487).

14 Sutterlin, M., Bussen, S., Rieger, L., et al. "Serum folate and vitamin B12 levels in women using modern oral contraceptives (OC) containing 20 mg ethynyl estradiol" (*European J. Obstet. Gynecol. & Reprod. Biol.* 2003, 107:57-61).

15 Lussana, F., Zighetti, M., Bucciarilli, P., et al. "Blood levels of homocysteine, folate, vitamin B6 and B12 in women using oral contraceptions compared to non-users" (*Thrombosis Research* 2003, 112:37-41).

16 Thane, C., Bates, C., and Prentice, A. "Oral contraceptives and nutritional status in adolescent British girls" (*Nutri. Res.* 2002, 22:449-462).

17 Berry, C., Montgomery, C., Sattar, N., et al. "Fatty acid status of women of reproductive age" (*European J. Clin. Nutr.* 2001, 55:518-524).

18 Thane, C., Bates, C., and Prentice, A. (2002).

19 Thane, C., Bates, C., and Prentice, A. (2002).

20 Grant, E. *Sexual Chemistry: Understanding Our Hormones, the Pill and HRT* (London: Cedar Press, 1994, pp. 12, 13, 103).

21 Fernando, S., Osianlis, T., Vollenhoven, B., et al. "A pilot double-blind randomized placebo-controlled dose-response trial assessing the effects of melatonin on infertility treatment (MIART): study protocol" (*BMJ Open* 2014, 4:e005986.

22 Barron, M. "Light exposure, melatonin secretion, and menstrual cycle parameters: An integrative review" (*Biological Research for Nursing* 2007, 9:49-69).

23 Barron, M. (2007).

24 Davis, S., Mirick, D., and Stevens, R. "Night shift work, light at night, and risk of breast cancer" (*J. National Cancer Institute* 2001, 93:1557-1562).

25 Barron, M. (2007).

26 DeFelice, J. "The Effects of Light on the Menstrual Cycle: Also Infertility, Clinical

Observations" (Spokane, Washington: The Natural Family Planning Program of the Sacred Heart Medical Center, 2003).

27 Barron, M. (2007).

28 DeFelice, J. (2003).

29 DeFelice, J. (2003).

30 Barron, M. (2007).

31 Whitaker, J. "Reset Your Biological Clock" (*Health and Healing* 2003, 13(2), pp. 6-8).

32 Takasaki, A., Nakamura, Y., Tamura, H., et al. "Melatonin as a new drug for improving oocyte quality" (*Reprod. Med. and Biol.* 2003, 2:139-144).

33 Whitaker, J. (2003).

34 Wilcox, A., Weinburg, C., and Baird, D. "Caffeinated beverages and decreased fertility" (*The Lancet*, Dec. 24/31, 1988, pp. 1453-1455).

35 Christianson, R., Oechsli, F., and van den Berg, B. "Caffeinated beverages and decreased fertility" (*The Lancet*, Feb. 8, 1989, p. 378); Bolumar, F., Olsen, J., Rebagliato, M., et al. "Caffeine intake and delayed conception: A European multicenter study on infertiltiy and subfecundity" (*Am. J. Epidemiology* 1997, 145:324-334); Derbyshire, E. "Dietary factors and fertility in women of childbearing age" (*Nutrition and Food Science* 2007, 37:100-104).

36 Caan, B., Quesenberry, C., and Coates, A. "Differences in fertility associated with caffeinated beverage consumption" (*Am. J. Public Health* 1998, 88:270-273).

37 Weng, X., Odouli, R., and Li, D. "Maternal caffeine consumption during pregnancy and the risk of miscarriage: a prospective cohort study" (*J. Obst. Gynecol.*, Jan. 2008, pp. 1e1-1e8).

38 Caan, B., Quesenberry, C., and Coates, A. (1998).

39 Pellicano, R., Astegiano, M., Bruno, M., et al. "Women and celiac disease: association with unexplained infertility" (*Minerva Medica* 2007, 98:217-219) de Souza Lobo Machado, A., Rodriquez Silva, L., Zausner, B., et al. "Undiagnosed celiac disease in women with infertility" (*J. Reprod. Med.* 2013, 58:61-64).

40 Hin, H., and Ford, F. "Celiac disease and infertility: making the connection and achieving a successful pregnancy" (*J. Family Health Care* 2002, 12:94-97).

41 Bradley, R., and Rosen, M. "Subfertility and gastrointestinal disease: 'Unexplained' is often undiagnosed" [CME review article] (*Obstet. Gynecol. Survey* 2004, 59:108-117).

42 Chavarro, J., Willett, W., and Skerrett, P. *The Fertility Diet* (New York: McGraw-Hill, 2008, pp. 129-131).

43 Han, K., Ko, Y., Park, Y., et al. "Associations between the periodontal disease in women before menopause and menstrual cycle irregularity" (*Medicine* 95(6) February, 2016).

44 Hart, R., Doherty, D., Pennell, C, et al. "Periodontal disease: a potential modifiable risk factor limiting conception" (*Human Reproduction* 2012, 27:1332-1342).

45 Papapanou, I. "Epidemiology of association between maternal periodontal disease and adverse pregnacy outcomes—systematic review" (*J. Clin. Periodontol.*, 2013, 40 [Suppl. 14]: S181-S194).

46 Shrim, A., Boskovic, R., Maltepe, C., et al. "Pregnancy outcome following use of large doses of vitamin B6 in the first trimester" (*J. Obstet. Gynecol.* 2006, 26: 749-751); Guy Abraham, M.D., also reports this upper level safe and beneficial during pregnancy when used as part of a multivitamin/multimineral containing other B vitamins and magnesium: Beck, S., Abraham, G. "Optivite PMT and Gynovite Plus Total Dietary Programs for Premenstrual Syndrome and Menopause" (Torrance, CA: Optimox Corp., 1992, p. 27).

47 Wilson, W. "Pre-conceptional vitamin/folic acid supplementation 2007: The use of folic acid in combination with a multivitamin supplement for the prevention of neural tube defects and other congenital anomalies." (Joint Society of Obstetricians and Gynaecologists of Canada-Motherisk Clinical Practice Guideline (*J. Obstetricians and Gynaecologists of Canada*, Dec. 2007, pp. 1003-1013). This organization recommends supplementing 5.0 mg (5,000 mcg) of folic acid for women with health risks, including epilepsy, insulin dependent diabetes, and obesity. Goh, Y., and Koren, G. "Folic acid in pregnancy and fetal outcomes" (*J. Obstet. & Gynaecol.* 2008, 28:3-13). Folic acid supplementation in amounts up to 5,000 mcg is recommended for all women to prevent neural tube defects. This amount does not mask vitamin B12 deficiency, according to these authors. Erickson, J., "Folic acid and prevention of spinal bifida and anencephaly: 10 years after the U.S. Public Health Service recommendation" (*MMWR Recommendations and Reports* 2002, RR13:1-3; www.cdc.gov/mmwr/preview/mmwrhtml/rr5113al.htm) My recommendation of 4,000 mcg is consistent with the amount recommended for preventing neural tube defects in high risk women.

48 Raffelock, D., Rountree, R., and Hopkins, V. *A Natural Guide to Pregnancy and Postpartum Health* (New York: Avery Press, 2002, p.131) These authors, one a medical doctor and the other a chiropractor, consider as much as 5,000 mcg of vitamin B12 safe during pregnancy and breastfeeding.

49 Fett, R., "The Power of Coenzyme Q10" in *It Starts with the Egg* (New York: Franklin Fox Publishing, 2014, pp. 123).

50 Shannon, M. "Down Syndrome and Folic Acid, Adoption Update, and Surprise Pregnancies" (*Family Foundations,* Jan.-Feb. 2000, pp. 6–7).

CHAPTER 11

1 Weng, X., Odouli, R., and Li, D. "Maternal caffeine consumption during pregnancy and the risk of miscarriage: a prospective cohort study" (*J. Obst. Gynecol.,* Jan. 2008, pp. 1e1-1e8).

2 Grieger, J., Grzeskowiak, L., and Clifton, V. "Preconception dietary patterns in human pregnancies are associated with preterm delivery" (*J. Nutr.* 2014, 144: 1075-1080).

3 Moore, A., Mundle, W., et al. "Pre-conception folic acid and multivitamin supplementation for the primary and secondary prevention of nerual tube defects and other folic acid-sensitive congenital anomalies" (*J. Obstet. Gynaecol.* Can. 2015, 36:534-549).

4 Glenville, M. "Nutritional supplements in pregnancy: commercial push or evidence based?" (*Curr. Opin. Obstet. Gynecol.* 2006, 18:642-647).

5 Fugh-Berman, A., and Kronenberg, F. "Complementary and alternative medicine (CAM) in reproductive-age women: a review of randomized controlled studies" (*Reprod. Toxicol.* 2003, 17:137-152).

6 Shrim, A. Boskovic, C., Maltepe, Y., et al. "Pregnancy outcome following use of large doses of vitamin B6 in the first trimester" (*J. Obstet. Gynecol.* 2006, 26:749-751).

7 Fugh-Berman, A., and Kronenberg, F. (2003).

8 Puotinen, C. "Preventing eclampsia: an interview with Tom Brewer, M.D." (*Townsend Letter for Doctors and Patients,* Nov., 2004).

9 Brewer, T. "If You Are Pregnant" (www.BlueRibbonBaby.org. If You Are Pregnant Subpages, c. 2007).

10 Puotinen, C. (2004, p. 6).

11 Davies, M. "Evidence for effects of weight on reproduction in women [Symposium: Diet, nutrition, and exercise in reproduction]." (*Reprod. BioMed. Online* 2006, 12:552-561); Kiel, D., Dodson, E., Artal, R., et al. "Gestational weight gain and pregnancy outcomes in obese women" (*Obstet. Gynecol.* 2007, 110:752-758).

12 Oken, E., Ning, Y., Rifas-Shiman, S., et al. "Diet during pregnancy and risk of preeclampsia or gestational hypertension" (*AEP* 2007, 17:663-668).

13 Frederick, I., Williams, M., Dashow, E., et al. "Dietary fiber, potassium, magnesium and calcium in relation to the risk of preeclampsia" (*J. Reprod. Med.* 2005, 50:332-344).

14 Duvekot, E., de Groot, C., Bloemenkamp, K., et al. "Pregnant women with a low milk intake have an increased risk of developing preeclampsia" (*European J. Obstet. & Gynecol.* 2002, 105:11-14).

15 Duvekot, E., de Groot, C., Bloemenkamp, K., et al., (2002).

16 Duvekot, E., de Groot, C., Bloemenkamp, K., et al., (2002).

17 Grieger, J., Grzeskowiak, L., and Clifton, V. (2014).

18 Papapanou, I. "Epidemiology of association between maternal periodontal disease and adverse pregnacy outcomes—systematic review" (*J. Clin. Periodontol.*, 2013, 40 [Suppl. 14]: S181-S194).

19 Beck, S., and Abraham, G. *Optivite PMT and Gynovite Plus Total Dietary Programs for Premenstrual Syndrome and Menopause with Answers to the Most Commonly Asked Questions* (Torrance, CA: Optimox Corp., 1992).

20 Kwock, D., The Daily Wellness Co. "Upon a physician's evaluation and recommendation to do so, FertilityBlend for Women can be continued during pregnancy for the purpose of sustaining improved progesterone levels and overall health." (Personal communication to M. Shannon, Feb. 6, 2009).

21 Kim, M., Hong, S., Han, J., et al. "Homocysteine, folate and pregnancy outcomes" (*J. Obstet. Gynaecol.* 2012, 32:520-524).

22 De la Calle, M., Usandizaga, R., Sancah, M., et al. "Homocysteine, folic acid and B-group vitamins in obstetrics and gynaecology" (*European J. Obstet. & Gynaelcol.* 2003, 107:125-134).

23 Wen, S., Chen, X., Rodger, M., et al. "Folic acid supplementation in early second trimester and the risk of preeclampsia" (*Am. J. Obstet. Gynecol.* 2008, 198:45-e1–45-e7).

24 De la Calle, M., Usandizaga, R., Sancah, M., et al. (2003).

25 Kim, M., Hong, S., Han, J., et al., 2012; Makedos, G., Papanicolaou, A., Hitoglou, A., et al. "Homocysteine, folic acid and B12 serum levels in pregnancy complicated with preeclampsia" (*Arch. Gynecol. Obstet.* 2007, 275:121-124).

26 De la Calle, M., Usandizaga, R., Sancah, M., et al. (2003); Ray, J., and Laskin,

C. "Folic acid and homocyst(e)ine metabolic defects and the risk of placental abruption, pre-eclampsia and spontaneous pregnancy loss: A systematic review" (*Placenta* 1999, 20:519-529).

27 De la Calle, M., Usandizaga, R., Sancah, M., et al. (2003).

28 Juarez-Vazquaz, J., Bonizzoni, E., and Scotti, A. "Iron plus folate is more effective than iron alone in the treatment of iron deficiency anaemia in pregnancy: a randomised, double-blind clinical trial" (*Br. J. Obstet. Gynaecol.* 2002, 109:1009-1014).

29 Lee, K., Zaffke, M., and Baratte-Beebe, K. "Restless legs syndrome and sleep disturbance during pregnancy: the role of folate and iron" (*J. Women's Health and Gender-Based Medicine* 2001, 10:335-341).

30 De la Calle, M., Usandizaga, R., Sancah, M., et al. (2003).

31 Goh, Y., and Koren, G. "Folic acid in pregnancy and fetal outcomes" (*J. Obstet. & Gynaecol.* 2008, 28:3-13).

32 Raffelock, D., Rountree, R., and Hopkins, V. *A Natural Guide to Pregnancy and Postpartum Health* (New York: Avery, 2002, p. 131).

33 Ellis, J., and Presley, J. "B6 and Pregnancy" in *Vitamin B6: The Doctor's Report* (New York: Harper and Row, 1973, pp. 90, 96-97).

34 Ellis, J., and Presley, J. (1973, pp.112-113).

35 Scalf, R., personal communication to M. Shannon (March, 1990).

36 Hibbeln, J., Davis, J., Steer, C., et al. "Maternal seafood consumption in pregnancy and neuro-development outcomes in childhood (ALSPAC study: an observational cohort study)" (*The Lancet* 2007, 369:578-585).

37 Bloomingdale, A., Guthrie, L., Price, S., et al. "A qualitative study of fish consumption during pregnancy" (*Am. J. Clin. Nutr.* 2010, 92:1234-1240).

38 Olsen, S., Secher, N., Tabor, A., et al. "Randomized clinical trials of fish oil supplementation in high risk pregnancies. Fish Oil Trials in Pregnancy [FOTIP] Team" (*Br. J. Obstet. Gynaecol.* 2000, 107:382-395).

39 Raffelock, D., Rountree, R., and Hopkins, V. (2002, p. 146).

40 Rothman, K., and Moore, L. "Teratogenicity of high vitamin A intake" (*NEJM* 1995, 333:1369-1373).

41 Raffelock, D., Rountree, R., and Hopkins, V. (2002, p. 146).

42 Casey, B., and Leveno, K. "Thyroid disease in pregnancy" (*Obstet. Gynecol.*, 2006, 108:1283-1292)

43 Casey, B., and Leveno, K. (2006).

44 Shomon, M. The Thyroid Hormone Breakthrough (New York: Collins, 2006, p. 231).

45 Raffelock, D., Rountree, R., and Hopkins, V. (2002, p. 221) .

46 Lee, J., and Hopkins, V. *Dr. John Lee's Hormone Balance Made Simple* (New York: Wellness Central, 2006, pp. 139-140).

47 Raffelock, D., Rountree, R., and Hopkins, V. (2002, pp. 199-203).

CHAPTER 12

1 George, L., Granath, F., Johansson, A., et al. "Risks of repeated miscarriage" (*Paediatric and Perinatal Epidemiology* 2006, 20:119-126).

2 Roberts, C., and Murphy, A. "Endocrinopathies associated with recurrent pregnancy loss" (*Seminars in Reproductive Medicine* 2000, 18:357-362).

3 George, L., Granath, F., Johansson, A., et al. (2006).

4 Maconochie, N., Doyle, P., Prior, S., et al. "Risk factors for first trimester miscarriage —results from a UK-population-based case-control study" (*BJOG* 2007, 114:170-186).

5 Maconochie, N., Doyle, P., Prior, S., et al. (2007).

6 Morrison, J., Glueck, C., and Wang, P. "Dietary trans fatty acid intake is associated with increased fetal loss." (*Fertil. Steril.* 2008, 90:385-390).

7 Maconochie, N., Doyle, P., Prior, S., et al. (2007).

8 Bennett, M., "Vitamin B12 deficiency, infertility and recurrent fetal loss" (*J. Reprod. Med.* 2001, 46:209-212).

9 Weng, X., Odouli, R., and Li, D. "Maternal caffeine consumption during pregnancy and the risk of miscarriage: a prospective cohort study" (*J. Obst. Gynecol.*, January 2008, pp. 1e1-1e8).

10 Rice, H., and Baker, B. "Workplace hazards to women's reproductive health" (Minnesota Medicine, Sept. 2007, http://www.minnesotamedicine.com/PastIssues/September2007/tabid/2209/Default.aspx).

11 Nepomnaschy, P., Welch, K., McConnell, D., et al. "Cortisol and very early pregnancy loss" (*PNAS* 2006, 103:3938-3942).

12 Fritz, M., Adamson, G., Barnhart, K., et al. "Progesterone supplementation during the luteal phase and in early pregnancy in the treatment of infertility: an educational bulletin" (*Fertil. Steril.* 2008, 89:789-792); Dendrinos, S., Makrakis, E., Botsis, D., et al. "A study of pregnancy loss in 352 women with recurrent miscarriages" (*Arch. Gynecol. Obstet.* 2005, 271:235-239); Potdar, N., and Konje, J. "The endocrinological basis of recurrent miscarriage" (*Curr. Opin. Obstet. Gynecol.* 2005, 17:424-428); George, L., Granath, F., Johansson, A., et al. (2006).

13 Ohara, N., Tsujino, T., and Maruo, T. "The role of thyroid hormone in trophoblast function, early pregnancy maintenance, and fetal neurodevelopment" (*J. Obstet. Gynaecol. Can.* 2004, 26:982-990).

14 Abalovich, M., Gutierrez, S., Alcaraz, G., et al. "Overt and subclinical hypothyroidism complicating pregnancy" (*Thyroid* 2002, 12:63-68).

15 Potdar, N., and Konje, J. (2005).

16 Roberts, C., and Murphy, A. (2000).

17 Davies, M. "Evidence for effects of weight on reproduction in women [Symposium: Diet, nutrition and exercise in reproduction]" (*Reprod. BioMed. Online* 2006, 12:552-561).

18 Maconochie, N., Doyle, P., Prior, S., et al. (2007).

19 Martinelli, P., Troncone, R., Paparo, F., et al. "Celiac disease and unfavorable outcome of pregnancy" (*Gut* 2000, 46:332-335).

20 Rossi, E., and Costa, M. "Fish oil derivatives as a prophylaxis of recurrent miscarriage associated with antiphospholipid antibodies (APL): A pilot study" (*Lupus* 1993, 2, 319-323); Carla, G., Iovenitti., P., and Falciglia, K. "Recurrent miscarriage associated with antiphospholipid antibodies: prophylactic treatment with low-dose aspirin and fish oil derivatives" (*Clin. Exp. Obstet .Gynecol.* 2005, 32:49-51).

21 George, L., Granath, F., Johansson, A., et al. (2006).

22 Dendrinos, S., Makrakis, E., Botsis, D., et al. (2005).

23 Leridon, H. "A new estimate of permanent sterility by age: Sterility defined as the inability to conceive" (A paper presented at the Annual Meeting of the Population Association of America, Philadelphia, PA, Mar. 31-April 2, 2005, reviewed in Billari, F., Kohler, H., Andersson, G., et al. "Approaching the limit: Long-term trends in late and very late fertility." (*Population and Development Review* 2007, 33:149-170).

24 Maconochie, N., Doyle, P., Prior, S., et al. (2007).

25 Goh, Y., and Koren, G. "Folic acid in pregnancy and fetal outcomes" (*J. Obstet. Gynaecol.*, 2008, 28:3-13).

26 Sotres-Alvarez, D., Siega-Riz, A., Herring, A., et al, "Maternal dietary patterns are associated with risk of neural tube and congenital heart defects" (*Am. J. Epidemiol.* 2013, 177:1279-1288).

27 Wang, M., Wang, Z., Gao, L. et al. "Maternal body mass index and the association between folic acid supplements and neural tube defects" (*Acta Paediatrica* 2013, 102:908-913).

28 Wilson, R. "Pre-conception folic acid and multivitamin supplementation for the primary and secondary prevention of neural tube defects and other folic acid-sensitive congenital anomalies" [Society of Obstetricians and Gynaecologists of Canada] (*J. Obstet. and Gynaecol. Can* 2015, 37:534-549); Goh, Y., and Koren, G. (2008).

29 De la Calle, M., Usandizaga, R., Sancah, M., et al. "Homocysteine, folic acid and B-group vitamins in obstetrics and gynaecology" (*European J. Obstet. & Gynaelcol.* 2003, 107:125-134).

30 De la Calle, M., Usandizaga, R., Sancah, M., et al. (2003).

31 Goh, Y., and Koren, G. (2008).

32 Erickson, J., "Folic acid and prevention of spinal bifida and anencephaly: 10 years after the U.S. Public Health Service recommendation" (MMWR Recommendations and Reports 2002, RR13:1-3; www.cdc.gov/mmwr/preview/mmwrhtml/rr5113al. htm).

33 Wilson (2015).

34 Wilson, W. (2007).

35 Rothman, K., and Moore, L. "Teratogenicity of high vitamin A intake" (*NEJM* 1995, 333:1369-1373).

36 Goh, Y., and Koren, G. (2008).

37 MRC Vitamin Study Research Group, "Prevention of neural tube effects: Results of the Medical Research Council Vitamin Study" (*Lancet* 1991, 338:131-137).

38 Schorah, C. "Commentary: From controversy and procrastination to primary prevention" (*International J. Epidemiology* 2011 (40:1156-1158).

39 Czeizel, A., Metneki, J. And Dudas, I. "Higher rate of multiple births after periconceptional vitamin supplementation" (*NEJM* 1994, 330:1687-1688). [Note that a 40% increase in twinning is actually a very small increase in the actual number of twins, since twinning is an uncommon event. If, for example, twins occur in 2% of births, then instead of 20 per 1,000 births, a 40% increase would translate into 28 per 1,000.]

40 Bailey, L., and Berry, R. "Folic acid supplementation and the occurrence of congenital heart defects, orofacial clefts, multiple births, and miscarriage" (*Am. J. Clin. Nutr.* 2005, 81suppl.):1213S-1217S).

41 Li, Z., Gindler, J., Wang, H., et al. "Folic acid supplements during early pregnancy and the likelihood of multiple births: a population-based cohort study" (*The Lancet* 2003, 361:380-384).

42 Kallen, B., "Use of folic acid supplementation and risk for dizygotic [fraternal] twinning" (*Early Human Development* 2004, 80:143-151).

43 Czeizel, A., and Vargha, P. "Periconceptual folic acid/multivitamin supplementation and twin pregnancy" (*Am. J. Obstet. Gynecol.* 2004, 191:790–794).

44 Ray, J., and Laskin, C. "Folic acid and homocyst(e)ine metabolic defects and the risk of placental abruption, pre-eclampsia and spontaneous pregnancy loss: A systematic review" (*Placenta* 1999, 20:519-529).

45 Hook, E., and Czeizel, A. "Can terathanasia explain the protective effect of folic-acid supplementation on birth defects?" (*The Lancet* 1997, 350:513-515).

46 Windham, G., Shaw, G., Todoroff, K., et al. "Miscarriage and the use of multivitamins or folic acid" (*Am. J. Med. Genetics* 2000, 90:261-262).

47 Hook, E., and Czeizel, A. (2002).

48 Bailey, L., and Berry, R. (2005) 41 Windham, G., Shaw, G., Todoroff, K., et al. "Miscarriage and the use of multivitamins or folic acid" (*Am. J. Med. Genetics* 2000, 90:261-262).

49 Maconochie, N., Doyle, P., Prior, S., et al. (2007).

50 Vial-Nova, C., Wehby, G., Queiros, F., et al. "Periconceptual use of folic acid and risk of miscarriage—findings of oral cleft prevention program in Brazil" (*J. Perinatal. Med.* 2013, 40:461-466).

51 Whitaker, J. "Down Syndrome Can Be Treated" (*Health and Healing* 2007, 17:1-3); www.nutrivene.com/view (11/11/17).

52 Leichtman, L. "Targeted nutritional intervention (TNI) in the treatment of children with Down syndrome: principles behind use, treatment protocols, and an expanded bibliography" (www.lleichtman.org/tni 2002).

53 Gueant, J., Gueant-Rodriguez, R., Anello, G, et al. "Genetic determinants of folate and vitamin B12 metabolism: A common pathway in neural tube defect and Down syndrome?" (*Clin. Chem. Lab. Med.* 2003, 41:1473-1477).

54 Meiosis I is called the reduction division, because of the reduction of the chromosome number from 46 to 23. However, each of the chromosomes at the end of meiosis I is complexed with an identical copy. In meiosis II, the two identical copies separate. It is possible that a small percentage of trisomy 21 occurs during meiosis II.

55 James, S., Pogribna, M., Pobribny, I., et al. "Abnormal folate metabolism and mutation in the methylenetetrahydrofolate reductase gene may be maternal risk factors for Down syndrome" (*Am. J. Clin. Nutr.* 1999, 70:495-499). ["The nondisjunction event is maternal in ~95% of cases, occurring primarily during meiosis I in the maturing oocyte, before conception."]

56 James, S., Pogribna, M., Pobribny, I., et al. (1999); Hobb, C., Sherman, S., Yi, P., et al. "Polymorphisms in genes involved in folate metabolism as maternal risk factors for Down syndrome" (*Am. J. Hum. Genet.* 2000, 67:623-630); Sheth, J., and Smeth, F. "Gene polymorphism and folate metabolism: a maternal risk factor for Down syndrome" (*Indian Pediatrics* 2003, 40:115-123); Eskes, T. "Abnormal folate metabolism in mothers with Down syndrome offspring: Review of the literature" (*European J. Obstet. Gynaecol. and Reprod. Biol.* 2006, 124:130-136); Coppede, F., Colognato, R., Bonelli, A., et al. "Polymorphisms in folate and homocysteine metabolizing genes and chromosome damage in mothers of Down syndrome children" (*Am. J. Med. Genetics* 2007, Part A 143A:2006-2015).

57 Takamura, N., Kondoh, T., Ohgi, S., et al. "Abnormal folic acid-homocysteine metabolism as maternal risk factors for Down syndrome in Japan" (*European J. Nutrition* 2004, 43:285-287).

58 Kauer, A., and Kauer, A. "Maternal MTHFR polymorphism(677C-T) and risk of Down's syndrome child: meta-analysis" (*J. Genetics* 2016, 95:505-513).

59 Ray, J., Meier, C., Vermeulen, M., et al. "Prevalence of trisomy 21 following folic acid food fortification" (*Am. J. Med. Genetics* 2003, 120A:309–313).

60 Whitaker, J. (Personal communication to M. Shannon, October 13, 1996).

61 For what it is worth, I (MMS) was tested in 2015 and in fact do have some degree of the genetic variation that causes impaired folate metabolism.

62 Whitaker, J. (Personal communication to M. Shannon, October 29, 1996).

63 Slama, R., Bouyer, J., Windham, G., et al. "Influence of paternal age on the risk of spontaneous abortion" (*Am. J. Epidemiol.* 2005, 161:816-823).

64 Eskes, T. (2006).

65 Tremellen, K. "Oxidative, stress and male fertility-a clinical perspective" (*Human Reproduction Update*, pp. 1-16, 2008).

66 Tremellen, K. (2008).

CHAPTER 13

1 ACOG Committee Opinion, "Age-Related Fertility Decline" (*J. Obstet. Gynecol.* 112 [No. 2, Part 1 Aug 2008]: 409–411).

2 Shomon, M. *The Thyroid Hormone Breakthrough: Overcoming Sexual and Hormonal Problems at Every Age* (New York: Collins, an imprint of HarperCollins, 2006, p. 37).

3 Badawy, A., Ostate, O., and Sherief, S. "Can thyroid dysfunction explicate severe menopausal symptoms?" (*J. Obstet. Gynecol.* 2007, 27:503-505).

4 Lee, J., and Hopkins, V. *Dr. John Lee's Hormone Balance Made Simple: The Essential How-to Guide to Symptoms, Dosage, Timing, and More* (New York: Wellness Central, 2006, p. 30).

5 Gittleman, A. *Before the Change: Taking Charge of Your Perimenopause* (San Francisco: HarperSanFrancisco, a division of HarperCollins Publishers, 2004, pp. 68-69).

6 Abraham, G. Personal communication to M. Shannon (1991).

7 Gittleman, A. (2004, pp. 78-79).

8 Lee, J. *What Your Doctor May Not Tell You About Menopause* (New York: Warner Wellness, 2004, p. 336).

9 Lee, J. (2004, pp. 81-82).

10 Lee J., and Hopkins, V. (2006, pp. 93-95).

11 Lark, S. "My Alkaline Power Plan for Healthy Bones" (*The Lark Letter*, July, 2006, pp. 1-6).

12 Lark, S. (2006).

13 Lerchbaum, E. "Vitamin D and menopause—A narrative review" (*Maturitas* 2014, 79:3-7).

14 Pilz., S., Kienreich, K., Tomaschitz, A., et al. "Vitamin D and cancer mortality: systematic review of prospective epidemiological studies" (*Anticancer Agents Med. Chem.* 2013, 13:107-117); Garland, C., Garland, F., Gorham, E., et al. "The role of vitamin D in cancer prevention" (*Am. J. Public Health* 2006, 96:252-261).

15 Cauley, J., Chlebowski, R., Wactawski-Wende, J. et al. "Calcium plus vitamin D supplementation and health outcomes five years after active intervention ended: The Women's Health Initiative" (*J. Women's Health* [Larchmt] 2013, 22:915-925).

16 Heaney, R. "Phosphorus nutrition and the treatment of osteoporosis" (*Mayo Clin. Proc.* 2004, 79:91-97).

17 Lark, S. (2006).

18 Sanson, G. *The Myth of Osteoporosis: What Every Woman Should Know About Creating Bone Health* (Ann Arbor, MI: MCD Century, 2003, p. 153).

19 McIlwain, H., M.D, and Bruce, D., Ph.D., et al. *Reversing Osteopenia: The Definitive Guide to Recognizing and Treating Early Bone Loss in Women of All Ages* (New York: Owl Books, 2004, p. 7).

20 Lee, J. (2004, pp. 162-171).

21 Fritel, X., Ringa, V., Quiboeuf, E., et al. "Female urinary incontinence, from pregnancy to menopause: a review of the epidemiological and pathophysiological findings" (*Acta Obstetricia et Gynecologica Scandinavica* 2012, 91:9010910); Mishra, G., Cardozo, L., and Kuh., D. "Menopausal transition and the risk of urinary incontinence: results from a British prospective cohort" (*BJU International* 2010, 106:1170-1175).

22 Mishra, G., Cardozo, L., and Kuh., D., 2010.

23 Lee, J. (2004, p. 336).

24 Loong, T., "Internal factors contributing to optimal skin health and rejuvenation" (*J. of Aesthetic Nursing*, 2015, 4:270-275).

25 Brandt, F. "Sugar: The Enemy Within" in *10 Minutes/10 Years* (New York: Free Press, a trademark of Simon and Schuster, Inc., 2007, pp. 35-51).

CHAPTER 14

1 Horowitz, B., Edelstein, S., and Lippman, L. "Sugar chromatography studies in recurrent Candida vulvovaginitis" (*J. Reprod. Med.* 1984, 29:441).

2 Falagas, M., Betsi, G., and Athanasiou, S. "Probiotics for prevention of recurrent vulvovaginal candidiasis: a review" (*J. Antimicrobial Chemotherapy* 2006, 58:266-272).

3 Horowitz, B. Edelstein, S., and Lippman, L. "Sexual transmission of Candida" (*Obstet. Gynecol.* 1987, 69:883).

4 Falagas, M., Betsi, G., and Athanasiou, S. (2006).

5 Kontiokari, T., Nuutinen, M., and Uhari, M. "Dietary factors affecting susceptibility to urinary tract infection" (*Pediatr. Nephrol.* 2004, 19:378-383).

6 Shorter, B., Lesser, M., Moldwin, D., et al. "Effect of comestibles on symptoms of interstitial cystitis" (*J. Urology* 2007, 178:145-152).

7 Lee, J., and Hopkins, V. *What Your Doctor May Not Tell You about Menopause* (New York: Warner Books, 2004, p. 97).

8 Abraham, G., personal communication to M. Shannon (1991).

9 Lee, J., and Hopkins, V. (2004, p. 396).

10 Ito, T., Polan, M., Whipple, B., et al. "The enhancement of female sexual function with ArginMax, a nutritional supplement, among women differing in menopausal status" (*J. Sex & Marital Therapy* 2006, 32:369-378).

11 Lark, S. "Lift Your Libido" (*Women's Wellness Today* 2008, 15(7):6-7).

12 Lark, S. (2008).

13 www.calvin.edu.pribeiro/DCM-Lewis-2009/Lewis/the-four-loves.pdf.

CHAPTER 15

1 Giahi, L., Mohammadmoradi, S., Javidan, A., et al. "Nutritional modifications in male infertility: a systematic review covering 2 decades" (*Nutrition Reviews* 2015, 74: 118-130).

2 Salma, U., Gill, H., Keith, L., et al. "Male subfertility and the role of micronutrient supplementation: clinical and economic issues" (*J. of Experimental & Clinical Assisted Reproduction* 2011, 8.1, p. 1).

3 Salma, U., Gill, H., Keith, L., et al.; Sheweita, S., Tilmisany, A., and Al-Sawaf, H. "Mechanisms of male infertility: Role of antioxidants" (*Current Drug Metabolism* 2005, 6:495-501).

4 Calogero, A., Condorelli, R., Russo, G., et al. "Conservative nonhormonal options for the treatment of male infertility: Antibiotics, anti-inflammatory drugs, and antioxidants" (*Biomed Res. Int.* Vol. 2017, Article ID 4650182, 17 pages).

5 Gaskins, A., Colaci, D., Mendiola, J., et al. "Dietary patterns and semen quality in young men" (*Human Reprod.* 2012, 27:2899-2907).

6 Jurewicz, J., Radway, M., Sobala, W., et al. "Dietary patterns and the frequency of disomy in human sperm" (*Urology* 2016 93:86-91).

7 Jurewicz, J., Radway, M., Sobala, W., et al. (2016).

8 Afeiche, M., Williams, P., Gaskins, A, et al. "Meat intake and reproductive parameters among young men" (*Epidemiology* 2014, 25:323-330).

9 Afeiche, M., Gaskins, A., Williams, P., et al. "Processed meat intake is unfavorably and fish intake favorably associated with semen quality indicators among men attending a fertility clinic" (*J. Nutr.* 2014, 144:1091-1098).

10 Afeiche, M., Williams, P., Mendiola, J., et al. "Dairy food intake in relation to semen quality and preproductive hormone levels among physically active young men" (*Reproductive Epidemiology* 2013, 28:2265-2013).

11 Afeiche, M., Williams, P., Mendiola, J., et al. (2013), p.2273.

12 Jensen, T., Heitmann, B., Jensen, M., et al. "High dietary intake of saturated fat is associated with reduced semen quality among 701 young Danish men from the general population. (*Am. J. Clin. Nutr.* 2013, 97:411-418).

13 Estamian, G., Amirjannati, N., Rashidkhani, B., et al. "Dietary fatty acid intakes and asthenozoospermia: a case-controlled study" (*Fertil. Steril.* 2015, 103:190-198).

14 Estamian, G., Amirjannati, N., Rashidkhani, B., et al. (2015).

15 Chavarro, J., Minguez-Alarcon, L., Mendiola, J., et al. "Trans fatty acid intake is inversely related to total sperm count in young healthy men" (*Human Reprod.* 2014, 29:429-440).

16 Chavarro, J., Toth, T., Sadio, S., et al. "Soy food and isoflavone intake in relation to semen quality parameters among men from an infertility clinic" (*Human Reprod.* 2008, 11:2584-2590).

17 Chavarro, J., personal communication to M. Shannon (Jan. 3, 2009).

18 Chiu, Y., Afeiche, M., Gaskins, A., et al. "Sugar-sweetened beverage intake in relation to semen quality and reproductive hormone levels in young men" (*Human Reprod.* 2014, 29:1575-1584).

19 Jensen, T., Swan, S., Skakkebaek, N., et al. "Caffeine intake and semen quality in a population of 2,554 young Danish men" (*Am. J. Epidemiol.* 2010, 171:883-891).

20 Tremellen, K. "Oxidative stress and male fertility–a clinical perspective" (*Human Reproduction Update* 2008, pp. 1-16).

21 Tremellen, K. (2008).

22 Sheweita, S., Tilmisany, A., and Al-Sawaf, H. (2005).

23 deSouza, G., and Hallak, J. "Anabolic steroids and male infertility: a comprehensive review" (*BJUI* 2011, 108:1860-1865).

24 Semet, M., Paci, M., Saias-Magnan, J., et al. "The impact of drugs on male fertility: a review" (*Andrology* 2017,5:640-663).

25 Agarwal, A., Deepinder, F. Sharma, R., et al. "Effect of cell phone usage on semen analysis in men attending infertility clinic: an observational study" (*Fertil. Steril.* 2008 89:124-128); Gutschi, T.al-Ali, B., Shamloul, R., et al. " Impact of cell phone use on men's semen parameters" (*Andrologica* 2011,43:312-316); Agarwal, A., Singh, A., Hamada, A., et al. "Cell phones and male infertility: A review of recent innovations in technology and consequences" (*Int. Braz. J. Urol.* 2011:37-432-454).

26 Sallmen, M., Sandler, D., Hoppin, J., et al. "Reduced fertility among overweight and obese men" (*Epidemiology* 2006, 17:520-523).

27 Dupont, C., Faure, C., Sermondade, N., et al. "Obesity lead to higher risk of sperm DNA damage in infertile patients" (*Asian J. Andrology* 2013 15:622-625).

28 Sermondade, N., Faure, C., Fezeu, L., et al. "BMI in relation to sperm count: an updated systematic review and collaborative meta-analysis" (*Human Reprod. Update* 2013, 19:221-231). In this study, BMI (body mass index, calculated by body weight in kg/ height in cm2) was used to define underweight as BMI <18.5; normal weight as BMI 18.5-24.9; overweight as BMI 25.0-29.9; obesity as BMI 30.0-39.9; and morbid obesity BMI > 40 as per World Health Organization 2000.

29 Sermondade, N., Faure, C., Fezeu, L., et al. (2013).

30 Kaukua, J., Pekkarinen, T., Sane, T., et al. "Sex hormones and sexual function in obese men losing weight" (*Obesity Res.* 2003, 11:689-694).

31 Frisch, R. *Female Fertility and the Body Fat Connection* (Chicago: University of Chicago Press 2002, p. 35). In referring to extreme weight loss in men, at the point of loss of sperm production, the late Dr. Frisch wrote, "They look like skeletons."

32 Sermondade, N., Faure, C., Fezeu, L., et al. (2013).

33 Tremellen, K. (2008).

34 Salma, U., Gill, H., Keith, L., et al. (2011).

35 Esmaeili, V., Shahverdi, A., Moghadasian, M., et al. "Dietary fatty acids affect semen quality: a review" (*Andrology* 2015, 3:450-461).

36 Comhaire, F., and Mahmoud, A. "The role of food supplements in the treatment of the infertile man" (*Reprod. BioMed. Online* 2003, 7:385-391).

37 Robbins, W., Xun, L., FitzGerald, L. et al. "Walnuts improve semen quality in men consuming a Western-style diet: randomized control dietary intervention trial" (*Bio. Reprod.* 2012, 87:101-108).

38 Comhaire, F., and Mahmoud, A. (2003).

39 Esmaeili, V., Shahverdi, A., Moghadasian, M., et al. (2015).

40 Ross, C., Morriss, A., Khairy, M., et al. "A systematic review of the effect of oral antioxidants on male infertility" (*Reprod. Biomed. Online* 2010, 20:711-723); Mendiola, J., Torres-Cantero, A., Vioque, J. "A low intake of antioxidant nutrients is associated with poor semen quality in patients attending fertility clinics" (*Fertil. Steril.* 2010, 93:1128-1133).

41 Harris, W., Harden, T., and Dawson, E. "Apparent effect of ascorbic acid medication on semen metal levels" (*Fertil. Steril.* 1979, 32:456-457).

42 Dawson, E., Harris, W., Rankin W., et al. "Effect of ascorbic acid on male infertility" (*Ann. New York Acad. Sci.* 1987, 498:312).

43 Dawson, E., Harris, B., Teter, M., et al. "Effect of ascorbic acid supplementation on the sperm quality of smokers." (*Fertil. Steril.* 1992, 58:1034-1039).

44 Song, G., Norkus, E., and Lewis, V. "Relationship between seminal ascorbic acid and sperm DNA integrity in infertile men" (*Int. J. Andrology* 2006, 29:569-575).

45 "Dietary intake of antioxidant nutrients is associated with semen quality in young university students" (*Human Reprod.* 2012, 37:2807-2814). These authors noted that the vitamin C intake of men in the lowest quartile of semen quality averaged 60 mg/day, the RDI for vitamin C.

46 Calogero, A., Condorelli, R., Russo, G., et al. (2017).

47 Boxmeer, J., Smit, M., Utomo, E. et al. "Low folate in seminal plasma is associated with increased sperm DNA damage" (*Fertil. Steril.* 2009, 92:548-556).

48 Wong, W., Merkus, H., Thomas, C., et al. "Effect of folic acid and zinc sulfate on male factor subfertility: a double-blind, randomized, placebo-controlled trial" (*Fertil. Steril.* 2002, 77:491-497).

49 Maret, W., and Sandstead, H. "Zinc requirements and the risks and benefits of zinc supplementation" (*J. Trace Elements in Medicine and Biology* 2006, 20:3-8).

50 Ebisch, I., can Heerde, W., Thomas, C., et al. "C677T methylenetetrahydroflate reductase polymorphism interferes with the effects of folic acid and zince sulfate on sperm concentration" (*Fertil. Steril.* 2003, 80:1190-1194).

51 Beckett G., and Arthur, J. "Selenium and endocrine systems" (*J. Endocrinol.* 2005, 184:455-465).

52 Keskes-Ammar, L., Feki-Chakroun, N., Rebai, T., et al. "Sperm oxidative stress and the effect of an oral vitamin E and selenium supplement on semen quality in infertile men" (*Archives of Andrology* 2003, 49:83-94).

53 Scott, R., MacPherson, A., Yates, R., et al. "The effect of oral selenium supplementation on human sperm motility" (*Br. J. Urology* 1998, 82:76-80).

54 Comhaire, F., Cristophe, A., Zalata, A., et al. (2000).

55 Suleiman, S., Ali, M., Zaki, Z., et al. "Lipid peroxidation and human sperm motility: protective role of vitamin E" (*J. Androl.* 1996, 17:530-537).

56 Calloway, D. "Nutrition and reproductive function of men" (*Nutrition Abstracts and Reviews/Reviews in Clinical Nutrition* 1983, 53:373).

57 Minguez-Alarcon, L., Mendiola, J., Lopez-Espin, J., et al. (2012).

58 Eskanazi, B., Kidd, S., Marks, A., et al. (*Human Reprod.* 2005, 20:1006-1012).

59 Tremellen, K. (2008).

60 Salma, U., Gill, H., Keith, L., et al. (2011).

61 Salma, U., Gill, H., Keith, L., et al. (2011).

62 Safarinejad, M. "Efficacy of coenzyme Q10 on semen parameters, sperm function and reproductive hormones in infertile men" (*J Urol.* 2009, 182:237-248).

63 Safarinejad, M. "The effect of coenzyme Q10 supplementation on partner pregnancy rate in infertile men with idiopathic oligoasthenoteratozoospermia: an open-label prospective study" (*Int. Urol. Nephrol.* 2011, 44:689-700).

64 Tisco, B., Gaskins, A., Hauser, R., et al. "Coenzyme Q10 intake from food and semen parameters in a subfertile population" (*Urology*, 2016).

65 Afeiche, M., Williams, P., Gaskins, A., et al. (2014).

66 Calogero, A., Condorelli, R., Russo, G., et al. (2017).

67 Lenzi, A., Lombardo, F., Sgro, P., et al. "Use of carnitine therapy in selected cases of male factor infertility: A double-blind crossover trial" (*Fertil. Steril.* 2003, 79:292-300); reviewed in Agarwall, A., Nallella, K., Allamaneni, S., et al. (2004).

68 Zhou, X., Liu, F., and Zhai, S. "Effect of L-carnitine and/or L-acetyl-carnitine in nutrition treatment for male infertility: a systematic review" (*Asia Pac. J. Clin. Nutr.* 2007, 16 (Suppl. 1):383-390).

69 Comhaire, F., and Mahnoud, A. (2003); Conhaire, F., El Garem, Y., Mahmoud, A., et al. "Combined conventional/antioxidant 'Astaxanthin' treatment for male infertility: a double-blind, randomized trial" (*Asian J. Andrology* 2005, 7:257-262). [Astaxanthin is a red pigment that gives the pinkish color to many seafoods. It is a carotenoid; that is, a fat-soluble nutrient related to beta-carotene. (www.astaxanthin.org)]

70 Sallmen, M., Sandler, D., Hoppin, J., et al. (2006).

71 Calogero, A., Condorelli, R., Russo, G., et al. (2017).

72 Whitaker, J., M.D. "Erectile dysfunction: What works/what doesn't" (*Health & Healing*, June 2016, 6-7).

73 Stanislavov, R., and Rohdewald, P. "Improvement of erectile function by a combination of French maritime pine bark and roburins with aminoacids" (*Minerva Urol. Nefrol.* 2015, 67:27-32).

74 Krassaa, G. "Male reproductive function in relation with thyroid alterations" (*Best Practice & Research in Clinical Endocrinology and Metabolism* 2004, 18:183-195).

75 Kumar, A., Chaturvedi, K., and Mohanty, B. "Hypoandrogenaemia is associated with subclinical hypothyroidism in men" (*Int. J. Andrology* 2007, 30:14-20).

76 Stogdill, B., M.D., personal communication to M. Shannon (July, 1989).

77 Balch, P. *Prescription for Nutritional Healing*, 5th ed. (New York: Avery Press, 2010, p. 671).

78 Balch, P. (2010, p. 671).

79 Rohrman, S., Giovannucci, E., Willett, W., et al. "Fruit and vegetable consumption, intake of micronutrients, and benign prostatic hyperplasia in U.S. men" (*Am. J. Clin. Nutr.* 2007, 85:523-529).

80 Pytel, Y., Vinarov, A ., Lopatkin, N., et al. "Long-term clinical and biologic effects of the lipido-sterolic extract of Serenoa repens in patients with symptomatic benign prostatic hyperplasia" (*Advances in Therapy* 2002, 19:297-306).

81 Pytel, Y., Vinarov, A ., Lopatkin, N., et al. (2002).

82 Fleshner, N., Zlotta, A. "Prostate cancer prevention" (*Cancer* 2007, 110:1889-1899.

83 Cheung, E., Wadhera, P., Dorff, T., et al. "Diet and prostate cancer risk reduction" (*Expert Rev. Anticancer Ther.* 2008, 8:43-50).

84 Cheung, E., Wadhera, P., Dorff, T., et al. (2008).

85 Vaishampayan, U., Hussain, M., Banerjee, M., et al. "Lycopene and soy isoflavones in the treatment of prostate cancer" (*Nutrition and Cancer* 2007, 59:1-7).

86 Chavarro, J., Stampfer, M., Campos, H., et al. "A prospective study of trans-fatty acid levels in blood and risk of prostate cancer" (*Cancer Epidemiol. Biomarkers & Prevention* 2008, 17:95-101).

87 Szymanski, K., Wheeler, D., and Mucci, L. "Fish consumption and prostate cancer risk: a review and meta-analysis" (*Am. J. Nutr.* 2010, 92:1223-1233).

88 Clark, L., Combs, G., Turnbull, B., et al. "Effects of selenium supplementation for cancer prevention in patients with carcinoma of the skin: a randomized controlled trial" (*JAMA* 1996, 276: 1957-1963); Combs, G., and Gray, W. "Chemopreventive agents: selenium" (*Pharmacol Ther.* 1998 79:179-182).

89 Heinonen, O., Albanes, D., Virtamo, J., et al. "Prostate cancer and supplementation with alpha-tocopherol and beta-carotene: incidence and mortality in a controlled trial" (*J. Natl. Cancer Inst.* 1998, 90:440-446).

90 Mettlin, C., Natarajan, N., and Huben, R. "Vasectomy and prostate cancer risk" (*Am. J. Epidemiol.* 1990, 132:1056-1061); Rosenberg, L., Palmer, J., Zauber, M., et al. "Vasectomy and the risk of prostate cancer" (*Am. J. Epidemiol.* 1990, 132:1051-1055); Giovannucci, E., Ascherio, A., Rimm, E., et al. "A prospective cohort study of vasectomy and prostate cancer in U.S. men" (*JAMA* 1993, 269:873-876); Giovannucci, E., Tosteson, T., Speizer, F., et al. "A retrospective cohort study of vasectomy and prostate cancer in U.S. men" (*JAMA* 1993, 269:878-882).

CHAPTER 16

1 Carmichael, A. "Can Vitex agnus castus be used for the treatment of mastalgia? What is the current evidence? (*ECAM* 2008, 5:247-250).

2 *The Art of Natural Family Planning Transitions Student Guide* (Cincinnati, OH: The Couple to Couple League, 2013 p. 109).

3 Cordain, L., Lindeberg, S., and Hurtado, M. "Acne vulgaris: a disease of Western civilization" (*Arch. Dermatol.* 2002, 138:1584-1590).

4 McIntosh, M.E. "Treatment of women with the galactorrhea-amenorrhea syndrome with pyridoxine (vitamin B6)" (*J. Clin. Endocrinol. Metab.* 1976, 42:1192).

5 Kapcala, L. "Galactorrhea and thyrotoxicosis" (*Arch. Intern. Med.* 1984, 144:2349).

6 Ryan-Harshman, M., and Aldoori, W. "Carpal tunnel syndrome and vitamin B6" (*Canadian Family Physician* 2007, 53:1161-1162).

7 Siega-Riz, A., Promislow, J., Savitz, D., et al. "Vitamin C intake and the risk of preterm delivery" (*Am. J. Obstet. Gynecol.* 2003, 189:519-523).

8 Prior, C., Vigna, Y., et al. "Spinal bone loss and ovulatory infertility" (*NEJM* 1991, 323:1221-1227).

9 Streeten, E., Ryan, K., McBride, D., et al. "The relationship between parity and bone mineral density in women characterized by a homogeneous lifestyle and high parity" (*J. Clin. Endocrinol. Metab.* 2005, 90:4536-4541).

10 Rothman, K., and Moore, L. "Teratogenicity of high vitamin A intake" (*NEJM* 1995, 333:1369-1373).

11 Bruchalsi, J. (personal communication to M. Shannon, October 6, 2008).

APPENDIX C

1 www. calvin.edu.pribeiro/DCM-Lewis-2009/Lewis/the-four-lives.pdf.

INDEX

Birth control pill 94, 105, 120, 178, 180, 184
Birth defects 57, 117, 124, 198–200, 208, 218, 229–230, 232–233, 235, 239–240, 308
Black currant oil 251
Bladder infections 18, 182, 248, 257, 264–265, 273
Bloating 21, 106, 108, 117, 179
Blood clotting 122, 147, 222, 226
Blood glucose 4–5, 9, 16–17, 19, 24, 85, 88, 166, 168–170, 188, 198, 200–201, 223, 249–250, 258, 267, 299
Blood glucose levels 5, 9, 17, 85, 88, 168–170, 198, 200, 249–250, 258, 267, 299
Blood pressure 18, 170, 200, 202, 206, 211, 270
Blood sugar 3–5, 8–12, 16, 21, 23–24, 84–85, 93, 110, 168, 198, 200–201, 218, 249, 299
Blood sugar levels 3–4, 8, 11–12, 16, 21, 168, 201, 249, 299
Blue Ribbon Baby 203, 207, 321
BMI. *See* Body Mass Index (BMI)
Body fat 9, 83, 120–121, 127, 133, 139, 141, 151, 156–161, 173–174, 177, 225–226, 241, 244–248, 250, 254, 268, 270, 281–282, 289
Body hair 164, 173, 248. *See also* Hirsutism
Body Mass Index (BMI) 158, 225–226
Body weight 83, 89, 115, 117, 133, 136, 157–160, 167, 170, 177–178, 221–222, 225–226, 229, 245, 248, 251, 254–256, 260, 270, 275
Bone Builder 253
Bone density test 307
Bone health 252–256, 260, 307
Borage oil 251
Brain cancer, childhood 240
Brain development 5, 50, 212
Brain fog 26, 166, 211, 217, 249–250
Brain function 8, 12, 30, 92
Brandt, Frederic, M.D. 258
Breadmaker 39–40, 42, 89
Bread recipe 40
Breakfast 4, 6, 14, 23–24, 32–33, 43, 56, 61, 84, 86, 89, 110, 204, 300
Breakthrough bleeding 120

Breast cancer 174, 178, 185, 233, 253
Breastfeeding 5, 18, 26, 55, 86, 122, 138, 141, 153, 186–187, 194, 199, 213–218, 232, 269–270, 274, 301, 306
Breastfeeding and Natural Child Spacing 26, 312
Breast pain 108, 110, 299
Breast self-examination 305
Brewer, Gail Sforza 319
Brewer, Tom, M.D. 203, 318–319, 322, 372
Broda O. Barnes, M.D., Research Foundation, Inc., The 322
Bromelain 134
Bromocriptine 304
Brown bleeding 140, 153
Brown, Marilyn 318
Bulimia 158, 160
B vitamins 13, 16, 19, 48, 50–51, 55, 59, 85, 90, 92–93, 107–108, 111, 117, 124, 126, 142, 149, 160, 169, 184, 188, 190, 193, 199, 207, 209, 211, 217–218, 230, 236, 240, 250, 268, 283, 286, 290–291, 297, 299, 301, 306

C

Caffeine 19–20, 28, 84–85, 93, 110, 187–189, 193, 196, 198, 215, 223, 250, 253, 258, 262, 272–273, 279, 299–300
Calcium 56, 58, 86, 92–93, 109, 111, 113, 117, 122–123, 128, 130, 133, 135, 160, 187, 200, 203, 207, 252–254, 284, 306
Calcium carbonate 113, 200
Cancer 8, 148, 154, 174, 178, 185, 233, 240, 253, 258, 280, 294–295, 297
Candida albicans 180, 261. *See also* Yeast overgrowth
Canisters 44, 46
Canola oil 10, 15, 32, 49, 123, 303
Capsicum 124
Carbohydrate intolerance as symptom of PCOS 164
Cardiovascular disease 8, 55, 169, 230, 308
Carpal tunnel syndrome 305
Catholic Church 129, 310
Cayenne pepper 124, 126

Celiac disease 55, 158, 189–191, 196, 226, 232
Celiac Disease Foundation 191–192, 322
Chasteberry extract 113, 144, 299
Chavarro, Jorge, M.D. 53
Ccheese 4, 6, 10, 14–15, 23–25, 29–30, 39, 86–88, 113, 168, 204, 278–279, 296, 300
Childbirth 122, 148, 161, 206, 218, 246, 256–257, 269, 271
Childhood obesity 26
Children 5, 25–27, 37, 39, 44, 50, 52, 88, 90, 92–93, 116, 126, 147, 152–153, 172, 179, 182, 192, 211–213, 217, 228, 234–242, 260, 295, 306–307, 310
Chlorophyll 124, 126
Chocolate 17, 19, 85, 110, 265, 272, 290, 302–303
Cholesterol 10–11, 88, 166–167, 184, 270
Christianson, Alan 78, 84, 311
Chromium 16, 48, 112, 169–170, 174
Chronic candidiasis 182, 312
Cleft palate 230, 232
Cod liver oil 49–50, 90, 92, 129, 134, 182, 213, 248, 284, 286, 288, 293, 296
Co-enzyme Q10 194, 236
Coffee. *See* Caffeine
Comhaire, Frank 283
Community Supported Agriculure (CSA) 34
Constipation 21, 92, 179, 189, 291
Containers 10, 18, 44, 94
Cookbooks 22, 29, 38
Corn syrup 17
Corpus luteum 108, 131–132, 138, 140–141, 143, 148, 173, 224, 301
Cortisol 84, 115, 146–148, 151, 217, 221, 223, 250
Cortisone 180–181, 268
Couple to Couple League, The iii–v, x, xii, 53, 59, 105, 107, 143, 172, 180, 194, 242, 265, 275, 289, 323
Cramps 106–107, 116, 126, 128–129, 134, 210, 263
Crook, Elizabeth B. 320
Crook, William G., M.D. 54, 134, 178, 182, 263, 268, 292, 320, 368
Cycle irregularities 99, 137–139, 146, 155–156, 158–159, 167, 184–185, 188, 191, 239, 260, 306

Cycles, long 120–121, 145, 147, 158, 160, 163, 172–173, 177, 191, 244, 301, 304
Cycles, short 155
Cysts 110, 164–165, 167

D

Daily values 54
Dairy products 17, 30, 35, 86, 109–110, 113, 128, 130, 181, 203, 207, 215, 222, 253, 262, 285
Davis, Adelle 88, 315
Dean, Carolyn, M.D., N.D. 171, 179, 320
Deep freezer 38
DeFelice, Joy, R.N. 186, 314
Depression 16, 50, 86–87, 106, 158, 166, 170, 217, 245
Depression-free, Naturally 312
Dessert 9, 23, 38, 259
Developmental problems 88, 212, 224
Dexa Scan 255
DHA 12, 30–32, 49–50, 52, 88, 90, 92–93, 123–124, 129–130, 132–133, 136, 170, 212–213, 215, 227, 250, 283–284. *See also* Docasahexaenoic acid
Diabetes 50, 55, 166, 168, 170, 211, 308
Diabetes, gestational 50, 170
Dietary fiber 107
Diet, inadequate 52
Dihydrotestosterone (DHT) 293
Dinnerware 44, 46
Diploid cells 100, 277
Docosahexaenoic acid (DHA) 49
Dopamine 108, 293
Down syndrome 57, 100–102, 193, 235–240
Dr. Atkins' New Diet Revolution 312
Dr. David Reuben's Quick Weight-Gain Program 313
Dreams 92
Dr. John Lee's Hormone Balance Made Simple 249, 313, 368, 375, 380
Drugs ix, 51, 97, 128–129, 172, 180–182, 187, 189, 234, 255, 268, 280, 295
Dry mouth 87
Dysmenorrhea 126–130, 135–136. *See also* Menstruation, painful

E

255, 266, 269. *See also*
Progesterone cream
Natural Resources Defense Council
31, 88
Nausea 77, 116, 127, 189, 199–201, 208, 211
Neural tube defects 198–199, 209, 229, 231, 233–237, 240
New England Journal of Medicine 306
NFP chart 99, 114, 137, 139, 154, 216–217, 224, 244, 249, 289
Nicotine 72, 280, 296
Night lighting 67, 186–188, 194, 196, 223, 228, 302
Night sweats 246–247
Nonsteroidal anti-inflammatory drugs 128
Norepinephrine 70, 71, 73–75, 249
Nowosadzka, Marta, M.D. 315
Numbness of hands 179, 210–211, 305
Nurses' Health Study 11, 110, 132, 167–168
NutraSweet 87, 110, 168–169, 193, 302, 304
Nutritional counselor 308–309
Nutrition Almanac 317
Nutritious food 41, 202
Nutrivene-D 235–236

O

Obesity 26, 121, 127, 164, 166, 168, 171, 174, 178, 229, 240, 248, 254, 257, 268, 281–282, 296–297
Older mother 116, 199, 209
Olive oil 7, 10, 15, 31, 110, 214–215, 258, 303
Omega-3 essential fatty acid 130, 171, 283
Omphalocoele 230
Optimox Corporation 112, 317, 327
Optivite PMT 59, 107–108, 111, 113, 133, 143, 145, 161, 174, 208, 330
Optivite PMT® and Gynovite® Plus Total Dietary Programs for Women With Answers to the Most Commonly Asked Questions 317
Oral contraceptives 114, 133, 180–181. *See also* Birth control pill
Oral thrush 180
Organic farms 35
Organic foods 32–33

Orgasm 257, 270–271, 274
Osteoporosis 50, 158, 251, 253–256, 306–307
Ovarian cysts 167
Ovaries 16, 19, 21, 77, 98, 100–101, 114, 127, 164–166, 175, 241, 245, 248, 267–268
Overweight 21, 83–84, 115, 127, 141, 145, 158, 163–165, 167, 170–175, 177–178, 184, 188, 193, 198, 203, 206, 222, 247–248, 268, 273, 277, 279, 282, 289, 296, 302, 306
without PCOS 83, 164, 173–175
Ovulation xi, 57, 63, 83, 98–102, 104, 113–114, 120–121, 127, 131, 138–141, 143, 145, 152, 156, 159–161, 163, 165, 172, 177, 183, 185, 193, 221, 224, 226, 236, 240, 242–244, 249, 254, 265–266, 268, 276, 301–302, 307
delayed 139, 159, 183, 185, 226, 268, 302
Ovum xi, 57, 98, 100–104, 138, 140–142, 193, 196, 220–221, 224, 236, 239–240, 242, 276–277, 283, 301
blighted 101, 224
Oxidative stress 52, 102, 104, 131, 143, 236, 239, 277, 279, 282, 286, 296

P

Pain 18, 21, 50–51, 70, 72, 81, 108, 110, 119–121, 126–136, 178–179, 189, 208, 228, 250, 255, 263, 265, 267, 271, 291, 299–300, 305
breast 108, 110, 299
low back 263
pelvic 263
with intercourse 178, 291
with urination 263
Painful Bladder Syndrome 265
Panax ginseng 269
Pancreas 16, 20, 75–76, 165
Pans 42–43, 46
Papain 134
Parlodel 304
Pelvic pain 127, 130, 134, 263
Perimenopause 63, 105, 187, 241–245, 247–248, 250–251, 254–256, 260, 269, 306. *See also* Premenopause
Period, menstrual. *See* Menstruation
Phytonutrients 8, 10, 16, 20, 30, 55, 90, 283, 293

Yogurt maker 41

Z

Zinc 16, 48, 50, 52, 56, 73, 93, 102–104,
108–109, 111, 117, 124–126, 133,
143–144, 182, 184, 191, 193, 217,
222, 230, 237, 239, 248, 250, 254,
264, 268, 283–285, 289–291, 297,
303

ABOUT THE AUTHOR

Marilyn McCusker Shannon holds a Master's degree in human physiology with a minor in biochemistry from Indiana University's Medical Sciences Program. In 2019 she retired from Purdue University Fort Wayne, Indiana, where she taught human anatomy and physiology to health professions majors for over thirty years.

Marilyn and her husband Ron have been a Teaching Couple for the Couple to Couple League for Natural Family Planning (NFP) since 1982. Her interest in the impact of nutrition on reproductive health is an outgrowth of her educational background and her experience as an NFP instructor.

Ron and Marilyn are the parents of nine children—five daughters and four sons. Their seventh and ninth children were adopted as babies, and their eighth was born to them shortly before Marilyn's 48th birthday. The Shannons live on a small farm in Indiana, where the family interests include raising dairy goats and poultry, and gardening. They have been a homeschooling family since their oldest son started grade school. Their homestead is also the birthplace of several of their children.

Made in the USA
Monee, IL
04 December 2023

48136084R00230